The Harvard Medical School
Guide to Tai Chi

Harvard Health Publications
HARVARD MEDICAL SCHOOL

THE

Harvard Medical School Guide to Tai Chi

12 WEEKS TO A HEALTHY BODY, STRONG HEART, AND SHARP MIND

Peter M. Wayne, PhD

Assistant Professor of Medicine, Harvard Medical School
Director of Research, Osher Center for Integrative Medicine
Brigham and Women's Hospital and Harvard Medical School

WITH Mark L. Fuerst

Shambhala
Boston & London
2013

This book is dedicated to my parents and family,
for their love, support, and encouragement all along the way
and to all my teachers and mentors, East and West,
for their wisdom, generosity, and inspiration.

Shambhala Publications, Inc.
Horticultural Hall
300 Massachusetts Avenue
Boston, Massachusetts 02115
www.shambhala.com

The information in this book is not intended as a substitute for personalized
medical advice. The reader should consult a physician before beginning this or
any exercise program. The author and the publisher assume no responsibility
for pain or injury experienced from the practice of exercises presented here.

9 8 7 6 5 4 3

Printed in the United States of America

♾ This edition is printed on acid-free paper that meets
the American National Standards Institute Z39.48 Standard.
♻ This book is printed on 30% postconsumer recycled paper.
For more information please visit www.shambhala.com.

Distributed in the United States by Random House, Inc.,
and in Canada by Random House of Canada Ltd

Designed by James D. Skatges

Library of Congress Cataloging-in-Publication Data

Wayne, Peter.
The Harvard medical school guide to tai chi: 12 weeks to a healthy body,
strong heart, and sharp mind / Peter Wayne, with Mark Fuerst.
p. cm.
Includes bibliographical references and index.
ISBN 978-1-59030-942-1 (pbk.: alk. paper)
1. Tai chi—Therapeutic use. 2. Health. I. Fuerst, Mark. II. Title.
RM727.T34W39 2012
613.7'148—dc23
2012025187

Contents

PART THREE
Integrating Tai Chi into Everyday Life

Foreword

Health care has always undergone change. Old diseases disappear or are conquered; new ones take their place. New cures sometimes bring unexpected problems. Personal and societal expectations for health and longevity shift tremendously. Western patients now are asking for more prevention and health sustenance. Many want "soft-touch" in addition to hard technology. While many acute problems seem to be under control, it seems that there are not enough solutions for living with or gracefully managing chronic illness. New discoveries and directions are continually being examined.

Part of the quest for new answers is re-examining older approaches to illness. Have therapies that can provide answers to new problems withstood the test of time? Certainly, the popularity and recent scientific research into acupuncture and Ayurvedic medicine suggest that, in parallel with globalization, there is a new opening to non-biomedical systems. I've had a ringside seat on this emergent global perspective with my own work building links between Asian medicine and modern medicine. Sorely missing has been a book that bridges the wisdom of Tai Chi with the scientific insights of biomedicine. This exceptional book has finally been written, remarkably within the context of a leading medical school; it provides the needed platform to link East and West.

The Harvard Medical School Guide to Tai Chi is a wonderful, elegant book that embraces the tensions between science and art, modern research and traditional wisdom, movement and stillness, and effort and effortlessness. The authors have written a Tai Chi book that embodies the gracefulness of Tai Chi. Ideas, insights, concepts, overviews, and details, based on, for example, neuroimaging of the brain and Lao Tzu, move and swirl around in an elegant, rhythmic mixture that feels like Tai Chi. They make the Tai Chi movement called "Waving Hands Like Clouds" into both a visualization and an intuition, as well as a precise, measurable movement with quantifiable physiological effects.

This book connects ancient traditions that look to the past with fast-paced, cutting-edge science that constantly re-envisions a new future. It respects both wisdom and experience from the East and science and experiments from the West. Separations become opportunities to see connections. Boundaries are seen just as convenient signposts to keep a conversation on a linear topic (for at least a while).

Peter Wayne himself is an embodiment of these tensions. His background—as a Harvard academician and medical researcher originally trained as an evolutionary biologist, an esteemed and revered Tai Chi teacher, and a down-home, no-nonsense Brooklyn guy with immigrant parents—has written an evidence-based book that captures the poetry of Tai Chi. This book is audacious. Ideas intersect, methodologies switch, and tensions nourish each other. Tai Chi is broken down into component therapeutic parts, while science is used to demonstrate the intersection of mind and body and the importance of the imagination and ritual. The natural world seen through the lens of evolution connects with the cosmological notions of yin and yang. Nature and culture are separate and yet still merge. Just as the book knows no boundaries, you will be gently guided to new, unexpected places. In the end, you will have tasted and experienced the vastness of a poem with limitless implications. Inspiring ideas about meditative stillness are balanced with information from randomized controlled trials. Both are enveloped by practical, nitty-gritty advice, such as how to find a good Tai Chi teacher.

Peter has written a timely book that is accessible and relevant to many audiences. This book nourishes many needs. If you want to learn Tai Chi and integrate it into your personal life, you will find this book to be an enticing adventure. If you are an experienced Tai Chi and mind-body practitioner interested in understanding the relevant emergent science, you will find a supportive guide. Physicians, allied health professionals, and alternative practitioners looking to advise their patients will find a fount of knowledge. Finally, health policy people with questions about Tai Chi will find their answers.

Chapter 1 is a clear, readable overview of Tai Chi's history and current developments. The chapter goes beyond the mythic (though it tells us some of the myths) and presents Tai Chi as a constantly evolving practice that necessarily undergoes changes as it reaches the Western world and must engage science and medical research.

Chapter 2 introduces a particularly unique contribution of this book—the articulation of what Peter has coined the "Eight Active Ingredients of Tai Chi." With links to Tai Chi classics and modern science, the chapter offers a clear explanation of the therapeutic components of Tai Chi. The discussion dissects Tai Chi into unexpected components, and yet somehow manages to recombine them into an elegant whole. It allows you to test the territory and encourages you to make some new movements.

In Chapter 3, the eight active ingredients are integrated into a very practical Tai Chi training program, similar to programs employed in Peter's clinical trials. Throughout this chapter, you can hear Peter's calm, embracing teaching voice. You're actually in his class.

Chapters 4 through 9 present a very readable, exciting summary of medical and basic science research on Tai Chi. In a balanced, objective way, the research covers what is known about Tai Chi's impact on health, ranging from fall prevention and cardiovascular risk factors to how it helps manage chronic pain and depression. In some cases, Peter creatively reaches outside of Tai Chi research to show potential and future directions. For example, Chapter 8, his discussion of clinical and physiological studies of motor imagery research is beautifully linked with the traditional Chinese concept of intention (*yi*). Here, the evidence is presented not so much to document what science knows so far, but rather to open doors for innovative discussion.

In Chapters 10 through 14, Peter realigns and brings together all the previous discussions of science and situates them into practical activities of everyday life. Tai Chi now informs the social interactions you navigate at work and at home, as well as your creative endeavors, including in the arts and sports. Finally, he provides practical information about developing a regular Tai Chi practice, finding Tai Chi classes, and knowing what to look for in a good Tai Chi program.

This book provides powerful insights and messages from multiple angles that somehow are pertinent to many different kinds of people. What is more amazing, Peter Wayne weaves these different perspectives into a single dance that is the essence of Tai Chi—an embrace of the flow and movement of the cosmos itself.

TED KAPTCHUK
Associate Professor of Medicine
Harvard Medical School
Author, *The Web That Has No Weaver:*
Understanding Chinese Medicine

Acknowledgments

This book would not be possible without the teachings, support, and feedback of so many people, more than I can possibly list here.

The Osher Center for Integrative Medicine at the Harvard Medical School and Brigham and Women's Hospital has been an amazing incubating ground for many of this book's ideas. I am indebted to my mentors and friends Julie Buring, Ted Kaptchuk, Sally Andrews, and David Eisenberg for supporting my academic transition from evolutionary biology to integrative medicine research, for their vision, and for exemplifying and demanding the highest scientific standards; to my colleagues and research collaborators, many of whom provided feedback on book sections or directly contributed to the original research on which it is based, including Andrew Ahn, Gloria Yeh, Paolo Bonato, Helene Langevin, Richard Hammerschlag, William Stason, Eric Jacobson, Cathy Kerr, Brad Manor, Ge Wu, Rebecca Wells, Suzie Bertisch, Ellen Connors, Mary Anne Ryan, Andrea Hrbek, Gurjeet Birdee, Donald Levy, Rosa Schnyer, Russell Phillips, Doug Kiel, Harriet Samuelson, Adi Haramati, Steven Wolf, Jeff Hausdorff, Lew Lipsitz, Vera Novak, C. K. Peng, Ary Goldberger, and Weidong Lu; and to my mentors and colleagues who shaped my thinking in evolutionary biology and ecology, including William Drury, Craig Greene, John Connolly, Fahkri Bazzaz, Tim Sipe, David Ackerly, Suzanne Morse, and David Folger.

Much of the research this book draws from would not have been possible without the generous support of the Bernard Osher Foundation; federal grant support from the National Center for Complementary and Alternative Medicine at the National Institutes of Health; support from the Kohlberg Family Foundation; and the personal vision and trust of two mentor-patrons, Elizabeth McCormack and Betsy Aron.

Equally invaluable have been my many teachers of Tai Chi and related healing arts. I am grateful for their inspiring, unswerving commitments to their own journeys that generated the expertise and wisdom they so generously shared. I am especially indebted to my two root Tai Chi and internal martial arts teachers, Robert Morningstar and Arthur Goodridge, for their remarkable insights into Tai Chi and multitudes of related practices, and to their encouragement to think independently and share these practices with others; to Charles Genoud, whose teaching in Gesture of Awareness transformed my understanding of Tai Chi; to Mantak Chia, Michael Winn, and Marie Favarito for their teachings in Qigong and inner alchemy; to Calvin Chin for his patience in teaching me Kung Fu; and to Carol Caton, whose wisdom and teaching defy categorization. I am also thankful for my teachers in the healing arts, many of whom have helped keep me healthy on my journey, including Xiaoming Cheng, Weidong Lu, Eric Jacobson, Randall Ferrell, Kuei Kuahara, Matthew Kowalski, Art Madore, and Edgar Miller.

My Tai Chi and Qigong students, past and present, including all of our study volunteers, have inspired me through their practice and commitment, kept me honest, and motivated me continuously to explore and enrich my own practice, which makes it fun and easy to keep showing up to teach. I wish to acknowledge especially the camaraderie and friendship of my senior students. Many of them have helped teach in our clinical trials and have contributed meaningfully to the material in this book; they include Jane Moss, Stanwood Chang, Regina Gibbons, Chris Lavancher, Deborah Cake, Marty Heitz, Pam Cobb, and Chris Zarza.

Most personally, I wish to thank my parents for their bravery, strength, and love, and my big sister Debbie for her unswerving support. And, finally, I am grateful beyond words to Liz, my life partner and best friend, and Sam, my son, the richest sources of joy I have known. Thanks to both of you for tolerating my often too busy life, and reminding me every day what it's really all about.

It has been great working with my coauthor, and now friend, Mark Fuerst. This book would never have happened without his deft writing skill, commitment to learning Tai Chi while writing this book, and remarkable patience, generosity, and optimism. We would also like to thank our Shambhala editor, Beth Frankl; the Chief Editor of Books at Harvard Health Publications, Julie Silver; and our agent, Linda Konner; for sharing their wisdom of the publishing industry and for their total support of this book project. Thanks also to C. J. Allen for his excellent photographic skills, and to Dan Litrownik for his assistance with footnotes.

In addition, Mark Fuerst would like to acknowledge the love and support of his wife Margie, son Ben, and daughter Sarah during the time spent away from them while he was writing and editing; the continuing love of his mother, Peppy; the camaraderie, brainstorming, and encouragement of the writers of the Brooklyn Brown Bag Lunch Group; and the wisdom, kindness, and patience of his two Tai Chi teachers, Phil Catapano and Rebecca Wolf.

The Harvard Medical School
Guide to Tai Chi

Introduction

East Meets West at Harvard Medical School

In July 2009, along with six other Tai Chi and mind-body researchers representing leading US medical schools, I found myself sitting on a panel with five of the most renowned living grand masters of Tai Chi—the equivalents of Dalai Lamas of Tai Chi. This unprecedented meeting between Tai Chi researchers and masters was part of the First International Tai Chi Symposium on the campus of Vanderbilt University Medical School, a landmark event for the world of Tai Chi. For the first time, masters representing all major Tai Chi styles convened in one place to teach and personally share their passion for Tai Chi, show unity across all styles, and speak with one voice about the future of this ancient martial art. More than 500 Tai Chi enthusiasts, medical researchers, policy makers, and health-care lobbyists sat in the audience awaiting this historical event.

For me, the fact that this evening's symposium was devoted to exploring the role that Western scientific research might play in informing Tai Chi's development and integration into Western health care was even more remarkable. Working by day as a medical researcher objectively studying the science of Tai Chi and at night as a community-based Tai Chi instructor, for many years I have walked the metaphorical S-shaped line dividing the more rational and intuitive halves of the Tai Chi yin and yang symbol. Both as a scientist and a teacher/practitioner, I have explored how best to bridge the wisdom underlying my two vocations, or in the lingo of Tai Chi, how the yin and yang can inform one another.

In many ways, the symposium was very successful. Some rich exchanges between the masters and researchers highlighted the promise of Tai Chi for improving health in our aging population; for example, by preventing heart disease and fall-related fractures. Other exchanges centered on the potential for cutting-edge scientific instrumentation to elucidate the impact of Tai Chi on physiological processes in the brain, heart, and musculoskeletal system. A brief discussion suggested how modern technology might help understand better the traditional Chinese medicine concepts foreign to most Westerners, such as Qi, or energy flow in the body.

Yet, despite these unprecedented exchanges of ideas, toward the end of the evening, I found myself a little dissatisfied and wanting much more. On a very simple level, I felt as if a few hours' time was far too little to devote to such rich topics. However, even more fundamentally, I felt that the depth of the discussions was limited by the huge cultural, linguistic, and epistemological barriers between the Tai Chi masters and the scientists. We do not yet have a well-developed language or framework to facilitate the bridging between the practice and the science of Tai Chi. As I sat on stage at the interface of two very different cultures—Eastern healing arts and Western science—I saw clearly how much work still was needed to build bridges. Part of my calling, and a central purpose of this book, is to explore this interface between the East and West through Tai Chi.

The science of Tai Chi is just now catching up with and substantiating what Tai Chi practitioners have known for centuries—Tai Chi often leads to more vigor and energy, greater flexibility, balance and mobility, and an improved sense of well-being. Cutting-edge research now lends support to long-standing claims that Tai Chi favorably impacts the health of the heart, bones, nerves and muscles, immune system, and the mind. This research also provides insight into the underlying physiological mechanisms that explain how Tai Chi works. This knowledge has enabled researchers like my Harvard Medical School colleagues and me to shape the essential elements of Tai Chi into programs that are well suited for a modern Western lifestyle and to integrate Tai Chi training efficiently into the rehabilitation and prevention of many health conditions.

"Yin and Yang—The Mother of Ten Thousand Things"

As this quote from Lao Tzu suggests, Tai Chi derives its name from the concept of yin and yang ☯, also known as the Tai Chi symbol. Yin and yang is a central concept in traditional Chinese medicine, philosophy, and science, and it is one of the deepest pillars of Chinese culture. The yin-yang symbol, now a very popular symbol in the West as well, depicts two complementary polar opposites that, together, create a dynamic, balanced, integrated, and inter-dependent whole.

Tai Chi training embodies this yin-yang concept at multiple levels. At the most obvious, physical level, Tai Chi is an exercise that aims to strengthen, stretch, balance, and coordinate and integrate the left and right halves of the body, the upper and lower halves of the body, and the extremities of the body with the inside or core. At a more subtle level, Tai Chi integrates body and mind. Body movements are coordinated with rhythmic, conscious breathing and multiple cognitive and emotional components—including focused attention, heightened self-awareness, visualization, imagery, and intention.

At perhaps an even more subtle level, Tai Chi sensitizes and integrates you with your social and physical environment. At an interpersonal level, being in tune with other people in your social environment helps you to learn to read and appropriately respond to their cues. This internal/external integration is one of Tai Chi's secrets as a martial art—by becoming extremely sensitive to your opponent's moves, you learn to lead by neutralizing and following. Connecting with nature can also be an integral part of Tai Chi training. Practicing outside in a park may provide a sense of being recharged or nourished by the natural environment. For some, heightened conscious awareness of oneself, and our connection to and integration with the greater natural world, can also afford a spiritual dimension—enhancing a sense of being part of some larger vital, unfolding natural process.

To an outsider watching a master practice or perform Tai Chi, successful yin-yang integration is reflected in the seamless connection of graceful movements, with one flowing into another, as well as a sense of focus, calmness, and peacefulness. You can sense that the master has both inner and outer integration and awareness, and is in tune with himself or herself and the surrounding environment. In Tai Chi, as with yin and yang, everything is interconnected. The Tai Chi master reflects what Professor Ted Kaptchuk, my Harvard Medical School colleague and scholar on Chinese medicine, calls a "Web that has no Weaver."[1]

This Eastern holistic and ecological view of the body, mind, and health now is becoming increasingly appreciated and adopted within the Western medical community. Elements of this holistic perspective have been implicit throughout the history of what we now call conventional medicine, or biomedicine, but the modern Western medical community increasingly has relied on a reductionist framework for defining health, managing disease, and training physicians. The central tenet of this modern reductionist model is to focus on root causes of disease, for example, infectious agents, genetic or developmental abnormalities, or injuries. The reductionist approach assumes that complex problems can be solved by dividing them into smaller, simpler parts, or into more tractable units. Another Harvard Medical School colleague and collaborator, Dr. Andrew Ahn, has called this strategy "divide and conquer."[2]

Of course, reductionism in modern medicine has led to tremendous successes, including the development of medications, genetic markers, imaging, and curative surgery. However, reductionism has its limits and downsides. As Ahn says, "Reductionism becomes less effective when the act of dividing a problem into its parts leads to a loss of important information about the whole."[3]

This limitation inherent in dividing a problem is especially the case in complex chronic diseases such as diabetes, coronary artery disease, or recurrent low-back pain, where a single factor rarely is implicated as being solely responsible for the disease development or presentation. Rather, multiple factors are often identified, and the disease evolves through complex interactions between them. In addition to missing the forest for the trees, some other concerns of reductionism include the loss of the whole person, depersonalization of medicine, lack of communication among specialists, and even greater costs due to lack of coordinated care.

HARVARD LOOKS TO THE EAST

At Harvard Medical School, as well as at many other academic medical centers across the United States, signs of holistic thinking are evident in medicine at all levels, from clinicians to researchers to educators, including a vibrant program evaluating the medical benefits of Tai Chi and related mind-body practices. In 2000, the Harvard Medical School Council of Academic Deans established the Division for Research and Education in Complementary and Integrative Medical Therapies. The program was charged with facilitating interdisciplinary and inter-institutional faculty collaboration for purposes of: (1) research evaluation of complementary and integrative medical therapies; (2) delivering educational programs to the medical community and the public; (3) and investigating the design of sustainable models of complementary and integrative care delivery in an academic setting. Since its inception, and now under the auspices of the Osher Center for Integrative Medicine jointly based at Harvard Medical School and Brigham and Women's Hospital, faculty and collaborators have received dozens of National Institutes of Health grants, published hundreds of peer-reviewed scientific papers, and are affecting significantly the care received across Harvard hospitals. Today, nearly all of the Harvard hospitals have programs that provide some form of integrative medicine. At both Brigham and Women's Hospital's Osher clinic and Massachusetts General Hospital's Benson Henry clinic, physicians and complementary alternative medicine practitioners see patients, and prescriptions might include a course of Tai Chi, meditation, yoga, and counseling on diet and lifestyle, alongside conventional medicine. Harvard Medical School hospitals are examples of how insight and credible research supporting the therapeutic promise of Tai Chi and related mind-body practices can catalyze the integration of these practices into conventional medical practice.

This book seeks to show, in a scientifically balanced and objective manner, the clinical promise for Tai Chi and to provide insights into the underlying physiological processes that explain how Tai Chi improves health. Tai Chi includes a rich mixture of therapeutic components––what I've organized as the "Eight Active Ingredients." Articulating knowledge of these ingredients has enabled my Harvard Medical School colleagues and me to sharpen the focus of Tai Chi for our modern Western lives and target more efficiently rehabilitation and prevention for many health conditions. With this knowledge, we have formulated a variety of simplified Tai Chi protocols that have been tested in numerous clinical trials at Harvard Medical School and affiliated hospitals, the essential elements of which I share in this book.

My Life in Tai Chi

My interest in Tai Chi research has grown out of a long-term personal passion for martial arts and Eastern philosophy, which started when I was in high school, around the same time my interests in science started forming. My Tai Chi training, which is still ongoing, has included many great teachers—from both the East and the West. While I have been studying for more than 35 years, it still feels as if I have only touched the surface of this rich, ancient art. Since 1985, I have taught in the Boston area at a community school that I founded, which gives me an opportunity to share what I have learned with a wide range of people and to think about the best ways to transmit this information; teaching there also provides a place to integrate what I learn from my Harvard Medical School research. I loosely view my Tai Chi classes as the equivalent of my medical colleagues' clinical practice.

My journey to becoming a scientific Tai Chi researcher has not been a linear one, but rather one that has taken many twists and turns. After doing an undergraduate interdisciplinary study in human ecology and two years in plant-population biology research in Europe, I completed a PhD in Evolutionary Biology at Harvard University. In 2000, following a trip to China and additional formal training in Tai Chi and Qigong, I decided to make a significant career shift, bringing my two worlds together and employing my research skills and ecological framework to study the clinical and basic aspects of Chinese medicine, including Tai Chi. My first position was as founding Research Director at the New England School of Acupuncture. I obtained National Institutes of Health grants, and then established and led a formal collaboration with Harvard Medical School centered on Asian medicine. In 2006, I formally became a faculty member at Harvard Medical School. As director of the Tai Chi and Mind-Body Research Program, and more recently, as overall Research Director for the Osher Center for Integrative Medicine, I have found my dream job. Both as a scientist and a Tai Chi thinker, I love looking for connections and building bridges.

Being both a researcher at Harvard Medical School and a community-based Tai Chi practitioner is a yin-yang balancing act. As a scientist during the day at Harvard Medical School, I adhere to the rules of objective, unbiased, rigorous scientific research. My work is not to find results to prove that Tai Chi is good; in other words, I am not an advocate researcher. Rather, I seek dispassionately to understand what works, what doesn't work, what is safe, and if there is promise for a certain population or medical condition, to explore how best to integrate Tai Chi with state-of-the-art health care. My colleagues and I use rigorous research designs that minimize bias, and we follow strict scientific codes. This assures that bias does not affect the research.

In my own Tai Chi practice and when teaching Tai Chi classes, my research informs my experience and teaching, but sometimes I need to abandon the framework of science. Part of the practice of Tai Chi and other meditative arts requires turning off rational thinking and tapping into other, less understood processes, like intuition and imagination. For example, Tai Chi classics say, "Belief or mind moves internal energy (Qi) and Qi moves the body." At this point in my Tai Chi training, on a good day, this idea is very clear to me. I can readily shift into a meditative Tai Chi flow. But the scientific community is still far from defining or quantifying Qi, or knowing all the neurophysiological pathways involved in mind-body-energy connections.

My primary goal as a teacher is to use whatever tools I can to help students have meaningful experiences, so to teach only from pure science would be inefficient and unethical. The practitioner half of me remains skeptical of science and thinks maybe science can never address some issues. Nevertheless, my two jobs, one as a daytime researcher and the other as an evening Tai Chi teacher, involve a dynamic dance between yin and yang, both informing one another and incubating rich thoughts, and they have led to my unique style of teaching and practicing Tai Chi.

Throughout this book, I will be clear which half of me is talking. When scientific evidence exists, I will provide the link to published research. I will distinguish this evidence from my personal experiences or experiences my students share, or principles that Tai Chi classics purport or my teachers and other masters espouse.

About The Harvard Medical School Guide to Tai Chi

The Harvard Medical School Guide to Tai Chi grew out of my long-standing training in Tai Chi, my interest in mind-body research, and my balance as both a practitioner and a researcher. Through my Tai Chi classes and research studies, I have been fortunate enough to help people in their twenties and thirties improve their athletic abilities and martial arts practices, provide an outlet for those in their forties and fifties to reduce the stresses of the work world, and help people in their sixties, seventies, eighties, and nineties find a gentle form of restorative exercise.

This book puts down on paper how to use the concepts of Tai Chi to enhance your health. It shows, step by step, how the Eight Active Ingredients of Tai Chi can heighten bodily awareness and inner focus, make body movements more graceful and efficient, enhance natural breathing and heart health, and help attain peace of mind. The growing problems associated with our fast-paced, multitasking, overstimulated, more-is-better, Western lifestyle can be counteracted by the "meditation in motion" of Tai Chi. The dynamic changes derived from a regular Tai Chi practice provide a practical strategy for navigating life with less stress and more balance. I assemble and integrate in this book a diverse set of knowledge from both the East and the West—from the simplified Tai Chi exercises outlined to the ancient roots of Tai Chi and the modern science substantiating its health claims—with the sincere intention and hope that it will enrich your life and help provide you with a roadmap for your own Tai Chi journey.

One explicit goal of this book is to make Tai Chi more accessible and easier to practice regularly. Just like having a doctor's prescription for a medication, a diet, or an exercise regimen, these therapies only work when you adhere to them. In addition, despite your best intentions, because of a busy lifestyle—whether it's being an overworked executive, a fast-moving soccer mom, or an athlete with limited time for cross training—you may need a program that is not only effective, but also practical. The simplified program this book introduces is very easy to learn and allows you to focus on the essential principles of Tai Chi. What's more, in addition to a formal program, you will learn numerous simple exercises that you can easily sneak into your everyday life at home or at work, adding a little more energy and flow to help you think and perform all your tasks better.

In this book, you will find:

- An introduction to the traditional principles of Tai Chi, as viewed through the lens of modern medical science
- A simplified Tai Chi protocol, including extensive descriptions and photos of the exercises that you can do on your own, similar to regimens that a number of clinical trials have demonstrated to work
- Insight into the underlying physiological processes that explain how Tai Chi can improve your health
- State-of-the-art, objective summaries of the research literature that highlight what is and what is not yet known about the health benefits of Tai Chi
- How the Eight Active Ingredients of Tai Chi can be integrated into personal and professional relationships, improve work productivity, enhance creativity, and boost sports performance

We hope that, in reading this book, you will come to the conclusion that Tai Chi addresses a critical need for novel approaches in today's health care and, most importantly, that the integration of Tai Chi into the medical world can help prevent the progression and personal and economic burden of chronic diseases.

Part of the goal of mixing scientific evidence with Eastern wisdom—again, this yin-yang concept—is that knowledge gives you power. If you understand how the body works and the amazing degree to which it can regulate itself, and you understand how Tai Chi accentuates multiple self-healing processes, this knowledge can allay much of the fear associated with illnesses as they arise and empower you to play a leading, central role in your own health. Gaining a more intimate knowledge of how your body works may even catalyze your progress in Tai Chi training. My hope is that this knowledge will also intrigue Tai Chi instructors to become more interested and knowledgeable about the research so they are better able to communicate and collaborate with the conventional medical community and better serve their students.

The Harvard Medical School Guide to Tai Chi also offers you information about developing a regular Tai Chi practice, locating Tai Chi classes, and knowing what to look for in a good Tai Chi program. My hope is that by following the instructions this book provides, you can achieve the same positive changes I see every day in my students and in the volunteer participants in our studies; they provide their stories in their own words, describing what it's like to learn Tai Chi and how it has affected their lives. I also provide my personal experiences working with Tai Chi masters to show how you, too, can improve your health, strengthen your heart, and sharpen your mind.

PART ONE

Tai Chi and Its Essential Elements

1

The Ancient Promise of, and Modern Need for, Tai Chi

"You don't have to have a health issue to do Tai Chi. But if you do, you should find a way to incorporate Tai Chi into some part of your life," says Faith, age 54, an attorney who began Tai Chi to manage her back pain. "You can do it anywhere and practice it with no special equipment. Whether it's 10 minutes a day on your own or 60 minutes in class a few times a week, you will be better for it. There's something with these ancient arts. They don't last for centuries for nothing."

One challenge I face in my academic talks on Tai Chi simply is how to define Tai Chi. I'll sometimes begin my talk with a slide of a large lightbulb with the title "What Is Tai Chi?" I'll then admit that Tai Chi is hard to define and explain that a common Tai Chi lightbulb joke helps us understand why: How many Tai Chi players does it take to change a lightbulb? Answer: 100. One to change the bulb and the other 99 to say, "We do not do it that way in our style of Tai Chi."

The diversity and richness of Tai Chi derives from a few reasons. First, Tai Chi is made up of multiple components, including many physical, cognitive, and psychosocial ingredients. Just like making soup, the more ingredients you begin with, the greater is your potential for diverse recipes. Second, because Tai Chi's long history is embedded within an ever-changing social and cultural background, many Tai Chi styles have developed that emphasize slightly different characteristics.

I often use some variation of the following broad definition: Tai Chi is a mind-body exercise rooted in multiple Asian traditions, including martial arts, traditional Chinese medicine, and philosophy. Tai Chi training integrates slow, intentional movements with breathing and cognitive skills (for example, mindfulness and imagery). It aims to strengthen, relax, and integrate the physical body and mind, enhance the natural flow of Qi, and improve health, personal development, and self-defense.

TAI CHI: WHAT'S IN A NAME?

What we refer to as Tai Chi throughout this book is a simplified abbreviation of the more formal name *Tai Chi Chuan,* variously written as t'ai chi ch'uan, taijiquan, tai ji quan, or tai ji chuan, depending on the styles of transcription.[1]

Tai translates literally as "great" or "large." *Chi* is used as a superlative, for example, "biggest" or "most ultimate." Together, they are used to characterize the philosophical concept of the all-encompassing yin-yang principle, often translated as Supreme Ultimate.

Chuan generally is translated as "fist" or "boxing." Sometimes, it is described as a manifestation, as the closing fist expresses a sense of practical materialization.

Together, Tai Chi Chuan is variously translated as Supreme Ulti-mate Boxing, Great Extremes Boxing, and Grand Ultimate Fist. It describes a form of boxing or exercise that is based on the principles of yin and yang, dynamic change and transformation, integrating the body and mind, and the internal and the external.

Chi vs. Qi and Tai Chi vs. Qigong

The character for "Qi" is different from the "chi" of Tai Chi. Qi is like the word *snow* in the Eskimo language—it means many things, and yet it is hard to define. "Qi" refers to vital energy, information, breath, or spirit. Qi is not unique to humans, but rather is what per-vades the whole universe.

Qi is the first part of a very diverse set of mind-body practices called Qigong. Broadly speaking, Qigong translates as the cultiva-tion or mastery of Qi. Some styles of Qigong are oriented more to-ward health and spirituality, in which you sit and do breathing and meditative exercises. Other styles are more vigorous and are designed to enhance your martial art skills. Most people think of Tai Chi as a form of Qigong because it cultivates, moves, and helps manage Qi.

THE HISTORICAL ROOTS OF TAI CHI

Tai Chi has a relatively stable nucleus of movement principles and inter-nal energetics, but a cell membrane that interacts with great fluidity to its environment.[2]

—DOUGLAS WILE, TAI CHI HISTORIAN AND SCHOLAR

Tai Chi is viewed best as a diverse set of living and evolving practices—practices that have been informed by the insights of a long lineage of de-voted practitioners, molded and adapted over time to ever- (and still-) changing cultural needs and social landscapes. This diversity is enhanced further by Tai Chi's rich and intertwined historical origins, including threads linking it to Asian martial arts, healing arts, philosophy, and spiritual practices that span thousands of years. Even within its relatively recent history over the past three centuries, Tai Chi has shown dynamic adaptation to changing cultural needs and opportunities in China. It has evolved from a secret, orally transmitted self-defense system in the 1700s to the early 1800s; to a more widely shared fighting art used to train the military; to a publicly shared method for personal development and longevity exercises in the mid-1800s to mid-1900s; to a national exercise, sport, and performing art the government promotes and showcases to the rest of the world as a national treasure.

Tai Chi's expansion into the West over the past 50 years, including its interface with science and evidence-based biomedicine, along with Westerners' hunger for holistic health and philosophical wisdom from the East, has dramatically catalyzed its evolution. Tai Chi is now taught in hospitals, sports clubs, colleges, and community centers across the United States, and hundreds of Tai Chi books are available to the Western public. Tai Chi has blended and mixed with other practices, including Qigong, yoga, meditation, and contemporary mind-body practices, such as Feldenkrais and the Alexander Technique. Like the philosophy of Taoism that animates it, the art and practice of Tai Chi continues to evolve and "go with the flow."

Like many ancient traditions, the early history of Tai Chi is a mixture of fact and myth. This history includes the interweaving of three deep influences of Chinese culture. Those three influences are martial arts, healing arts, and philosophy.[3]

MARTIAL ARTS INFLUENCE

Chinese culture is notorious for its long, diverse history of martial arts. Hand-to-hand combat and weapons practice were important in training ancient Chinese soldiers and rival clans. Skilled fighters also were highly valued as bodyguards, providing protection to wealthy government leaders and traveling merchants or messengers. China's rich diversity of martial arts often is depicted in Kung Fu movies, usually set in old temples and depicting battles between warring states or feuding families seeking revenge.

Martial arts also have played a prominent role in Chinese performing arts and theater. Demonstrations of martial arts prowess, fixed sparring routines, acrobatics, and lion dances have been a key component of public performances. These continue today and have recently reached Western and international communities through tours by the Shaolin monks and Peking acrobats.

An important landmark in the history of Chinese martial arts is the Shaolin Temple in Henan Province, considered the cradle of Chinese martial arts. Legend has it that the Bodhidarma, who brought Chan (Zen) Buddhism to China in the sixth century, arrived to find the monks at the Shaolin temple in extremely poor health and fitness. He taught them a series of exercises to strengthen their minds and bodies for meditation. These exercises evolved into what are now called Shaolin Boxing, Wushu, or Kung Fu.[4]

A key semi-mythical figure in the history of Tai Chi, often called the father of Tai Chi, is Chang San-feng, generally thought to have lived in the thirteenth century C.E. It is widely told that Chang San-feng was a Shaolin monk who decided to leave the monastery to become a Taoist hermit. In the Wudang Mountains, he gave up the harder Kung Fu fighting style he had learned and formulated a new art based on his observations of nature and Taoist principles of softness and yielding. Legend has it that he had an "aha" moment after watching a fight between a snake and a crane. Every time the crane would try to attack the snake's head, the snake would yield, evade, and hit the crane with its tail. When the crane would try for the snake's tail, the snake would yield and bite the crane. This process resulted in the emphasis of the basic Tai Chi (yin-yang) concepts of evading, yielding, and attacking. Chang developed a martial art based on natural principles that used softness and internal power to overcome brute force.[5] For this reason, Tai Chi and related martial arts that emphasize yielding and mindful or intrinsic strength, or Jin, are commonly classified as internal (or inner) styles. In contrast, many forms of karate and Kung Fu that typically rely on muscular strength and speed are classified as external (outer) styles.[6]

The early history of how core principles and movements attributed to semi-mythical characters, such as Chang San-feng, became codified into today's formalized Tai Chi forms is not agreed upon fully or understood. Some historians and scholars believe that many of the distinctive postures and names associated with contemporary Tai Chi may be attributable to Ming dynasty general Ch'i Chi-kuang (1528–87), author of the "Boxing Classic." Many of the movements this text describes are included in the martial art systems that were subsequently developed in the Chen family village of Henan—the home of Chen-style Tai Chi. Chen style is the oldest of all formal Tai Chi systems and the one back to which all other contemporary styles can be traced. Specifically, Chen-style Tai Chi is attributed to Chen Wang-ting (1580–1660) in the mid-seventeenth century. Similar to the legend of Chang San Feng, Chen Wang-ting is thought to have combined contemporary boxing techniques with meditative and health-promoting Qigong exercises, resulting in a more internalized martial art that emphasized softness, circular movements, and Jin.

Another key figure in Tai Chi's martial development is Yang Lu-ch'an (1799–1872), who learned this art in Chen village. Some accounts suggest Yang Lu-ch'an was an aspiring young martial artist who witnessed Chen masters apply their secret art and was so impressed that he had to learn it. So, he moved to Chen village to be a servant and learned by clandestinely watching family disciples train under master Chen Chang Shing. After watching these lessons, he practiced diligently on his own in secret. Apparently, one day when master Chen Chang Shing was not home, a troupe of martial artists visited the village and challenged the Chen family practitioners to a fighting match. After the troupe defeated Chen's family members, Yang emerged, defeated the troupe, and defended the Chen family's honor. This earned him the respect of Master Chen, who accepted Yang as his first "outside" (non-family) student. Master Chen also gave Yang permission to leave the Chen village and teach others.[7] In 1852, Yang Lu-ch'an moved to Beijing to teach what he called "soft boxing" or "cotton boxing." His high martial skills earned him the title "Yang the Invincible." In addition, among other teaching activities, he was appointed to teach his art to the Imperial Guards and members of the Qing court. Yang also adapted his teaching methods for a broader growing public audience who was increasingly interested in health and personal development; this approach included a less-strenuous regimen with less emphasis on martial applications.

Yang's teaching, along with the teachings of his children, and especially one of his grandsons, Yang Cheng Fu, laid the foundation for what is now called Yang-style Tai Chi, the most widely practiced style in the world today. Many of Yang's senior students and disciples also played a significant role in the evolution of numerous other prominent Tai Chi lineages, including the Wu, Wu/Hao, and Sun styles (see "Tai Chi Styles and Forms" below).

While the majority of practitioners today practice Tai Chi for health, the martial arts aspect is still popular and is central to the art's evolution. Martial skills are no longer tested in hand-to-hand battles to the death, but they are tested in regulated sports competitions. Some events include full-contact sparring, like boxing and contemporary mixed-martial arts. More commonly, martial skills are tested in two-person events called "Push Hands," where the goal is to uproot physically an opponent while keeping one's own feet rooted. Almost as if by magic, the highest-level practitioners appear to exert no apparent effort in pushing hands. When pushed, they are able to relax, evade, and deflect an opponent's incoming force, and sometimes, send their uprooted opponent flying a great distance.

However, even for students not interested in self-defense training or Push-Hands competition, many teachers, including myself, consider it essential to teach functional, martial applications of Tai Chi, such as rooting, structural connectedness, and yielding. Developing these interactive skills can provide students with critical kinesthetic experiences that catalyze the comprehension and integration of the core principles of Tai Chi into their solo practice routine. This training can also provide students with functional benefits to more general everyday activities, such as lifting heavy objects, maintaining balance in a fast-moving, crowded marketplace, or staying centered during emotionally challenging interactions.

TAI CHI STYLES AND FORMS

Over time, various Tai Chi styles have evolved. These styles share many basic or core Tai Chi principles. As Tai Chi has evolved, some of the principles, and the manner in which they are expressed practically in practice regimens, also have evolved. In a sense, Tai Chi is like the kid's game of telephone where one person whispers a phrase into another's ear, and after many whispers, the phrase often becomes quite different. Tai Chi has morphed with insights and specific emphases of each master and the students who carry on the tradition. Among the most common styles today are the

Chen, Yang, Wu, Hao, and Sun. Each of these five styles is named after the founder's family name. Many other less popular styles exist, and new ones continue to evolve, including shortened and simplified protocols for research similar to the one found in this book.

Forms and Movements

Within each style, you will find many choreographed routines. The language used to describe these routines may vary, but they are most commonly called forms or sets. Each form, whether done with bare hands or weapons (for example, sword, staff, or spear), has a certain number of movements or postures. For example, within Yang-style schools, some teach a form having as many as 150 movements, while others teach as few as eight movements.

HEALING ARTS INFLUENCE

Tai Chi shares a common historical pathway with the development of traditional Chinese medicine, which explicitly includes prescriptions of exercise and lifestyle, along with herbs, diet, acupuncture, massage, and other modalities for maintaining health and longevity. One of the earliest texts of traditional Chinese medicine, "The Internal Canon of the Yellow Emperor" (c. 2000–1600 B.C.E.)," mentions how the Yellow Emperor practiced health-promoting exercises based on the movements of animals. A later famous physician, Hua Tuo (c. 145–208 C.E.), is credited with developing a fitness training regimen also patterned after animal movements. Often called the five animal frolics, Hua Tuo's exercises apparently were developed so that each exercise targets a specific internal organ within the framework of traditional Chinese medicine.[8] For example, the tiger exercise targets the energetic functioning of the lungs, and the bear exercise targets the kidneys. The fundamental goal of these exercises, as is the case with Chinese medicine in general, is to enhance and balance the circulation of Qi among the organ systems and throughout the body as a whole. Movements in contemporary Tai Chi forms, such as "Snake Creeps Down," "Crane Cools Its Wings," and "Step Back to Repulse the Monkey," reflect and extend this tradition of observing nature, mimicking elements of naturalistic, animal-like movements, and applying them to health and self-defense.

To be a successful, enduring, high-level martial artist, practitioners needed to be healthy in body and mind. During Tai Chi's evolution as a martial art, practitioners likely recognized and appreciated its health benefits because it emphasizes internal development, and for some, but not all, also was associated with health-promoting philosophies and lifestyles.[9] However, only after Yang Cheng Fu began teaching Tai Chi more widely in the early- to mid-1900s, drawing students interested in martial arts as well as the elite intelligentsia, did Tai Chi begin to be practiced more widely for health promotion and self-development. This growing public interest in Tai Chi for health coincided with a national "self-strengthening" movement the government advocated, which sought to improve Chinese society and its self-image by preserving Chinese values yet adopting, when appropriate, ideas and technology from the West. A line in a Tai Chi classic poem entitled "Thirteen Posture Song" reads, "What is the purpose of this discipline? To lengthen one's life, extend one's years, and to give one an ageless springtime."[10]

A noteworthy development in Tai Chi's widespread promotion for health was the development of a 24-posture simplified form, or the Beijing Form. This form was developed in 1956 by the National Physical Culture and Sports Commission of the People's Republic of China as part of the drive to standardize Tai Chi training for social reform and sport. This form was part of a national fitness program.[11] Today, you can go to parks across China and see millions practicing Tai Chi. This practice is clearly part of the country's health maintenance system, and many Chinese hospitals integrate Tai Chi into rehabilitation. The recent development of shortened forms of all major styles of Tai Chi has made it easier to teach and to learn Tai Chi, and learning one of these short forms is now mandatory for most Chinese college students.

Philosophical Influence

Tai Chi's roots also are intertwined with multiple Eastern philosophies and religions, among which Taoism is the most prominent. The oral tradition of Taoism is believed to extend back in Chinese history to 3,000

B.C.E. One of earliest and most seminal Taoist writings, the "Tao Te Ching," is attributed to Lao Tzu and is dated about 2,500 years ago.[12] At the core of Taoism are multiple principles for guiding a person's path through life. In fact, one literal translation of *Tao* means "way" or "path." Exactly how principles of Taoism and other Eastern philosophies were infused into Tai Chi is not clear due to its long, complex history and the poorly written records. Nevertheless, it is very clear when reading Lao Tzu and other Taoist texts that several key principles of Taoism resonate with the practice, philosophy, and spirit of Tai Chi.

One example is Tai Chi's emphasis on softness and yielding. Lao Tzu wrote, "Nothing in the world is as soft and yielding as water. Yet for dissolving the hard and inflexible, nothing can surpass it. The soft overcomes the hard; the gentle overcomes the rigid." A second example is self-awareness and responsibility for one's self, which applies to health, relationships, and martial interactions. Lao Tzu wrote: "Knowing others is intelligence; knowing yourself is true wisdom. Mastering others is strength; mastering yourself is true power."[13]

Some branches of Taoism also offer a cosmological framework, a way of seeing oneself as connected to something larger and as part of nature. Nature and its organic forces and processes offer us a kind of inspiration for life, something we continuously can be nourished by and learn to grow from if we listen and observe. Lao Tzu wrote: "When you realize where you come from, you naturally become tolerant, disinterested, amused, kindhearted as a grandmother, dignified as a king. Immersed in the wonder of the Tao, you can deal with whatever life brings you."[14]

This philosophical influence contributes to the richness of Tai Chi as an exercise sought after for body, mind, and spirit, and these philosophical aspects likely contribute to its therapeutic effects. Importantly, many teachers explicitly refer to these teachings in their classes, and some have calligraphy wall hangings, books, and other expressions of these principles around the Tai Chi studio to remind students of these ideas and to create a larger context for the practice of these exercises. This influence may be as relevant in China as it is in the West. Tai Chi scholar Douglas Wile wrote that "for the tens of millions of practitioners in China today, Tai Chi fills the spiritual vacuum left by the collapse of socialist idealism."[15]

On the front door of my Tai Chi school, I have a copy of a poem entitled "Hall of Happiness," written by one of my teacher's teachers, Grand Master Cheng Man Ching—a poem he hung on the front door of what was one of the first Tai Chi studios established in the West.

HALL OF HAPPINESS

May the joy that is everlasting gather in this hall. Not the joy of a sumptuous feast, which slips away even as we leave the table; nor that which music brings—it is only of a limited duration. Beauty and a pretty face are like flowers; they bloom for a while, then die. Even our youth slips swiftly away and is gone.

No, enduring happiness is not in these . . . . We may as well forget them, for the joy I mean is worlds away from these. It is the joy of continuous growth, of helping to develop in ourselves and in others the talents and abilities with which we were born—the gifts of heaven to mortal men. It is to revive the exhausted and to rejuvenate that which is in decline, so that we are enabled to dispel sickness and suffering.

Let true affection and happy concourse abide in this hall. Let us here correct our past mistakes and lose preoccupation with self. With the constancy of the planets in their courses or of the dragon in his cloud wrapped path, let us enter the land of health and ever after walk within its bounds.

Let us fortify ourselves against weakness and learn to be self-reliant, without ever a moment's lapse. Then our resolution will become the very air we breathe, the world we live in; then we will be as happy as a fish in crystal waters. This is the joy which lasts, that we can carry with us to the end of our days. And tell me, if you can; what greater happiness can life bestow?

CHENG MAN CHING
New York City, 1973[16]

TAI CHI IN THE WEST

While historians have shown that many aspects of Chinese medicine and culture, including Tai Chi, came to the United States in the 1800s during the building of railroads, the main entry was in the 1960s. One of the earliest and most prominent teachers to bring Tai Chi to the West was Cheng Man Ching.[17] A student of Yang Cheng Fu, Cheng Man Ching was the perfect ambassador of Tai Chi for the West. Master Cheng was classically trained in painting, poetry, philosophy, Chinese herbal medicine, and martial arts, the so-called five excellences. Prior to and throughout his Tai Chi training and teaching, he maintained many distinguished academic positions in universities, as well as governmental leadership positions related to the development and dissemination of Chinese culture. In 1964, he came to the United States and started Shr Jung Center for cultural arts in New York, and later, the Shr Jung Tai Chi School.[18]

In the early 1960s, even in large cities such as New York, Eastern practices were hard to find. There were some martial arts (karate and judo), but most mind-body Eastern practices, even yoga, were still considered cult-like and in conflict with Judeo-Christian beliefs, and many were kept somewhat underground. This period was also a time of significant cultural change, with the Vietnam War and broad questions of materialism, nonviolence, and the hippie movement. The Beatles could be seen on TV with Maharishi Mahesh Yogi, and transcendental meditation was becoming popular.

When Cheng Man Ching arrived and launched his Tai Chi school, this was a landmark event and struck many chords. As photos and black-and-white videos of the early days at Shr Jung reveal, he attracted very diverse groups, from ex-patriot Chinese seeking an opportunity to study under a traditional master and martial artists seeking new internal secrets, to people of all races and genders seeking insight into Eastern wisdom. As the Chinese historian and scholar Professor Douglas Wile wrote, even to this day, "Tai Chi is China's cultural ambassador to the world . . . Touching lives of more westerners, and perhaps more deeply, than books, films, museums or college courses, Tai Chi is often an entrée to Chinese philosophy, medicine, meditation, and even language."[19]

Many of Cheng Man Ching's senior students in Asia, including Benjamin Peng Lo, William Chen, and T. T. Liang, followed him to the United States and continued to study with him and help him teach new students. They went on to become significant teachers and helped further spread Tai Chi throughout the United States.

Since the 1960s, many new teachers, including leading representatives from all major Tai Chi lineages, have come to the United States and set up schools or have taught seminars at New Age centers such as Omega and Esalan. Some ran summer camps and held annual Tai Chi festivals, which furthered the spread and diversity of Tai Chi in the United States. Parallel expansions occurred throughout North and South America, Europe, and Australia. This growth happened concomitantly with the rapid infusion of other Eastern arts, including teachings from many schools of Qigong, yoga, and Buddhism, as well as healing mind-body therapies originating in the West (for instance, Feldenkrais and the Alexander Technique).

A reflection of how successful the invasion has been is World Tai Chi Day, organized by Bill Douglas. One of the purposes of this day is "to bring together people across racial, economic, religious, and geo-political boundaries, to join together for the purpose of health and healing, providing an example to the world." Millions of people around the world—65 nations participated in 2011—gather one day each year to celebrate the health and healing benefits of Tai Chi and Qigong.[20]

In China, the opportunity to learn an internal art and work closely with a high-level master was a rare, once-in-a-lifetime event for most people. Westerners now have unprecedented access to teachings from all traditions through classes, books, videotapes, and the Internet. This access has led to comingling of practices, which some scholars believe has led to a greater infusion of energetic, spiritual, and martial principles into training, which were not always emphasized in contemporary, widely taught, and sometimes-censored nationalized forms.[21] This comingling also has led to new hybrids, sometimes repackaged with new names, such as Tai Chi Yoga and Mindful Tai Chi. Because no single, sanctioned national organization currently is responsible for monitoring the development of Tai Chi training and teacher credentialing and, in the West, there is little political control over teaching practices prohibited in China due to political reasons, it is likely that the West will continue to serve as an important cradle for the development and evolution of Tai Chi.

Tai Chi Meets Western Science

One final and highly significant factor to mention in Tai Chi's evolution and increasing popularity in the West is its interface with biomedical science. Biomedical research has been especially important in attracting Western middle-aged and older-aged adults into Tai Chi, and drawing the attention of health-care providers, insurance companies, and policy makers.

The scientific method was not foreign to ancient Taoists, who as alchemists and physicians are credited with the development of anesthesia and many other medicinal discoveries.[22]

But, Western, peer-reviewed research has made the biggest impact on communicating the health benefits of Tai Chi. The first Western randomized, controlled trial, published in 1987, evaluated Tai Chi for balance and range of movement in older adults.[23] Today, more than 700 peer-reviewed papers have been published, and this number is growing at an exponential rate.

We maintain a Tai Chi research database in our research group at the Osher Center for Integrative Medicine that, as of fall 2012, contains more than 400 clinical studies (including 180 randomized trials) that have been conducted in the West alone. This research includes compelling, but in many cases not yet definitive, data that Tai Chi may improve aspects of balance, cardiovascular health, the immune system, sleep, psychological well-being, and other dimensions of health. This research also has begun to characterize the physiological mechanisms underlying the observed clinical effects, adding further credibility to the research findings. This research also is making a difference in Westerners' perception of Tai Chi. Recent surveys suggest three million Americans practice Tai Chi specifically for health.[24]

This evidence-based research also has catalyzed Tai Chi into the biomedical setting. For example, Tai Chi is taught at several hospitals affiliated with Harvard Medical School, as it is at many other major medical centers around the country. The evidence for Tai Chi is leading to more awareness within the medical community. In my own community-based school, an increasing number of students come because their physicians or other health-care providers have referred them. Tai Chi classes seem to fill a need for a form of therapy that touches body, mind, and spirit—what the medical community calls a biopsychosocial approach—for prevention and rehabilitation.

MEDICALIZATION OF TAI CHI

One interesting byproduct of the biomedical research and evolution of Tai Chi forms is the development of simplified protocols amenable to short, clinical trials. These protocols make it easier to learn Tai Chi in a safe way and even allow people who are older or whose bodies are deconditioned to experience the essential elements of Tai Chi and participate in clinical trials. The first one to be used in a randomized, controlled trial was developed by Tai Chi Master Tingsen Xu as part of the landmark trial published by researchers at Emory University to evaluate Tai Chi for balance in the elderly.[25] The protocol included 14 moves, done independently and without sequencing. For each move, there was a clear hypothesis of the impact of the movement patterns for the development of balance. Since then, multiple protocols, some with as few as five movements, and most including a suite of warm-up and cool-down exercises, have been evaluated in clinical trials.

Perhaps due in part to this research, a trend of using Tai Chi protocols in medical work has evolved. A quick search on the Internet can identify trademarked programs entitled Tai Chi for Balance, Tai Chi for Parkinson's, Tai Chi for Multiple Sclerosis, Tai Chi for Arthritis, and Tai Chi for Depression. While some of these protocols are based on evidence from scientific studies, it is not yet clear that the unique characteristics of these forms are uniquely therapeutic for the specified conditions. No Western studies to date have compared any one Tai Chi form to another and demonstrated whether any specific protocol is better than any other, or better than Tai Chi programs available in the community. This represents an important future area of interest for the Tai Chi research community.

Biomedical research on Qi and Qigong is also a growing field. Scientists are studying the bioelectric properties of acupuncture points and meridians, using space-age technology to monitor the characteristics of energy waves emitted from the bodies of Qigong masters and healers. This technology ranges from sensitive infrared sensors and infrasonic sound detectors to photon-emission spectroscopy and superconducting quantum-interference devices (which measure extremely subtle magnetic fields). In addition, researchers are examining the biological impact of emitted Qi on cultures of cells in petri dishes and in controlled human clinical trials.[26]

The interface between Western science and Eastern healing arts is a very rich and exciting one, with the promise of discoveries equally relevant to medical scientists, and teachers and practitioners of traditional mind-body practices.

2

The Eight Active Ingredients
of Tai Chi

Based on my research and years of Tai Chi training, I share in this chapter what I have come to appreciate as Eight Active Ingredients of Tai Chi. Like the components of a multi-drug combination to lower cholesterol and blood pressure, each ingredient is believed to have a unique impact on the physiology of the body. However, Tai Chi has many more ingredients, and most of these therapeutic factors are inseparable from, and synergistic with, one another. Perhaps what makes Tai Chi so special is that this holistic, multicomponent exercise affects us at physical, psychological, social, and philosophical levels. Its multilevel effects are especially important for complex chronic diseases that involve many systems throughout the body; for example, the nervous, respiratory, endocrine, and immune systems all interact with the cardiovascular system to affect how well the heart functions.

The Eight Active Ingredients of Tai Chi are as follows:

1. Awareness (including mindfulness and focused attention)—Perhaps the most fundamental ingredient underlying Tai Chi, the slow,

deliberate movements and attention to breathing, body positions, and sensations, fosters acute self-awareness, a prerequisite to all other ingredients. The emphasis on moment-to-moment awareness results in mindfulness and improved focus.

2. Intention (including belief and expectation)—Additional active ingredients of imagery, visualization, and related cognitive tools alter intention, belief, and expectation, and contribute significantly to the therapeutic and physiological effects of Tai Chi.

3. Structural Integration (including dynamic form and function)—Enhanced integration within and between multiple structural and physiological systems is another key active ingredient that underlies Tai Chi's therapeutic effect. Biomechanically efficient shapes and patterns of movement have functional consequences across many systems.

4. Active Relaxation—Tai Chi's circular, flowing motion helps shift the body and mind into deeper levels of relaxation, and is a form of meditation in motion.

5. Strengthening and Flexibility—Tai Chi provides moderate aerobic training equal to levels obtained in walking at a moderate pace. The integrated movements result in less strain, greater power with less effort, and better balance. The slowness of the Tai Chi movements, in combination with slightly flexed stances and placing weight on one leg at a time for sustained periods, leads to significant lower extremity strength training and increased loading on the skeleton, which promotes strong bones. In addition, slow, continuous, relaxed, and repetitive movement also results in dynamic stretching, which enhances overall flexibility.

6. Natural, Freer Breathing—More efficient breathing improves gas exchange, massages body tissues, including internal organs, helps regulate the nervous system, improves mood, and balances and moves Qi within the body and between the body and the environment.

7. Social Support (including interaction and community)—Being part of a group has proven therapeutic value for various medical conditions, including cancer, heart disease, depression, and anxiety. In ongoing Tai Chi classes, students develop a strong sense of com-

munity, and with rich interactions and support from teachers and peers, often undergo a profound journey of self-discovery.

8. Embodied Spirituality (including philosophy and ritual)— Tai Chi creates a practical framework for practicing living with a more holistic, Eastern philosophy that integrates body, mind, and spirit. It can also be a powerful vehicle to add a spiritual dimension to your life. Also, the ritualistic practice of Tai Chi may help amplify and sustain its therapeutic benefits.

The complexity of Tai Chi, however, makes it a challenge to study scientifically. This chapter highlights how the emerging field of systems biology and the ecological principles underlying traditional Chinese medicine (TCM) complement one another and provide a framework for studying and understanding how complex interventions like Tai Chi can affect health.

How the Eight Active Ingredient Framework Was Developed

In modern medicine, drugs are prescribed because of their active ingredients. Well-defined, laboratory-synthesized chemical compounds, such as ibuprofen, the active ingredient in Advil or Motrin, are specifically designed to impact physiological pathways to elicit a predictable, desired effect—in the case of ibuprofen, blocking the sensation of pain and reducing inflammation and fever.

Other nonspecific factors, such as your belief that the drug will work, advice from your doctor or pharmacist, and the color and shape of the pill generally are thought to play a smaller role in the drug's therapeutic benefits. Researchers generally try to study the impact of a single, active ingredient while controlling for all other nonspecific effects. This way of thinking has led to the gold standard of the double-blind, placebo-controlled randomized trial in which one group of people receives the active ingredient and another group receives an inactive ingredient (with all other factors identical except the active ingredient), which in drug trials is usually a simple sugar pill. Neither the people receiving the experimental drug nor the people administering it know whether the pill has the active or inactive ingredient.

Tai Chi is obviously different from drug therapy. It has no well-defined, single chemical ingredient and is more a mixture of exercise and meditative and psychosocial components. Yet, for various reasons, I have found it useful to think of and teach Tai Chi within a framework of Eight Active Ingredients. My colleagues and I use this conceptual framework to evaluate the clinical benefits of Tai Chi, explore its underlying mechanisms of action, and shape the way we teach Tai Chi in our trials.

My personal training in different styles of Tai Chi and related martial and healing arts over the past 35 years has also helped shape the active ingredients framework. Like most Tai Chi "cross-trainers," at first, I noticed the difference between styles. But, after a few styles and multiple teachers, I started to appreciate what the styles had in common, that is, the key principles or active ingredients. Additionally, my training branched out beyond Tai Chi and martial arts into other internal-healing arts systems, including Qigong and various styles of meditation. Some of these practices focus on postural alignment or internal-energy sensation while standing still in one posture for a long time, while others focus exclusively on the pattern of breathing and observations of thoughts. My curiosity led me to formal training in Eastern manual and energy-based therapies such as Shiatsu, tuina, and Reiki, which highlighted principles of body alignment, energy flow, and the links between body and mind.

Learning the various elements of these therapies helped me recognize their implicit role in Tai Chi. I came to appreciate that Tai Chi is composed of exquisitely designed, multiple components, that is, a rich set of integrated active ingredients. Rather than teaching outer choreography, I was inspired to teach more from the inside out. I wanted to develop these principles further. I wanted to use relatively easy-to-learn, simplified Tai Chi movements as a means to deliver the active ingredients.

The catalyst to put a formal structure to the Eight Active Ingredients came with the invitation to evaluate Tai Chi scientifically in a short clinical trial. I was asked to design a 10-week study to compare Tai Chi to a traditional physical therapy control group for patients with inner-ear balance disorders. My goal as a scientist was not to "prove" that Tai Chi would be helpful. In fact, I was dubious we could significantly help this highly impaired group in just 10 weeks. However, I was committed to developing a Tai Chi protocol that gave as full a "dose" of Tai Chi as possible in 10 weeks so that the study would be a scientifically credible test of Tai Chi's potential.

I knew that focusing on the traditional sequenced choreography of Tai Chi, which has a long learning curve, would not work. Even short forms of Tai Chi can take months to memorize and learn well enough to have a therapeutic effect. What's more, these balance-disorder patients were quite old, frail, and physically deconditioned due to limited physical activity. Given their concerns about balance and falling, trying to teach them a relatively complex sequence of movement was more likely to create stress and fear.

Instead, we developed a Tai Chi protocol based on a handful of movements, along with a simple set of Tai Chi warm-up exercises.[1] The patients could learn each Tai Chi movement or warm-up exercise in a few minutes with no memorization and practice alone. The ease and safety of the movements allowed the study participants to focus on self-awareness, relaxation, proper alignment, and breathing almost immediately, and to drop quickly into a state of moving meditation. We chose Tai Chi movements that could easily be adapted to the patient's abilities and limitations, and designed the sequence to become more challenging as the patient progressed. The new Tai Chi protocol was not a one-size-fits-all, rigid set of movements, but rather thoughtfully chosen, adaptable Tai Chi movements that afforded the participants the opportunity to experience deeply the fundamental principles (active ingredients) of Tai Chi.

Over time, we have used this approach and adapted Tai Chi movements and warm-up exercises for different groups of people in different clinical trials, including heart failure, chronic obstructive pulmonary disease, bone health, Parkinson's disease, and depression. Our study participants report to us that they feel stronger and healthier, and, maybe more importantly, they also say they appreciate being taught in a way that helps them logically understand how the active ingredients of Tai Chi physiologically impact their health. If it makes sense to them, then they are more likely to sustain their practice.

After we started reporting the results of our clinical trials in journal articles and lectures at conferences, certain questions emerged from our academic peers: What are the physical and physiological mechanisms that seem to underlie the improvements we observed in balance, strength, exercise capacity, mood, and quality of life? How do we know it's not just placebo? Is one main component of Tai Chi responsible for the effects? Is Tai Chi the same as exercise or relaxation techniques alone—or does its multiple active ingredients synergistically impact many different health-related processes?

This questioning further encouraged us to think about and shape our Tai Chi training around the active ingredients. It also shaped our research. We began to focus more on exploring the mechanisms of how Tai Chi works. We began to include physiological and psychological measures that would help us interpret the role of the active ingredients. Ultimately, we used these questions and emerging research results from our group and others to refine and improve our protocols for populations with specific needs and symptoms.

Finally, after observing success in our clinical trials, I began to teach using the Eight Active Ingredients approach in my community classes. People were coming to community classes for the same reason they volunteered for clinical trials—to get healthier and feel better. After 30 years of teaching entry-level Tai Chi classes centered around traditional Yang-style forms, I realized our beginning curriculum was inefficient and often frustrating, for both students and teachers. Many students do not have the patience required to learn the choreography easily, and if in a group, they often become frustrated and feel bad about falling behind. For me, and other teachers, it is hard to watch students with memory or balance issues struggle with the movements and fail to receive much of what Tai Chi has to offer. Inevitably, we lose a large number of these students before they ever get a real taste of the deeper Tai Chi experience.

When I began teaching students the simplified movements similar to those used in our clinical protocols, emphasizing the Eight Active Ingredients, I saw quicker results and students kept coming to class. Among students who studied for only a few months and did not learn the formal Tai Chi choreography, I observed improved balance, strength, and greater sense of well-being. They also quickly learned enough simple exercises to practice on their own and more readily integrate Tai Chi principles in other physical activities. Students who moved on to learn the sequences of traditional Tai Chi forms were stronger and more grounded in Tai Chi principles, and they could safely take on more complex moves. To my surprise, people continue to attend basics classes, even 10 or more years into their Tai Chi training and after they have progressed into various solo, weapon, and two-person Tai Chi exercises. The basics class seems to be a place where they can add insight and deepen their experience of what they already "know" about Tai Chi.

I introduce the Eight Active Ingredients in this chapter in the same way as in my classes and clinical trials. I will elaborate on and link evidence in the medical research to these ingredients, and their potential therapeutic effects, in the chapters in Part Two that address Tai Chi research for specific medical conditions.

Like any complex system, there are many ways to divide the subcomponents of Tai Chi. At the most basic yin-yang level, Tai Chi often is characterized as having two main sets of principles or active ingredients—mind and body. At the other end of the scale, you can probably differentiate dozens of subtle principles. Other Tai Chi systems may divide the principles

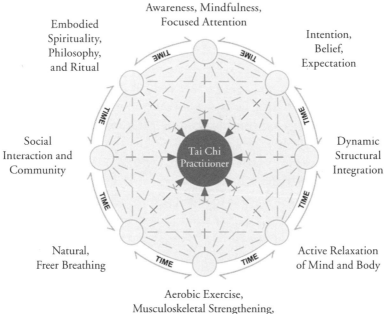

The Eight Active Ingredients of Tai Chi: A Systems Biology Framework
Arrows indicate how each ingredient can directly affect a Tai Chi practitioner, and they show the rich interdependence of the ingredients.

in other ways and include others not mentioned here. I hope this classification system encourages discussion and catalyzes you to mine the richness of Tai principles in your own Tai Chi practice.

In describing the Eight Active Ingredients, I have tried to distill and articulate essential components of Tai Chi. In practice, each of these eight ingredients is interdependent and interwoven with the others. For example, you cannot change your breathing substantially without altering your posture, neuromuscular dynamics, inner awareness, intention, and mood. Just as white light shining through a prism leads to a rainbow of colors, the Eight Active Ingredients allow you to appreciate the multiple components that make up the whole of Tai Chi.

1. Awareness (including Mindfulness and Focused Attention)

Tai Chi is commonly known as "meditation in motion." One of Tai Chi's active ingredients relates to becoming more aware of, and at greater ease with, what is happening within your body and mind at any given moment. Awareness of moment-to-moment sensations allows you to train and hold your attention or mental focus, providing you with a tool to manage distracting thoughts and incessant mental chatter. As a result, you are more fully engaged with physical tasks at hand and more in the moment. Unlike other Eastern practices, in Tai Chi training, you are not taught meditation within the context of sitting on a pillow, but through practical body-centered exercise. This practice may make what you learn more translatable to practical, everyday activities of daily living. Cheng Man Ching was fond of saying, "The difference between sitting meditation and Tai Chi is that even if you get it (for example, relaxation or awareness) studying meditation, there is nothing you can do if someone tries to knock you off your cushion."[2]

EXPERIENCING AWARENESS

I commonly begin all my Tai Chi classes standing in a circle with an invitation to be aware of, or mindful of, what's going on in the body at the present moment. I'll say, "Before you begin to *do* anything in this session, allow yourself to more fully 'arrive' into the present moment and simply notice what you are sensing right now. Can you feel your feet on the ground? Can you notice how you are breathing? Do your best not to 'think' too much about or judge what you are sensing or experiencing, and try not to rush to fix or improve how you are standing or breathing. Simply notice."[3]

Then I might add a few more suggestions to focus attention further and engage inner awareness. "As you stand, does one leg feel more or less weight bearing on it than the other? Is there more pressure on the inner edges versus the outer edges of your feet? Can you sense where inside your body your breath easily goes and where it does not go? Just simply notice."

After a minute or two of standing still, slowing down, and noticing, we then typically begin the simplest Tai Chi movement—what I call Tai Chi Pouring. As a setup for Tai Chi Pouring, I explain that the body is literally 70 percent liquid. In evolutionary terms, we humans brought solutions similar to the ocean into our bodies to survive on land; that is, we internalized the ocean, literally. We are filled with an inner ocean of water, blood, and lymph. I suggest sensing body movement more as a pouring, wave-like phenomenon rather than as a solid object changing shape or position.

Tai Chi Pouring also exemplifies the genius of Tai Chi, which is that slow, conscious movement (in comparison with stillness) helps you to become aware, sense, and feel what is happening within your body in the present moment. Often, I'll start with a focus on the dynamic sensations in the soles of the feet. "Begin to pour your weight gently from side to side, and notice the sensations in the soles of the feet. As you shift and pour your weight from side to side, tune in to your liquid nature or inner ocean. How juicy do the soles of your feet feel? Does one foot feel juicier than the other does? Is the arch or toe region more sensitive or aware of being bathed by this inner ocean than the heel? Are there parts of your feet where you do not feel any juiciness at all?"

After dwelling in the feet for a minute or so, we move to other parts of the body, using the subtle movements generated by Tai Chi

Pouring to sense and explore the ankles, knees, hips, abdomen, spine, neck, head, and arms. This initial exercise serves as a kind of scanning or inventorying of the whole body, like an internal roll call. Feet . . . present; ankles . . . present; left hip . . . absent. Importantly, throughout this exercise, the goal is to notice or feel a body part or sensation, not to think, judge, or react to a sensation. One of my teachers used to say that focusing on and sensing any part of your body would move Qi there, whereas "thinking" about that part of your body more often than not moves Qi to your head.

The very simple exercise of Pouring, or shifting the body from side to side with awareness, illustrates the connection of cognitive, active ingredients of Tai Chi. They play a key role in all Tai Chi movements and related exercises—heightened body awareness, focused attention, and greater integration of mind and body. On one level, this combination of ingredients almost seems obvious, like a simple truism. But just showing up and being present without trying to change anything is also one of the most challenging, deepest principles of Tai Chi. These ideas are reflected in a quote of Lao Tzu's, commonly cited in Tai Chi writings, "In non-doing, nothing is left undone."

Heightened Body and Sensory Awareness

Heightened body and self-awareness, and an ability to sustain focused attention without overthinking or judging, are profound components of Tai Chi. A growing body of research suggests that significant therapeutic effects result from these ingredients alone, in and of themselves.[4]

Through slow, deliberate movements and attention to breath and mental quality, Tai Chi fosters acute self-awareness—of bodily sensation, thoughts and emotions, and the connection between mind and body. Increasing bodily awareness allows you to sense the inner landscape of your body and better discriminate areas with or without strain or tension, stronger or weaker regions, as well as movements that feel graceful or fearful. This awareness may play a significant role in the prevention and rehabilitation of multiple medical conditions. For example, in Chapter 4

"Improve Your Balance and Bones," you will read how sensation in the soles of the feet is a critical component of balance and how Tai Chi improves balance even in patients with peripheral neuropathy who have nerve damage that causes pain, numbness, and loss of sensation in the hands and feet.[5]

Heightened body awareness might also play a role in improving musculoskeletal conditions, such as back pain, by helping to discriminate which postures and movement patterns alleviate or exacerbate pain. Tai Chi training may safely guide therapeutic stretching and strengthening, as well as balance out the musculoskeletal system. Research shows that long-term Tai Chi practitioners have better ability to sense or locate their limbs as they are moved, which is called a kinesthetic sense.[6]

Developing this sensitivity is a key component of the martial-arts application of Tai Chi. You become highly sensitive to the very beginning of your opponent's movement so you can react quickly and take advantage of it before the attack fully takes place. Quotes from Tai Chi classics illustrate this sensitivity: "If others move slightly, I move first" and "Use four ounces to deflect a thousand pounds."

More generally, Tai Chi's effect to enhance focus, awareness, and sensitivity helps you more clearly and effectively respond to any situation, such as walking on an uneven path, lifting heavy groceries or a young child, or thoughtfully responding to a spouse during an argument. Having a clearer state of mind at any one moment informs your next response.

Focused Attention

Tai Chi's emphasis on moment-to-moment awareness also trains mental focus. A gift of human evolution is that we can think about and plan for the future to be better prepared, or re-evaluate what happened yesterday so we don't make the same mistakes over and over again. But, especially in today's hyper-busy, multitasking society with so many demands, plans, and distractions, very rarely do we take time to slow down to notice fully what's happening in the present moment. Our ability to sustain focus on tasks in the present moment has greatly atrophied. During Tai Chi practice, you continuously are required to notice what is happening at any given moment, paying attention to certain qualities of movement, posture, breath, balance, and the impact of the environment around you (including other individuals). This training helps keep in check what the Asian meditative traditions call "monkey mind," or excessive distraction or focus on external, past, or future events.

Some other types of meditation encourage the complete clearing or emptying of the mind of all thoughts. In contrast, Tai Chi is more of an active, focused meditation. During practice, when the mind wanders, you gently refocus it back to noticing practical and functional bodily sensations in the present moment. One metaphor I commonly use during resting meditations is to think of the fabric of the body as a paper towel. Just as a paper towel naturally absorbs and holds water in its highly absorbent pores without expending effort, let the mind rest into and be held in or cradled by the fabric of the body. The spirit of this active ingredient is captured nicely in a clever phrase I saw on a bumper sticker and that I commonly cite in Tai Chi class, *"Meditation—it's not what you think."*

One of the issues with "monkey mind" for many people is that the mind wanders and gets lost down dark alleys of thinking and endless ruminating on negative thoughts and what-ifs. The mind wanders because bodily sensations are deeply interwoven with cognitive processes related to appraisal and interpretation, beliefs, memories, conditioning, attitudes, and affect. A highly innovative study conducted by Harvard professors Killingsworth and Gilbert in 2010 (discussed in Chapter 8, "Sharpen Your Mind") supports the notion that the more your mind wanders, the less happy you are.[7]

With practice, Tai Chi draws your attention to the present moment and helps you develop a state of mindfulness, openness, and acceptance. Tai Chi literally fosters peace of mind. A rich body of research shows that meditative exercises like Tai Chi can change the brain's structure and function, and that focused concentration and non judgmental, moment-to-moment awareness in and of itself (without overt exercise) may modulate multiple aspects of health, including pain, immune function, and mood.[8]

Finally, this active ingredient is also essential to allow you to gain the benefits of other active ingredients, such as efficient posture, effective breathing, and active relaxation. Greater inner awareness, for example, might bring attention to restricted breathing patterns or excessive tension in certain standing positions, which in turn foster more internal sensitivity and increased awareness.

2. Intention (including Belief and Expectation)

Tai Chi training typically draws images or metaphors from nature. Phrases from the Tai Chi classics such as "Be still as a mountain," "Move like a great river," and "Stand rooted like a tree," as well as the names of many Tai Chi movements themselves (for example, "Wave hands like clouds") include images that guide you toward certain kinesthetic, emotional, and energetic states. The additional active ingredients of imagery and visualization, and related cognitive tools that alter intention, belief, and expectation, complement the cognitive active ingredients related to awareness, mindfulness, and focused attention, and contribute significantly to the therapeutic and physiological effects of Tai Chi.

In sharp contrast to conventional biomedicine where the active ingredient (for example, ibuprofen) is believed to do nearly all the work, in Tai Chi, intention and belief are considered highly active and specific ingredients. In fact, Tai Chi classics emphasize that all embodied movement begins with belief, thought, or intention: The mind (*yi*, intention) leads the Qi, and the Qi moves the body. This central role of belief and expectation precludes the possibility of designing placebo-controlled studies of Tai Chi.[9]

FOLDING INTENTION INTO TAI CHI POURING

In the Tai Chi Pouring exercise, once students settle into, become aware of, and make contact with the entire body, I add intention to the awareness. I might enrich or elaborate with various images or simple metaphors. "As you pour your weight from side to side, remember that your inner ocean is a warm, tropical one, about 98.6 degrees, and filled with lots of nourishing salts and other therapeutic compounds. Imagine these juices more fully seeping into, permeating, rehydrating, and bathing all the tissues of your feet—the ligaments, tendons, muscles, and penetrating networks of connective tissues. As you pour or rock from side to side, imagine you are kneading or folding Qi-filled juices deeper into the fabric of your body, gently and patiently dissolving 'glued-up' tissues, melting tensions, and flushing out toxins and old 'issues' embedded in tissues."

In her landmark book *Imagery and Healing*, Dr. Jeanne Achterberg writes, "Imagery has always played a key role in medicine. Imagery is the thought process that invokes and uses the senses; vision, audition (hearing), smell, taste, the senses of movement, position, and touch. It is the communication mechanism between perception, emotion, and bodily change. A major source of both health and sickness, the image is the world's oldest and greatest healing source."[10]

The use of active imagery and expectancy has multiple therapeutic effects.[11] Simply visualizing movements without physically practicing them can improve recovery of motor function in stroke survivors, as well as encourage learning of new complex movements. Growing evidence suggests that brain areas engaged in the actual performance of movements are, to a significant extent, also active during motor imagery. That is, just thinking about a movement uses the same parts of the brain as when actually moving.[12] Meditation research shows that positive intention and imagery can significantly influence the brain and many physiological functions.[13] The rapidly growing field of placebo research also supports the diverse, often robust therapeutic effects of belief and expectation, which are central to Tai Chi.[14]

Tai Chi takes advantage of this power of belief. The highly accomplished Tai Chi master T. T. Ling commonly used the phrase "imagination becomes reality," which is also the title of a fantastic book documenting his 103-year-long life.[15]

WASHING YOURSELF WITH QI

One of my favorite moments in teaching new Tai Chi students, both in clinical trials and community-based classes, is introducing a Qigong warm-up exercise called "Washing yourself with Qi from nature." This very simple exercise, done either standing or seated, is designed to gather in healing, rejuvenating, peaceful energy from nature and guide this energy through every cell of the body, starting at the crown of the head and moving down through the chest, shoulders, spine, all the internal organs, through the legs and feet. I ask students—commonly older housewives and retired blue-collar workers with little or no exposure to New Age practices—to imagine doing this exercise while standing on a mountaintop, a beach, or wherever they feel they would be surrounded by nourishing energy. I invite them to trust the energy to permeate and revitalize every cell of the body, while at the same time filtering out tired, sick energy and washing it out through the soles of the feet into the earth.

Then I'll abruptly stop, smile, and acknowledge with them how odd or weird these ideas all sound. They typically agree, and we all laugh together. I'll then share with them some of the research my colleagues and I have done related to the placebo effect; our research supports the Tai Chi principle that what you think and believe affects your physiology and how you feel. If asthma patients believe they are breathing in ragweed (but actually, it is just saline mist), the majority have an asthma attack, and if they believe they are breathing in a rescue medication (again saline mist), they quickly recover.[16] After this brief interlude, I return to "Washing yourself with Qi from nature" and jokingly say, "So as we wash with Qi from heavens, you can go to your special place and imagine breathing in and bathing every cell in your body with healing energy, or you can breathe in ragweed or other toxic substances. It's your choice!"

The exercises this book presents employ various images and cognitive tools to achieve functional outcomes. For example, I might use the image of feeling rooted like a tree to enhance balance, or "waving the hand like clouds" to elicit a lighter, more open quality of movement. However, these images and ideas are tools to be explored in a playful, open-minded way. An image that works for you may not work for another, and an image that elicits a response at an early stage of your training may not be helpful at a later stage of practice. Rigidly clinging to any technique, cognitive or physical, can be inhibit your progress, because it limits experiencing what is really happening in your body and impedes the organic evolution you are gently shepherding along in Tai Chi training.[17]

3. Structural Integration
(including Dynamic Form and Function)

One translation of the essential meaning of Tai Chi, which is reflected in the yin-yang symbol, is dynamic integration. The integration of complementary components results in a more balanced, creative whole. Tai Chi, and more generally traditional Chinese medicine, does not emphasize the body as a machine-like assemblage of autonomous parts—separate muscles, bones, and organs. Rather, it assumes an intricately coordinated, dynamic living system. Enhanced integration within and between multiple structural and physiological systems is another key active ingredient contributing to Tai Chi's therapeutic effect.

Western biomedicine acknowledges multiple systems that integrate and sustain living functions. For example, the circulation system's major arteries and fine capillaries transport blood, nutrients, and communication compounds to every cell from head to toe. Similarly, the nervous system, with the brain and spinal cord as its central hub, uses electrochemical waves conducted along an intricate network of nerve cells to coordinate all sensory, motor, and behavioral functions. Two additional interrelated, interconnected systems central to Tai Chi are the TCM network of meridians, or energy channels, and the all-pervasive network of the body's connective tissue, or what the Tai Chi classics call the sinews. These two systems help conceptually to appreciate and experience greater integration.

According to TCM, a continuous, integrated flow of information and energy, or Qi, exists in the body. This information and energy moves along pathways called *jinglou* (or meridians) that link the viscera with different parts of the body, making the human body an integrated whole. When Qi flows freely through the meridians, the body is balanced and healthy. But, if the Qi becomes blocked, stagnated, or weakened, it can cause physical, mental, or emotional ill health.

Exciting research is beginning to explore potential anatomical bases for meridians and employ state-of-the-art technology to characterize biophysical and bioenergetic correlates of energy flow.[18] Becoming sensitive to all yin-yang parts of the body and using sensations of the internal flow of energy to integrate them—the bottom with the top, the left with the right, the inside with the outer surface—is a key training tool and active ingredient in Tai Chi.

A second framework many of my Tai Chi teachers emphasized, and one that I am focusing on increasingly in my teaching and research, is the body's network of connective tissues embedded within the larger extracellular matrix—the so-called "filler" substance existing between cells. Connective tissue forms a continuous, anatomical network throughout the body, and it has become increasingly appreciated as a communication system. It's all pervasive.

Connective tissue comes in many forms, all containing collagen, plus other macromolecules, and it has different levels of organization. Dense connective tissue, such as tendons, connects bone to muscles, while the more-fibrous ligaments connect bones to other bones. Fascia, a less densely organized and more elastic connective tissue, surrounds the outside of every muscle, as well as the surfaces of the smaller muscle-fiber bundles that make up the muscle. Fascia also wraps nearly all blood vessels, nerves, and internal organs. Fascia serves to bind structures together in much the same manner as plastic wrap holds the contents of sandwiches together.

Finally, loose connective tissue is the most common, but least understood or appreciated, connective tissue. Loose connective tissue holds organs in place and helps bind various types and layers of tissue to one another. Importantly, loose connective tissue is associated with a highly liquid environment that also binds water, ions, and other chemicals that together have been called the "living matrix."[19] The living matrix has properties that exquisitely connect all parts of the body (and maybe the mind), which is a perfect metaphor for the framework for Tai Chi![20]

Structural Integration

One of the core principles of Tai Chi relates to body posture. In fact, Tai Chi shapes what we typically call posture and alignment. Building on

ENHANCING INTEGRATION

I often draw on the biology of our connective tissue matrix to foster the integration between the body's parts and systems in the Tai Chi Pouring exercise. I'll say: "Be aware of the fabric of connective tissue and the living matrix that permeates and surrounds every cell in your body. As you pour from side to side, can you feel how the waves of your inner ocean connect the feet, ankles, and knees? Can you feel the 'juices' softening and nourishing the connective tissues? Do the liquid and bioelectric waves flow freely along these pathways, or are there blocks or dams to the flow?"

Movement of any one part of the body affects all others. Using sensitivity, you can realize that you can feel the movement of your arms all the way down to your toes. Or, feel how your breathing affects the shapes of your ribs and spine. The Tai Chi classics highlight this dynamic integration: "If any one part (of the body) should cease to move, then the movements will be disconnected and fall into disarray."[21]

phrases from the Tai Chi classics—for example, "Suspend the spine like a string of pearls from heaven"—Tai Chi trains you to maximize your body's physical potential and to find alignments that afford safe, unstrained, and graceful postures.

One alignment principle that informs most Tai Chi movements is verticality; that is, the head is centered over the torso, the torso rests over the hips, and the hips are centered over the base of support, the legs and feet. Other alignment principles include the centering of the knee joint over the central axis of the foot and the relaxed suspension of the elbows between the shoulders and wrists. Practitioners believe the use of proper alignment translates into more efficient movement patterns and decreased levels of muscle coactivation, which in turn is likely to lead to decreased stress on the joints and improved balance. (See research presented in Chapters 4 and 5.) This principle of structural integration and alignment is reflected in a quote from Master Cheng Man Ching: "Every joint in your body must be strung together. This allows Qi to pass smoothly through your body and benefits both form and application."[22]

Another central principle in Tai Chi is the emphasis on slow, coordinated, integrated movements. Changes from one posture to another unfold through time. Phrases from the classics such as "Movements begin in the feet, are steered by the waist, and administered by the hand" reflect functional movement principles related to human biomechanics. In addition to postural alignment and highly specific neuromuscular sequences, the slowness of transitions gives you time to sense your body's position, make appropriate modifications, and organize the parts so that they work together. The classics sometime call this "seamlessness" or describe it as being like "reeling silk from a cocoon." If movements are too abrupt and disintegrated, or too slow, the silk thread is broken as it is drawn from the cocoon. Another quote from the classics says "Movements from beginning to end are continuous and in an endless circle, just like a river which flows on and on without end."

In Tai Chi, the *tan tien* is an important physical and energetic center of the body, one of the key places you center and focus your awareness during Tai Chi practice. Located just beneath and behind the navel, the tan tien is also close to the body's center of gravity. The process of "centering" in the tan tien helps with physical balance, integrating the upper and lower body, and also helps with energetic integration, creating a hub of sorts where the mind, emotions, and physical body can easily interact, stay connected, and keep in balance. You'll find some helpful tan tien centering exercises in Chapter 4, "Improve Your Balance and Bones."

The concept of integration is related to the evolutionary biology principle of form and function, that is, where shapes and patterns of movement have functional consequences across many body systems. For example, if you improve your structural organization, you will also likely improve your physiological function—if your chest and ribs collapse less, you breathe more efficiently; if you relax your muscles more, you lessen the load and stress on your heart each time it pumps. This concept of form and function is a theme you will see running throughout this book.

Form and function even extend to emotion. Charles Darwin and, more recently, Paul Eckman have written about how emotions often have evolved in concert with hardwired associated body shapes that help serve as a form of nonverbal communication; an example is when babies purse or pucker their lips to show they dislike a certain food.[23]

One of my "aha" moments related to this idea occurred while I served as a teaching fellow for Professor E. O. Wilson in his evolutionary biology course at Harvard. In one of his final lectures on the evolution of body language, Wilson showed a series of slides that included multiple species of primate all using the same gesture of hands gleefully and vigorously held above their heads in a posture that he called the "victory gesture." Then he showed similar images of humans—a marathon runner with arms raised high while crossing the finish line and breaking the tape, a football kicker with arms up signaling a field goal. He emphasized that these shapes were all hardwired with emotions, and he jokingly said, "It's hard to feel sad if you mimic this shape." His examples and comments made me realize that part of what Tai Chi may be doing is creating shapes that have positive effects not only on physiological function, but also on emotional function. Recent Harvard Business School research (discussed in detail in Chapter 9) supports the notion that body shape influences negotiations and even changes the body's endocrine function and mood.[24] By fostering balanced, open, and relaxed postures, Tai Chi affects the functionality of just about every body system.

4. Active Relaxation

Embedded within the Tai Chi symbol is the intrinsic wisdom to find balance in everything, including how much effort you expend in training. This notion contrasts with the dominant, more-is-better mentality in our Western culture. Popular motivational speakers and athletic coaches often ask you to "give it your all" or to "give 110 percent" or to "push the envelope." One of my favorites is "if you are not living on the edge, you are taking up too much room." These aggressive strategies are appropriate at times, but the potential benefit of tempered effort usually is not valued as highly. As the comedian/actress Lily Tomlin wondered, "How come no one ever says try softer?" She also suggested, "For fast-acting relief, try slowing down."

Balance is inherent in the philosophy of Tai Chi and is expressed in the yin-yang symbol. The lighter half of the yin-yang symbol—representing activity and doing—has a small, dark circle representing inactivity or non-doing. Similarly, the dark half of the yin-yang symbol—representing inactivity or non-doing—has a small, light circle of activity. The small circles in each half representing the opposite half maintain balance, keeping each energy in check. We should avoid both extremes in Tai Chi—overdoing without reservation or lifeless, limp relaxation. These two interrelated Tai Chi training principles—moderation in effort and active relaxation—are the two flip sides of an important active ingredient that underlies many of Tai Chi's therapeutic effects.

Moderation in Effort

Nearly everyone, young or old, has had an experience of overdoing it—reaching just a little too far and straining a back muscle, turning too fast and spraining a knee ligament, shoveling too much snow or working too hard in the garden and sustaining injury. Tai Chi develops strength, flexibility, and increased range of motion, but it does so gradually, which may help minimize injury. This cautious, more gradual approach perhaps explains why Tai Chi is safe even for those who start training quite late in life (even into their nineties) or those who have serious neuromuscular skeletal conditions, such as fibromyalgia and arthritis.[25] This training philosophy also can translate into allowing you to move more safely during daily activities.

When you "do less," your tissues respond with greater, longer-lasting relaxation and improved range of motion. Slow, gradual movement gives the tissues time to let go and unwind in a more organic way, happening more from within as opposed to being forced from without. Some of the positive advantages of not pushing the limit may be due to the more efficient mechanical processes that occur within tissues. The muscles, ligaments, tendons, and fascia have more time to adapt to stretching, become warmed up, can change shape, and can release without being torn or strained.[26]

Going more gradually may have a neurological advantage related to alleviating the fear of further injury. Tight areas, especially those that have been injured or traumatized before, typically have an altered pattern of movement, called kinesiophobia (fear of movement), to protect them from further injury. In going slowly, you may have time to sense and respect this psychophysical trauma, or what TCM practitioners would call Qi stagnation. Going slowly may allow your body time to recognize the trauma and figure out a way to deal with it. Not listening can further exacerbate existing traumas, and possibly superimpose new ones on top of existing ones. Sometimes I use the analogy of Tai Chi movements being like rocking a baby to sleep. You can't force it. Rather, the gentle, predictable rocking motions create a feeling of trust and comfort. From that place of trust and comfort, like a baby resting into sleep, the tissues feel safe and gradually release their holding patterns and tensions.

Finally, going slowly and gradually allows you to sense how tensions in one body part, say the neck, may not be independent of tensions in other areas (the shoulders, head, or pelvis). This notion of interdependency fits in with the active ingredients of mindfulness and integration. Slow, gradual, moderated effort ushers in more of a system-wide change rather than a compartmentalized, one-body-part-at-a-time change.

Active Relaxation

If you thought the idea of "less can be more" seemed like a paradox, then the idea that true relaxation is an active process might seem even more paradoxical. In my classes, I'll often say, half-jokingly, "Relaxation can be a lot of work—and exhausting!"

Relax is not an easy word to define, and it often means different things to different people, depending on the context. Often, the connotation is as a reward (like dessert) that follows and is separate from the main activity (dinner). The Oxford dictionary states that to relax is "to rest . . . especially after work or effort."

Relaxation in Tai Chi is a much more active concept, and more functional, too. Remember that Tai Chi was developed and is practiced as a martial art. Tai Chi classic texts, written largely as manuals for practical martial arts training, included phrases such as, "In practicing Tai Chi Chuan, the whole body relaxes." This idea of relaxation is not a go limp, be empty, drop your guard, kick back on the couch, or zone out kind. To relax while standing upright or doing simple movements as you contend with an opponent requires you to develop a more active relaxation.

One of the Tai Chi concepts that informs the idea of active relaxation is "Sung." Sung is considered a defining characteristic of Tai Chi. As a qualitative mind-body state, Sung is variously translated as relaxed, loose, or open, or as a quality that permits the natural flow of energy. Sung is also described as a process related to sinking—not necessarily physically sinking, as in bending the knees or sitting into a deeper stance, but energetically sinking. The Chinese character or pictogram for Sung depicts hair contained in a tight bun letting go and hanging freely. In my teaching, I often introduce the concept of Sung as the opposite of "being uptight," emphasizing the literal aspects of this uptight behavior, including physically being more "up and tight" in the body. I ask students to picture a stressed-out person who has a tight chest, raised stiff shoulders, a scrunched-up neck, and shallow breathing.

One metaphor I use to help students to experience the concept of Sung is honey in a jar. Imagine a see-through jar that you turn upside down and then right side up again. It takes a while for the viscous honey to ooze back down to the bottom. Similarly, physical and emotional tensions can constrain Qi in the upper body. In Tai Chi training, you learn to let things "relax" downward naturally. And, sometimes, as with honey, the Qi gets stuck, becoming literally crystallized in chronically inflamed, scarred body tissues. To be able to flow down more freely, the Qi needs to dissolve first. Just as you would run the honey jar under hot water to turn the crystalized honey back into liquid, with Tai Chi, you use gentle movements, breathing, imagery, emotional and behavioral changes, self-massage, and other techniques to soften and free the Qi so it can more naturally settle, or experience Sung.

When your body releases tensions and Qi, it feels lighter, looser, more rooted, and bottom heavy, almost like a clown punching bag that wobbles but doesn't tip over fully. Your body becomes more efficient physiologically. Yet your relaxed Tai Chi body does not shift to an empty, collapsed state, but rather to a more upright, three-dimensionally fuller, energized, dynamic, relaxed state. The removal of physical and emotional strains frees up the underlying functional structures.

The relevance of Sung and active relaxation in Tai Chi becomes even more obvious when you consider the misnomer of standing still. Even the most advanced Tai Chi master never truly stands still because maintaining any upright posture is an active, dynamic process. The dynamics of standing still exist for several reasons. First, standing upright involves coordinating the activation of muscles that keep the skeleton erect and in place. Activation of these muscles is not a continuous on/off switch. Muscle fibers change over time due to fatigue and other internal neurophysiological processes. Second, many core processes generate subtle, internal movement, including breathing, swallowing, and flow of blood and lymph, and sometimes not-so-subtle movement, such as passing gas. Through evolution, the human body's structure became inherently top-heavy and unstable (like an ice cream cone balanced on its narrow triangular base). That means even small movements, such as breathing, require your internal balance systems to make adaptations in the feet, legs, and trunk to stabilize muscles and prevent you from falling over. Third, while these reactions occur in less than a blink of the eye, time lags in neuromuscular adaptations can occur that require continuous oscillations to maintain balance.

As you can see, maintaining a relaxed, Sung-like, upright body structure takes a lot of effort. Tai Chi brings exquisite awareness to your tensions, strains, and internal dynamics, and offers you a set of biomechanical and psychophysical tools to manage changes in a more efficient, relaxed manner. Tai Chi does not try to stifle these subtle dynamics rigidly, but rather tries to coordinate them and help you relax in the flow.

MODERATION IN EFFORT AND ACTIVE
RELAXATION IN TAI CHI POURING

After weaving the first three active ingredients into the Tai Chi Pouring exercise, I typically fold in the principles of moderation in effort and active relaxation. "As you pour your weight from side to side, notice that as one leg bears weight and assumes the responsibility of holding you up, your other leg can rest. Given that the empty (non-weight-bearing) leg has no responsibility for holding you up, how relaxed can you let that leg be? You might even let the heel of the empty leg slightly float up off the ground (no more than one-quarter inch). How empty and insubstantial can you let this resting leg be?"

While you rock back and forth exploring this idea, I might point out that what you are doing is literally embodying (physically/energetically becoming) a dynamic yin-yang or Tai Chi symbol. "In this continuous shifting of your weight, one side becomes more active, substantial, doing, filling—or yang—while the other side becomes less active, insubstantial, non-doing, emptying—or yin."

I point out that one of the gifts of Tai Chi is the emphasis on the yin of non-doing—that is, that less can be more. So, I might jokingly say, "If you are more of a Type A personality and driven like I am, challenge yourself to let your emptying leg relax more deeply each time you shift away from it." To link to the concept of active relaxation, I say, "Every time you relax your emptying leg, it affords a resting period and deepens your awareness of that structure. Small, repeated resting states increase the efficiency with which the leg can serve its supportive yang role. Over time, you will feel that even when your leg fully bears weight and is holding you up, it still maintains relaxed, non-doing yin qualities." This moderation in effort and active relaxation animate every movement and meditation in Tai Chi.

5. Strengthening and Flexibility

One of the principal reasons Tai Chi is so therapeutic is simply that it serves as an effective form of physical exercise. Seamlessly, and sometimes deceptively, blended into the more meditative and integrative ingredients is a sophisticated physical workout, including moderate aerobic, strength, and flexibility training. An important quality of Tai Chi, because of mindful and moderated approaches, is that it's a safe, highly adaptable form of exercise for all populations, ages, and levels of conditioning.

The medical community increasingly is appreciating physical exercise and activity as a primary tool for health maintenance and rehabilitation. A National Blueprint Consensus Report published in 2001, entitled "Strategic Priorities for Increasing Physical Activities among Adults," stated: "There is a substantial body of scientific evidence indicating that regular physical activity can bring dramatic health benefits to people of all ages and abilities and that this benefit extends over the entire life course. Physical activity offers one of the greatest opportunities to extend years of active independent life, reduce disability, and improve quality of life for middle-aged and older people."[27]

Tai Chi as an Aerobic Exercise

People practicing Tai Chi may not seem as if they are getting any aerobic benefit, but they are. Numerous studies have measured the aerobic intensity of Tai Chi and—depending on the training style, how deep you sink into postures, how fast you move from one posture to the next, and the duration of your practice—Tai Chi appears to be an aerobic activity of low to moderate intensity. Studies report the physical activity of Tai Chi to be equivalent to 1.6–4.6 metabolic equivalents (METS). To put this measurement in perspective, 1 MET is considered equal to your resting metabolic rate while sitting quietly. The majority of studies report Tai Chi intensity at about 3.5 METS, which approximates the intensity of moderate-paced walking at about three miles per hour on level ground. Tai Chi can get your heart rate up to 50–74 percent of maximum, depending on the type and intensity of Tai Chi and your age.[28]

The ability to modulate the intensity of Tai Chi makes it highly adaptable to different populations. For example, the METS of a simplified form of Tai Chi practiced while seated is 1.5. Like our simplified version of Tai Chi, experience shows this form to be safe for those with chronic heart failure.[29]

Sound evidence summarized in Chapters 6 and 7 supports the idea that Tai Chi can improve aerobic capacity and delay its decline in healthy older adults, and can enhance exercise capacity in those who have chronic cardiopulmonary diseases, such as heart failure and chronic obstructive pulmonary disease. Tai Chi can be a safe, effective adjunct to rehabilitation following heart attacks and bypass surgery, and may be equal to or better than brisk walking or moderate aerobic interventions at improving exercise capacity.[30]

Tai Chi as Strength Training

Tai Chi won't help you build a muscular physique so that you can compete in Mr. or Mrs. America contests, but it can provide significant strength training for both the lower and upper body. Motion analysis studies reveal that the slowness of the Tai Chi movements, the longer periods committed to standing on a single leg, and the slightly flexed stances result in substantial loading of the leg muscles and bones, affording significant lower extremity strength training. Multiple studies show that Tai Chi training increases lower muscle extremity strength. Some evidence, including our studies, shows that Tai Chi may help maintain strong bones and retard rates of bone loss, especially in post-menopausal women.[31]

Improvement in strength is not limited to the lower body. Studies show Tai Chi training can increase grip strength, which is an important indicator for overall health, in addition to being relevant to everyday functions, like opening jars.[32]

Tai Chi as Flexibility Training

The slow, continuous, relaxed, repetitive movements of Tai Chi also result in dynamic stretching, which enhances overall flexibility. Studies support Tai Chi's influence on increased torso flexibility.[33] The ability to reach for an object without falling is increasingly important to our aging population. An estimated 40 percent of Caucasian American women age 50 and older will experience a hip, spine, or wrist fracture—most often due to a fall—sometime during their lives.

Tai Chi and its associated warm-up exercises help to loosen up the entire musculoskeletal system, lubricating joints and tendons and stretching muscles throughout the body.

The Tai Chi Swinging and Drumming the Body exercise described in Chapter 3 integrates the principles of mindful awareness, intention, and moderation of effort into an aerobic practice. In fact, I often refer to these exercises as aerobic meditation. These exercises increase the amplitude of movements in the waist and the extremities, foster greater weight shifts and more dynamic balance and loading in the legs, and add an important aerobic component to your Tai Chi practice.

6. Natural, Freer Breathing

Efficient, mindful breathing is a key element of Tai Chi and a fundamental pathway through which Tai Chi training affects health and well-being. In Tai Chi, and more broadly, in traditional Chinese medicine, the breath is important not only for efficient gas exchange—that is, oxygen in and carbon dioxide out—but also to serve additional key functions. These functions include massage of internal organs and tissues, regulation of emotions, and movement of internal energy within the body and between the body and the surrounding environment. Breathing also serves as a mechanism for accentuating or implementing other active ingredients of Tai Chi, such as awareness, intention, and structural integration.

Breath awareness and training exercises have played a prominent role in nearly all Eastern healing traditions, including Tai Chi, Qigong, yoga, and other meditative practices. Breathing is also a primary focus of numerous contemporary mind-body therapies developed in the West, such as Middendorf Breath Work, Breath Therapy, Sensory Awareness, and Holotropic Breathing.[34] Breath awareness and training also is being integrated increasingly into biomedical stress reduction programs and sports training, and Tai Chi and other mind-body research is informing this integration.

Tai Chi and the Efficiency of Breathing

Tai Chi employs a multipronged approached to improving gas exchange. First, by improving your posture and having a less braced, more flexible structure, your body can inhale and exhale with less effort, and also increase the gross volume of air you take in. Put simply, the volume of air inhaled in a relaxed, upright, and open Tai Chi posture is much greater than the volume you can inhale while seated in a slouched, tense posture typical of a stressed-out desk worker. Improve your breathing form, and your body will function better.

Some research supports the idea that Tai Chi and related mind-body exercises may positively affect the volume and efficiency of gas exchange, including in populations with asthma, chronic obstructive pulmonary disease (COPD), and other respiratory conditions.[35] Greater breathing efficiency is associated with a reduced risk of heart diseases, all-cause mortality, and cognitive decline.[36] Even a short course of preoperative breath training in patients undergoing coronary artery bypass surgery can reduce the incidence of postoperative pulmonary complications.[37]

The slow, regular, and deep breathing Tai Chi employs also positively affects your nervous system, which in turn can improve the efficiency of your breathing. Tai Chi's emphasis on relaxation causes changes in the nervous and endocrine systems. During times of emotional stress, our sympathetic nervous system is stimulated, resulting in numerous physiological changes, including faster heart rate and rapid, shallow breathing. Chronic stress can reduce significantly the efficiency of breathing; breathing-related conditions, such as COPD, are commonly associated with excessive sympathetic activity. The breathing practiced in Tai Chi is believed to activate the parasympathetic nervous system, resulting in relaxation and reversal of changes caused by sending the sympathetic nervous system into overdrive.[38]

Basic Tai Chi Breathing

Classic and contemporary Tai Chi and Qigong texts describe various breathing techniques. These techniques have different names, but the one people universally recognize, and one that we teach in our clinical trials, is diaphragmatic breathing, also sometimes called natural, abdominal, belly, or tan tien breathing.

One of the best ways to recognize diaphragmatic breathing is to watch a sleeping baby breathe. As the baby inhales, the belly effortlessly expands, and to a lesser degree, the middle and upper torso expand, too, like a balloon being inflated. As the baby exhales, the belly, and the whole body, relaxes. The deep, slow, and rhythmic breathing is natural and effortless. Detailed instruction in diaphragmatic breathing, along with a greater discussion of physiological effects, can be found in Chapter 7.

Internal Physical Massage

The Tai Chi and Qigong literature commonly mention breathing down to the floor of the pelvis, breathing up the spine, or breathing all the way out to the extremities—even though the lungs obviously do not extend to these tissues. A substantial amount of research on the physiology of breathing supports the idea that deep breathing generates measurable changes in abdominal and visceral pressure; that is, breathing creates an internal massage.[39] These breath-induced pressure changes and rhythms may also positively affect blood flow within organs, including the kidneys and the brain.[40] Trials have shown that regular, internally directed massage led by the breath has positive effects on pain and function in back pain patients, and may more broadly help explain how Tai Chi helps with musculoskeletal pain.[41]

Breathing and the Other Active Ingredients

The impact of breathing on physical and physiological function naturally leads to interactions with the other active ingredients. Breathing offers an excellent tool for developing your sensitivity to stimuli that come from inside your body, which in turn helps to increase sensory awareness, integration, and mental focus. As each breath stimulates the hairs in your nose, passes over the membranes of your windpipe, stretches the lungs and surrounding ribs, and creates pressure waves in your belly and lower back, it unleashes a set of sensations and internal awareness deep within your body.

THE BREATH AS AN INNER NAVIGATION DEVICE

I often use the analogy of the breath being like a little "inner spaceship or navigation device," like the one in the movie *Fantastic Voyage.*

It intimately explores every nook and cranny within the body, and, as might have been said in *Star Trek,* has the potential to go where no breath has gone before.

In my classes, I'll say: "Notice the parts of your inner environment that are 'awake' and sensitive to subtle pressure or physiological changes caused by breathing, and the parts that are less awake or less sensitive. How does each breath feel as it travels through your body? Does the internal movement of the breath help you sense how parts of the body are integrated, or how parts are not connected? Does the breath wave flow down the left side of the body more freely than the right; does it move through the front more easily than the back? Do certain postures and movement patterns allow breath to move through you more or less freely than others?"

The breath helps you feel physical sensations and tensions, and allows you to recognize where you might be holding tension and restricting movement, leaving parts of your body disconnected.

The intimate and rich kinesthetic qualities of breathing also serve as an excellent anchor to hold your attention, improve focus, and calm the monkey mind. Within the framework of just observing without trying to change anything, you can learn to develop focus and mindfulness by following your breath. Uniting your mind with your breath gives your mind one simple, quiet thing to focus on.

Breath and Movement of Qi

In Tai Chi and related practices, breath serves to both connect to and draw in energy from nature and the surrounding environment. According to Chinese medicine, you draw in some of the vital energy or Qi you need to sustain your existence through the breath. In fact, one of the literal translations of *Qi* is "breath," and sometimes the two terms are used interchangeably. In some meditative Tai Chi exercises, as you breathe in, you imagine drawing energy from nature to recharge and rejuvenate. Then, as you breathe out, you imagine letting go of negative energy, tiredness, or stress. The breath also moves energy within the body. For example, guiding and following the breath to the abdomen in diaphragmatic breathing moves Qi to that region. As the classics suggest, "The inhalation and exhalation are long and deep and the Qi sinks to the tan tien."

7. Social Support
(including Interaction and Community)

Training in Tai Chi includes significant psychosocial (how psychology ties into the social environment) interactions, including students interacting with their instructors, interacting with other students, and more broadly, feeling a sense of belonging and identifying with a larger Tai Chi community. A strong body of research suggests that these forms of social support and sense of connection have huge, positive impacts on health, in terms of disease prevention, recovery rates, and remission following events such as heart attacks and cancer diagnoses.[42] Simply stated, being and feeling connected to others makes you healthier and happier, and fosters a longer life. Thus, one of the active ingredients of Tai Chi is the rich psychosocial support it affords.

Conventional medicine increasingly is appreciating the therapeutic value of the quality of interaction between a patient and a care provider. Not only does the amount of time spent with a patient affect outcomes, but also, the quality of that time is important—including attentiveness, empathy, and fostering optimism.

Ted Kaptchuk and other colleagues at Harvard Medical School have studied the richness of this interaction in great depth. One landmark study on irritable bowel syndrome (IBS) patients compared long, warm-and-fuzzy interactions (that is, augmented with intentional warmth, attention, and confidence) with non-fuzzy and limited interactions (control group). All of the participants received fake acupuncture—that is, no real specific medical intervention. Not surprisingly, the researchers found a dose-like response related to attention—a 62 percent improvement in IBS symptoms occurred in the augmented attention group compared with 44 percent improvement in the limited-contact group, and 28 percent improvement in the control group. The bulk of this effect was due to a "connection" between the patient and the practitioner, which was confirmed by video analysis, qualitative interviews, and surveys of both patients and practitioners.[43]

In the course of learning, Tai Chi students often develop deep relationships with teachers that are, in some ways, analogous to relationships with physicians or physical therapists. Teachers evaluate students' exercise performance and prescribe modifications and new material to facilitate learning. In this capacity, they are loosely similar to physicians and health-care providers who diagnose patients and then prescribe medications or therapies. Models of health behavior and motivational health–coaching research show that material presented empathetically and nonjudgmentally can improve compliance and, ultimately, lead to changes in health.[44]

Tai Chi instructors also commonly play the roles of motivators, coaches, and sometimes even therapists. Teachers often develop a friendly personal relationship with longer-term students as they watch them grow in their Tai Chi practice and, at the same time, hear about how these students endure the natural challenges of life. In my personal experience, I have become very sensitive to the relationships I build with students. Beginning with my response to an initial phone call or e-mail inquiry, especially if a potential student has specific medical issues, I try to listen with care and honestly share any promising information I may have on whether Tai Chi may be of help. I never overstate what I believe to be true from personal teaching experience or research evidence, and if possible, I throw in a little humor if the new student is nervous. Even before the student gets to the first class, we have kindled some hope—which in TCM means Qi is already moving or primed.

Interactions among classmates are also very rich. In my community-based classes, people form strong friendships and social networks, and a few have even gotten married! I've also observed these interactions when traveling through China and talking to my Asian Tai Chi friends. Those who meet in parks and practice daily tend to form special bonds, even bringing one another food when someone is sick.

Social interactions can deeply impact health. Social activities, such as playing bingo, going to sporting events, and attending religious services together, as well as gardening, preparing meals, and participating in fitness activities, have all been associated with longer survival. Social support may offer protection against the negative health consequences associated with stressful events, such as the loss of a spouse or parent. The feeling of being part of something bigger is one reason for the positive relationship between religious involvement and social support. Support from religious groups appears to be more satisfying and more resilient than support from secular groups.[45]

One of my Tai Chi teachers, Arthur Goodridge, once told me that a key reason people do Tai Chi is to get together, hang out, and feel connected to one another. His school is called "Moving Together."

8. EMBODIED SPIRITUALITY
(INCLUDING PHILOSOPHY AND RITUAL)

The core Tai Chi principles provide a roadmap not only for maintaining health, but also, more generally, for guiding your path through life. Taoist philosophy espouses a more natural, holistic view of life that integrates body, mind, and spirit. This view includes an appreciation of balance in all activities and pursuits, for example, avoiding excesses; accepting change and the need for adaptability (going with the flow); and honoring the importance of individual responsibility and self-cultivation.[46] Importantly, the highly structured nature of Tai Chi practice, along with social support provided within Tai Chi community classes, creates an organized, sometimes ritualized, framework for tangibly practicing, developing, translating, and integrating these somewhat intangible philosophical principles into everyday life.

Some people initially are attracted to Tai Chi because of this added philosophical dimension, beyond its function as a physical exercise, a form of therapy, or a martial art. Not surprisingly, this attraction to Eastern philosophical principles is also evident among those who seek out complementary and alternative medicine (CAM) therapies. In a landmark article based on a national survey of why patients use alternative medicine, Stanford University researchers found that CAM therapies attract those who hold personal values and worldviews that are spiritually and philosophically in tune with CAM beliefs regarding nature and the meaning of health and illness.[47] Once you begin to practice and embody Tai Chi principles, the philosophical, spiritual, and ritualistic characteristics of practice can affect your health and, therefore, constitute a key active ingredient.

Philosophy and Health

The central theme of Taoism, as reflected in the yin-yang symbol, is the holistic view of life and the value of integrating body, mind, and spirit. As we have emphasized in many of the other active ingredients, Tai Chi's approach to health is not just through training physical and physiological processes; it fully integrates principles related to your psychological well-being, social relationships, and larger beliefs about nature. Some view this holistic perspective of health as an alternative to the reductionist, materialist paradigm of Western medicine.[48]

Tai Chi training also helps you become more sensitive and skillful in balancing the physical body's intimate dance with the mind. For regular practitioners, these practical experiences may begin to impact everyday activities. After a session of Tai Chi, you may be more likely to eat slower and more mindfully; less likely to drive aggressively, or react to another more aggressive driver; and less likely to respond immediately in a loud voice to a child or office mate. You may become more willing to explore what would happen if you let go for a while. In this way, Tai Chi's philosophy and regimen of mind-body training can help shape your behavior.

One central Taoist concept Tai Chi emphasizes is change. Change and transformation, as the dynamic yin-yang symbol reflects, are essential features of nature. According to Taoism, the interplay between yin and yang creates change everywhere. Taoism espouses that the way to health and happiness is to learn to "go with the flow." Change is inevitable, and resisting change can be much more difficult than adapting to and taking advantage of it.

This idea of adaptability or resilience now is being brought to the forefront of medicine. Systems biologists increasingly believe that the health of a physiological system, for example, as evidenced by heart rate or blood pressure, is based on inherently fractal-like complex dynamics due to the input of many interacting signals.[49] The richer and more complex a system's dynamics, the greater its ability to withstand insults or perturbations, for example, a rapid change in blood pressure when you stand up quickly. This new systems biology paradigm is defining health as resilience or an ability to adapt, that is, to go with the flow. In later chapters, we will discuss research my colleagues and I are doing in collaboration with other Harvard researchers to study how Tai Chi influences physiological complexity and health resilience in older adults.

A third key principle inherent in Tai Chi and Taoism is "knowing" yourself and more fully participating in, and taking responsibility for, your own health. Studies suggest that one of the features that attracts people to Tai Chi and other CAM therapies is a desire to participate more proactively in maintaining their health. They want to be more in control of the health decision-making process and not simply have doctors tell them what to do.[50]

Importantly, research from multiple clinical trials in older adults shows that practicing Tai Chi improves what is called "self-efficacy," or people's beliefs in their capabilities to exercise control over their own functioning and over events that affect their lives.[51] Self-efficacy, in turn, often is associated directly with psychological health, improved health behaviors, and the ability to manage chronic diseases, such as osteoarthritis, heart failure, and balance disorders.[52]

In summary, this philosophy not only affects the quality of your Tai Chi practice, but also how you deal with maintaining your health or managing a chronic disease. It also can spill over into everyday life, making you more aware of how you tolerate and manage stress, and generally helps you make better lifestyle choices.

Spirituality and Health

Throughout much of history, medicine has been imbedded deeply in spirituality. From ancient Greek physicians, to shamanic traditions, to Chinese medicine, many healing traditions have viewed remedies not as material tools for curing disease, but as a means to release or enhance the spirit. One of the strongest tools for healing has been prayer and belief. However, due largely to the emergence of the scientific method in the late 1500s, the relationship between spirituality and medicine changed dramatically. Science could not be readily applied to spiritual beliefs or religion, and a chasm emerged between the two.[53]

Nevertheless, according to numerous surveys, most Americans today consider spirituality or religion (or both) a significant part of who they are; 90 percent believe in God or a higher power.[54] And, when they face illness, many turn to spiritual beliefs and prayer for comfort and solace.

What's more, epidemiological data show strong relationships between spiritual factors and health outcomes; this connection has opened up the discussion of the role spirituality plays in health and medicine. Dozens of accredited US medical schools now offer courses in spirituality in medicine.[55] Interdisciplinary academic programs, such as the Religion, Health, and Healing Initiative at the Center for Study of World Religion at Harvard and the Center for Spirituality, Theology, and Health at Duke University, have become increasingly popular. The study of the spiritual dimensions of Eastern mind-body practices, such as Tai Chi, yoga, and meditation, also has contributed to this re-evaluation.

Spirituality may be a positive factor for coping with illness, preventing illness, and aiding treatments, according to systematic reviews. Epidemiological studies suggest that relationships exist between spiritual or religious practices (church attendance, prayer) and health (longer life span, reduced risk of heart disease).[56] Clinical trials show that prayer and meditation influence immune physiology and neurophysiology. A whole scientific field, called psychoneuroimmunology, exists to study the interaction between psychological processes, including spiritual beliefs, and the nervous and immune systems.[57]

For some, spirit and body comingle and create what William James (one of the fathers of experimental psychology) called "the religion of healthy mindedness."[58] This effect happens because Tai Chi fosters an intimate self-awareness and requires you to slow down and look within yourself at feelings and sensations. One of my Tai Chi students elegantly described it this way: "I don't practice Tai Chi every day, but when I do, I find that it keeps me honest in myself and *it provides a 'knowing' that just thinking can't provide.*" For her, like many others, Tai Chi is a tool for self-inquiry that transcends matter and logic and has a spiritual dimension.

Finally, Tai Chi can help you make the connection between spirituality and the larger universe. For many, deep breathing leads to an exchange of energy with nature. Also, Tai Chi is designed to give you a feeling of being grounded and connected to the earth. It affords you the opportunity to connect your essence or spirit with something that is part of a bigger whole. To feel connected with nature and each other may be why millions of people in China and around the world gather in parks to practice Tai Chi in the morning.

Rituals

Some aspects of Tai Chi, like other exercises or activities performed in a repetitive manner, assume the characteristics of a ritual. Long-term regular practice of the same Tai Chi forms becomes a daily, almost liturgical, act and can represent a journey to a sacred presence.

The ritual of Tai Chi begins to emerge after you've been practicing for a while. This ritual, whether it involves weekly group classes or daily early-morning or late-night practice by yourself, keeps you engaged. Knowing that you will join a group of like-minded others to practice Tai Chi two or three times a week helps you to keep mentally and physically involved with Tai Chi. This adherence can help you to learn more about Tai Chi, and eventually your practice may evolve into something that becomes therapeutic.

Certain Tai Chi programs also encourage regular practice regimens and environments, for example, daily morning practice in the park. Some schools have mandatory rituals, such as removing street shoes before entering the training space or saluting the teacher. For some, even putting on Tai Chi slippers has ritualistic qualities. Many training spaces also commonly contain Tai Chi–related art and symbolic icons, and play meditative music during classes.

Collectively, these rituals, icons, and environmental factors have the potential to create a culturally rich context for meaning, remembering, and perhaps even amplifying certain therapeutic experiences during Tai Chi practice.

3

Put the Principles into Practice: A Simplified Tai Chi Program

This chapter provides a simplified Tai Chi program, structured in an easy-to-learn format, similar to the approach we have used in our research studies at the Harvard Medical School. This 12-week exercise program includes traditional exercises handed down from my Tai Chi teachers and, in some cases, further shaped and informed by my medical research experience. I chose these exercises to deliver and maximize the "dose" of the Eight Active Ingredients of Tai Chi. This program emphasizes essential Tai Chi movements that anyone can easily learn and practice just about anywhere—at home, out in nature, or even in a small quiet corner at work. Growing out of the ancient Tai Chi tradition, these exercises integrate gentle, relaxed flowing movements, mindfulness, natural breathing, and imagery—with the net result being a unique meditative, yet invigorated, state.

The program is structured and introduced here as a 12-week program, but you can be flexible in how you use the program or move through it. The Tai Chi exercises are broken down into three main sections. The first section introduces seven traditional Tai Chi warm-up exercises and can last between 15 and 30 minutes. The Tai Chi warm-up exercises focus on loosening up and structurally integrating the physical body; reinforce Tai Chi principles of incorporating awareness, focus, and imagery into movement; and promote overall relaxation and natural deep breathing. These exercises can serve as a workout in and of themselves. The second section focuses on five core Tai Chi movements following the traditional Cheng Man Ching Yang-style short form. You progressively add these movements over the 12 weeks. The proportion of time allocated to the core Tai Chi movements increases from 5 to 25 minutes as the time allocated to Tai Chi warm-ups decreases slightly. The program concludes with five minutes of a simple set of cool-down exercises, including gentle self-massage techniques. The total exercise program takes about 45–60 minutes.

The design of this collection of exercises allows it to stand alone as a complete Tai Chi program. Because it emphasizes core principles, it also serves as an excellent foundation if you want to progress to longer, choreographed Tai Chi styles, or, if you are more experienced, to deepen your understanding of basic principles.

A 12-WEEK SIMPLIFIED TAI CHI PROGRAM

Week	Activities	Approx. Duration (in minutes)
1–2	Tai Chi Warm-Up Exercises	Total 20–35
	Tai Chi Pouring, Swinging, Drumming, and Standing	3–5
	Swinging to Connect the Kidneys and Lungs	3–5
	Hip Circles and Spiraling the Lower Extremities	3–5
	Spiraling the Upper Extremities	3–5
	Spinal Cord Breathing	3–5
	Fountain	3–5
	Washing Yourself with Qi from the Heavens	3–5
	Tai Chi Movement #1:	
	Raising the Power	5–10
	Tai Chi Cool-Down Exercises	5
	Tai Chi Self-Massage and Meridian Tapping	3–5
	Washing Yourself with Qi from the Heavens	3–5

WARM-UP EXERCISES

WARM-UP EXERCISE 1: TAI CHI POURING, SWINGING, DRUMMING, AND STANDING

The combination of these simple exercises brings awareness into the entire body and stimulates a freer flow of Qi and blood. Tai Chi Pouring, Swinging, and Drumming involves meditatively shifting your weight from side to side, turning your waist, and swinging your arms naturally around your body. These actions loosen up the entire musculoskeletal system, strengthen the legs, deepen breathing, and provide moderate aerobic activity. Tai Chi Standing meditation provides the body and mind time to relax, integrate, and reorganize, and employs the key Tai Chi principle of "non-doing."

Tai Chi Pouring

Tai Chi classics say "Flow like water." The human body is about 70 percent liquid. Using the image of pouring and making waves in your "inner ocean," this exercise helps you experience, through movement, how you can deeply nourish, bathe, and massage your body's internal environment. You learn to sense your energy-rich inner ocean lubricating and integrating all the tissues, joints, and tendons, from the soles of the feet to the tips of the fingers and the top of the head. This framework helps bring the mind's attention and healing intention deeply and fully into the body.

Begin by standing with your feet shoulder-width apart and parallel to one another. Before beginning any movement, take a moment to be still and to be more fully in the present moment. Feel your feet on the ground; notice how you are breathing; feel your whole body. Just simply notice and invite your body and mind to rest in the present moment. Of course, don't worry if you are having difficulty relaxing your body or mind; it makes no sense to get stressed about being stressed! Just proceed and let the practice do its work.

When you are ready to initiate Tai Chi Pouring, slightly bend one knee and allow your weight to shift to that side, and then gently bend the other knee and allow the weight to shift to the other leg. It should feel as if you are "pouring" your weight from one leg to the other. As you rock back and forth and the waves of your inner ocean start flowing, try to "let go," "stay out of the way," and allow the waves to flow increasingly more freely throughout your whole body.

For the first minute or two of Pouring, focus your attention on the soles of your feet. Can you feel the warm, nutrient-rich ocean bathing the tissues of your arches, heels, and the places between and around your toes? Can you feel it in your left foot as much as your right foot? Where do you not feel your energy-rich "juices" permeating? Can you adjust the way you are standing and moving in a way that leads to a deeper, fuller massage of your foot tissues?

After awakening, massaging, and infusing Qi into the soles of your feet, try to feel how the ocean helps integrate your feet with your ankles, calves, shins, and knees. Allow your awareness to penetrate to the deepest layers of these tissues. Then, after a few more rocking cycles, progressively notice if you also can sense these waves moving through your hips, groin, belly, lower back, chest, shoulders, and arms. Be patient; it may take time to develop this openness and sensitivity.

As you rock and feel the connections in your body, also be aware of the key Tai Chi principle of yin and yang. When your weight is on your right leg, really let your left leg rest; regularly remind your left leg that it has no responsibility to hold you up. When you are on your left leg, let your right leg rest. You always have one side that is empty, while the other side is full; one side that's doing, while the other side is not-doing; one side active and one side passive. Notice that after relaxing one side, the ocean may flow more deeply and easily through its tissues.

Rock, relax, feel your body, be aware of your breath, and breathe deeply and naturally. Do your best not to think very much and simply relax into the flow.

Tai Chi Swinging and Drumming

Once you are "in the flow," begin Tai Chi Swinging by adding a little more momentum to the movement, turning your waist, and freeing your arms into a natural swinging pattern. When you transfer your weight to the left leg, turn your waist (with your navel and eyes aligned and moving together, that is, no twisting of the neck or spine) slightly toward the left leg, closing the left *kwah* (groin or inguinal fold). Simultaneously, release the knee of the right leg toward the left side, freely hanging it and resting it between the right hip and toes. Similarly, as you transfer weight to the right leg, turn your waist toward your right leg, closing the right kwah, and hang the left knee between the left hip and the toes. While you are shifting and rotating your torso, allow your arms to relax and swing naturally (like rag doll arms), with your hands and arms gently striking the body at the end of each rotation. Despite the slightly faster, more coordinated nature of this movement, continue to feel your feet on the ground, and sense the inner ocean bathing and integrating your entire body, from feet to head and hands. Practice Tai Chi Swinging and Drumming as if you were doing an aerobic meditation.

Once swinging feels natural and relaxed, add in the gentle stimulation of Drumming the Body. Starting with your upper body, as you swing and turn to the left, steer the right palm's natural swing to tap or drum the upper-left side of the chest (just above the breast), and as you shift and turn to the right, steer the left palm's swing to tap or drum the upper-right side of the chest. Each tap/drum provides a little stimulation, like a little vibrational massage to that body region. The light contact of the palm with the body should feel lively, bouncing off after each contact, much as it would if you were playing a hand drum. Then sequentially target your swinging palms to the left and right sides of your rib cage, beneath the breasts and on both sides of the abdomen. Next, target your swinging palms to drum the midline of the torso, beginning with the breastbone and descending to stimulate the solar plexus, navel, and lower abdomen. Finally, broadly targeting the tan tien regions, simultaneously drum the navel and lower back, and then simultaneously drum the lower abdomen and sacrum. Repeatedly drum at each of these body regions for 10 to 20 seconds.

Tai Chi Standing Meditation

When you finish Drumming the Body, relax and simply stand still for a few minutes. You may feel the vibrations and energy continue to resonate throughout your body, like the reverberations following the banging of a gong or the ringing of a church bell. Notice where in your body you feel these vibrations or related sensations (warmth, tingling, liveliness). Where are they most palpable or most intense? Also notice which body regions feel the least vibrations. Passively, through simple patience and deepening re-laxation, invite your energy to spread from the more vibrant areas to those areas experiencing less vibration. While remaining relatively still on the outside, and without "thinking" too much, invite the energy to even out and flow more freely through every cell in your body. Sequentially explore, bringing awareness to and relaxing the following areas to help balance out energy: your eyes and the muscles that surround them; your temples; your mouth, tongue, and jaw; the rest of your head bones; your neck and throat; your shoulders and arms, down to the fingertips; your chest and heart area; your ribs and spine; your belly and lower back; your entire pelvic region; and your legs all the way down to your feet.

Finally, imagine that you are like a tree, and you have roots that extend beneath your feet and penetrate deeply into the earth. Use your roots as a structure for releasing your tensions. The more you patiently relax and let go of tensions in the upper body and legs, and allow the Qi to sink into your roots, the more grounded and less top-heavy (or "up tight") you will feel. As you release and surrender to gravity, you will feel as if you are standing taller. Your more relaxed upper body will allow your spine to decompress, as the Tai Chi classics state, "hanging like a necklace of pearls from heaven."

Thinking as if you are a mighty, wise tree, invite your entire body to relax. Enjoy feeling grounded while your upper body floats with increasing ease; maintain awareness of your breathing. Who knew that standing while "doing" very little could be such a profound meditation?

Key Points to Keep in Mind

- While Pouring, Swinging, and Drumming, allow the movements to flow naturally. Don't force or strain anything. Pay particular attention to avoid twisting your knees; emphasize the opening and closing of the kwah, and do not over-turn the torso. Also, do not use too much force or create any strain or discomfort with Drumming. Some parts of the body (for example, the solar plexus) may be more sensitive than others are, so you should only tap them lightly.
- During weight shifts, focus more on the emptying leg than on the filling leg (that is, focus more on the leg that is more non-doing than doing), allowing the feet, ankles, knees, and hips to relax and release a bit more deeply following each weight shift.
- While focusing attention to and relaxing the body, try to feel and experience more than think. Don't worry too much about getting it right.
- Try to experience Tai Chi Swinging and Drumming as a sort of aerobic meditation, more than a purely physical, aerobic workout.
- Use the Standing meditation to rest, deepen your mind-body connection, and give your body time and energy to rebalance. As your body (and patience) gets stronger, extend your Standing time to as long as 10 to 15 minutes.

WARM-UP EXERCISE 2:
SWINGING TO CONNECT THE KIDNEYS AND LUNGS

This gentle movement also loosens up the body, provides moderate aerobic activity, develops dynamic balance, and stimulates deep breathing.

Maintaining a comfortable shoulder-width stance, begin by raising up your arms overhead, and then release them down, surrendering to the simple pull of gravity. As your arms swing upward and slightly outward, allow a gentle opening of your chest and ribs, a lengthening of your spine, as well as a lengthening of your arms from the shoulder blades to the fingertips. Also, shift about 70 percent of your weight to the balls of the feet (stand a little more forward). And, if it's comfortable for you, lift your chin and the gaze of your eyes slightly as your arms swing up. Imagine your lungs opening and stretching with this shape, and breathe in during the upswing.

Each time your arms come down, bend the knees slightly and sit into the kwah, shift about 60 percent of the weight in your feet to your heels, and exhale. As you "sit" into this posture, relax your hips and pelvic area (kwah), feel the slight opening of the lower spine, and feel the gentle stretch and massage in your lower back muscles and kidney region.

Repeat the upward and downward swinging, stimulating and connecting the lung and kidney region, 9 to 36 times. If your balance is stable, and/or if you want gradually to challenge and improve your dynamic balance, slightly raise your heels off the ground during the upswing, and return to a flat-footed position (slightly more weighted in the heels) on the downswing.

Key Points to Keep in Mind

- Begin with smaller movements, and as your tissues and joints warm up, gently let the movements get larger. But never force any movements, and stay within 70 percent of your maximum range of motion. Do even less if you have shoulder or back injuries.
- Do not bend your knees more than 10 percent; this is not a deep knee-bending exercise. Focus more on folding or sitting into the kwah.
- If coordinating your breath with the movements creates any discomfort, such as shortness of breath or light-headedness, simply breathe naturally and focus more on the quality of the movements.

WARM-UP EXERCISE 3:
HIP CIRCLES AND SPIRALING THE LOWER EXTREMITY

Relaxed, mindful, circular movements are used in Tai Chi to promote natural movement, Qi and blood circulation, and to enhance flexibility. This next set of exercises is designed to loosen up, better integrate, and enhance circulation through lower body regions.

Hip Circles

Standing with feet parallel and shoulder-width apart, and keeping your head upright and centered over the feet, make gentle circles in a clockwise direction with your waist, inviting an organic opening of its full range of motion. Explore using some of the Active Ingredients of Tai Chi.

Begin by exercising your *awareness*. Notice how much of the circle you can feel intimately with your hip movement. At first, simply notice without attempting to change anything. For example, if you imagine the hip circles you are making as a clockface, can you feel your movement pass through all 12 of the five-minute points? How about each of the 60 one-minute points?

Now add *intention*. Invite the "inner ocean" to nourish and lubricate all the tissues that you engage in making your circle, and with a gentle and kind intention invite any kinks and strains to dissolve. Remembering the 70-percent rule, don't force through any tight area; instead, patiently invite restricted areas to relax and open up a bit more with each rotation.

Fold in *dynamic structural integration*—feel your feet on the ground, and feel the connection between your feet and the hips and waist; feel the impact of your hip circles on your whole body.

Finally, be aware of your *breathing*. Breathe naturally, freely, and deeply. Can you feel how the breath and the movement interact?

Complete 6 to 36 clockwise circles. Then repeat the same process of circling in a counterclockwise direction. Enjoy how rich and engaging even a simple movement can be when you do it using Tai Chi principles.

Spiraling the Lower Extremities

Now apply the same meditation-in-motion approach to each of the lower extremity joints. Begin by shifting your weight entirely to your left leg. Rest your right toes on the ground directly beneath your right hip, and let your right knee hang freely between your hip and toes (the right heel should come off the floor). Begin making circles with your right kneecap, horizontal to the ground, and activate the Active Ingredients of awareness, intention, structural integration, and breathing, as well as the 70-percent rule, to this movement. With each rotation of the knee, feel the inner ocean nourishing the ligaments, tendons, and cartilage of the entire knee, including behind the knee, the sides, and even under the kneecaps. Focus on the knee region for six to nine rotations.

Continuing the same movement, simply shift your attention down to the right ankle and foot. Feel how the same movement articulates and helps bring awareness to the ankle and entire foot. Invite the inner ocean to permeate these tissues deeply. Focus on the ankle and foot for six to nine rotations.

Finally, shift your attention one last time to your right hip and groin. Feel how the same movement articulates your upper leg bone and helps bring awareness to the hip socket and the entire right side of the pelvic region. Invite the inner ocean to deeply penetrate the right hip, groin, buttocks, lower abdomen, and tailbone region. Focus on the right hip and pelvis for six to nine rotations.

When you are done with the right leg, shift your weight so you can let your left knee hang between the hip and toe, and mindfully spiral the joints of your left leg.

Key Points to Keep in Mind

- When spiraling the lower extremity, feel free to use the back of a chair or stand near a wall if you find it difficult to balance.
- When rotating the waist or leg joints, take your time; the slower you go, the better. You will not get extra points for going around faster or more times! Going slowly makes it easier to feel the effects and decreases the chances of causing strain or injury.
- While loosening the joints of one leg, remain aware of your other supporting leg. Appreciate the strength and dynamic support it provides.

WARM-UP EXERCISE 4:
SPIRALING THE UPPER EXTREMITY

Now you are going to do some simple exercises to loosen up the upper part of the body. These exercises use similar circular movements to improve body awareness, promote relaxation, and enhance range of motion and circulation in the shoulders, elbows, wrists, and fingers. If you need a little break, you can perform these exercises just as easily while sitting.

Wrist Circles

Beginning with your hands, create soft gentle fists and hold them comfortably in front of your body. Just as you did with the ankles, you are going to make little circles with your wrists, this time circling both simultaneously (one clockwise, the other counterclockwise). Use the mindful, circling movements to help you feel your wrists and their connections into your hands and forearms. As you gently stretch the muscles, ligaments, tendons, and fascia, use relaxed, kind intention to encourage your Qi-filled inner ocean to soften and nourish these tissues. And, even though you are paying careful attention to the wrists, maintain awareness of the rest of your body. Feel your feet on the ground, and be aware of your overall posture and the states of tension in your shoulders and neck. Don't stop breathing! After six or nine rotations in one direction, repeat the same movements in the reverse direction.

Hand Stretches

Now switch to some very simple stretches for the hands and fingers themselves. Begin with the palms facing upward. Sequentially stretch and bend each of the fingers inward toward the body, beginning with the pinky and ending with the thumb. At the end of this spiraling movement, the palm faces downward and the fingers and palms are gently stretched both laterally and lengthwise. Be gentle with your stretching, and use attention and intention to invite your Qi-filled inner ocean into every knuckle of every finger and all the tissues of your palms and the back of your hands. Repeat 6 to 9 times, and feel free to improvise on the movement pattern. Notice how slight variations in movement patterns and hand shapes can help you feel, and nourish and integrate, all parts in your hands and wrists. Feel like a cat stretching its paw. Over time, explore feeling the stretch all the way up to your elbows and shoulders. Rest for a few moments after these stretches. Take time to feel your hands; do they feel different compared to when you started these stretches? (Also see the Hand Tai Chi exercise on page 149.)

Shoulder Stretches

Now you are going to do some simple shoulder stretches and coordinate these with your breathing. Slowly shrug both shoulders as you breathe in, and exhale and gently release your shoulders down. Let your shoulders, neck, chest, and back relax. Again, breathing in, raise your shoulders up and exhale, and release them back down. Do not force or strain. Raise your shoulders using no more than 70 percent of your maximum effort. Use your meditative attention and intention to feel as if you can breathe some Qi and life into these tissues, imagining the breath itself permeating the entire shoulder girdle, neck, and upper torso. As you exhale, melt any tensions, and let them flow down and out of your body through your arms and legs. Repeat this series 6 to 9 times.

Key Points to Keep in Mind

- In all stretches, do not force the stretch. Think of these exercises more as a moving meditation than as effortful stretches.
- Feel your feet on the ground throughout, and stay grounded. Feel the integration of the body part you are moving using the whole of your body.·
- Breathe deeply and comfortably throughout the exercise.

WARM-UP EXERCISE 5:
SPINAL CORD BREATHING

This exercise focuses on increasing flexibility in the spine and chest, building tone in the core muscles, and stimulating and balancing the flow of energy through the front and back of the body. By creating a little more flexibility in the spine, ribs, and whole torso, you free up your breathing.

Begin with a comfortable shoulder-width stance. You are going to create two different shapes with the spine and then go back and forth between the shapes. The first shape is an arch going backward. Lift your chest and chin slightly, and very gently lengthen your entire spine, including your neck, and slightly exaggerate the arch in your lower back. As you do this shape, also draw your shoulder blades toward each other and slightly downward, while raising your palms to face forward just to the outside of your shoulders. This should result in a nice stretch in the whole front of the body. As usual, go no more than 70 percent of your full range of motion.

Now you are going to create a rounded C-shape in your spine in the other direction. Release your arms, bring your elbows and wrists closer together, and tuck your chin downward slightly while rounding your whole back like a turtle. Feel as if your spine, including your neck and tailbone, are being stretched and lengthened.

Once you feel comfortable with these two shapes, go back and forth at a slow pace from one shape to the other, opening and closing, stretching and relaxing the front and back of your body. Try to bring awareness to each of the 33 vertebrae in your spine, and use your intention to get the Qi and juices to permeate all of the spine's tissues, including the muscles, ligaments, tendons, fascia, nerves, and the bones themselves.

Open and close your spine 6 or 9 times. You can also explore folding your breathing pattern into this exercise, depending on how slowly you move. Breathe in as you open your chest and raise your arms, exhale as you round your back, tuck your chin, and draw your forearms together. If you are moving very slowly and have not yet developed an ability to breathe slowly and deeply, simply breathe naturally and focus more on the meditative stretching.

Key Points to Keep in Mind

- If at any time your breathing feels uncomfortable, just breathe naturally and focus much more on the lengthening and relaxation of the spine, ribs, and torso.
- Do not stretch too far or strain your back. Be extra careful if you have a history of back or neck problems, stretching no more than 50–60 percent of your full range of motion.
- You may also do this exercise in a seated position. Whether standing or sitting, feel your feet on the ground and stay aware of your whole body.

WARM-UP EXERCISE 6: THE FOUNTAIN

This very traditional Qigong exercise balances the left and right sides of the body, opens and integrates all the joints, releases tension, and coordinates movement with breathing. The movement further strengthens and adds flexibility to the lower and upper body by coordinating gentle flexing of the ankles and knees with vertical movement of the torso and continuous circular arm movements. See photos 1.1–1.3 on page 80.

Stand in a comfortable shoulder-width stance, feet parallel. As you gently flex your ankles and knees, cross your wrists in front of your navel, palms facing your body. Then slowly straighten and extend your legs and torso, and at the same time, let your hands float up your midline and then separate and turn outward, around head height, in a circular motion. During this rising movement, sequentially open and gently stretch all the joints in your body, including your ankles, knees, hips, spine, ribs, and arms all the way out to your fingers. As your arms continue to circle outward to your side and relax downward, point the palms laterally in the direction your ears point. Then, as the arms and palms descend, relax all your joints and again gently flex your knees. Try to time the movement so that by the time you complete your small flexing of the knees, your wrists return to the starting position, crossed in front of your navel. Repeat this movement 6 or 9 times.

Take a few moments to rest, either sitting in a chair or standing, before you start the next movement.

Key Points to Keep in Mind

- As you stretch and open all the joints, never go past 70 percent of your full range of motion. Similarly, as you bend, do not sink too deeply.
- Have a sense of opening, letting go, and relaxing the whole body.
- Throughout the exercise, keep your body upright and your spine vertical; feel your feet on the ground.
- You can coordinate this gentle, intuitive stretch with your breath. As you breathe in, open upward, and as your arms descend, exhale and let your breath settle. Doing this movement slowly is preferable, so breathing at your natural pace, independent of the pace of your movements, may be best.
- Feel free to improvise the patterns of your fountain-like movements, for example, stretching on one side more than the other side. Imagine an infant waking up and stretching in the crib. It's as if the whole body stretches and yawns. Listen to how your body wants to stretch, and try to feel as if you are intuitively stretching from the inside out.

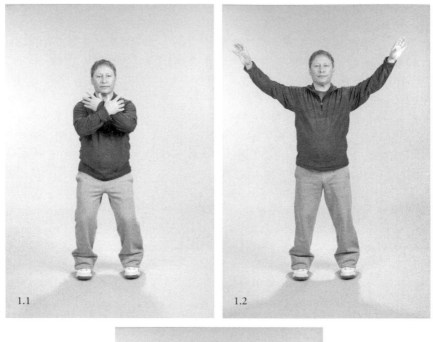

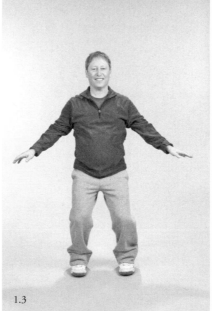

TAI CHI AND ITS ESSENTIAL ELEMENTS

WARM-UP EXERCISE 7:
WASHING YOURSELF WITH QI FROM THE HEAVENS

This very simple, enjoyable exercise relies greatly on imagery and intention. It's designed to gather in healing, rejuvenating energy from Nature and to guide this energy through every cell of the body, starting at the crown of your head and extending down through your legs and into your imaginary roots in the earth. See photos 2.1–2.5 on pages 82–83.

Begin by imagining yourself standing outside in nature surrounded by vibrant, healing, peaceful energy—perhaps a beach, peaceful garden, forest, or mountain top. Then circle your hands up the sides of the body and over the head. Imagine the hands can comingle with the surrounding natural energy, especially in the spacious sky (the "heavens"). Then, as the palms descend slowly, imagine you can guide this energy through every cell of your body—every blood cell, muscle, bone, nerve, and organ. Starting at the crown of the head, feel the energy seep into and relax all your face muscles and head bones, your eyes, and deep into the folds and glands of your brain. Sense that every place this energy reaches, deep relaxation and rejuvenation occurs. Continue down slowly through your neck and throat, shoulders, and chest. Let your body soak up this Qi. Guide this energy through all your organs, including your heart and lungs. Continue down through your abdomen, lower back, pelvis, and through both of your legs to the soles of your feet. And then, imagining you are like a tree with deep roots, guide the energy through your feet into your roots, anchoring you to the earth.

Once you are familiar with this first level of washing yourself with Qi, as you guide fresh healing energy through your body, simultaneously imagine a fine mesh that filters out any tiredness, tension, or uncomfortable "sicker" energy in your body. Have a sense of cleaning the body as well as recharging it. Both of these actions happen at the same time. Let this filtering include every cell from the top of your head to your feet, and then guide the negative energy through your roots into the earth where you imagine it will be recycled.

Each time you go through the exercise, feel fresh Qi penetrate just a little bit further. Feel as if you can clear out any tiredness, tension, or sicker, unbalanced energy. Don't think about it or judge it, just gently guide it out, almost as if you are purifying the body. Begin to feel a little more lightness in your body, as if your body is a little more awake. Feel free to breathe fresh energy into every cell. Repeat this 3 to 9 times. When you finish, rest for a minute, and breathe naturally.

Key Points to Keep in Mind

- Be playful and patient in exploring which images, if any, are more effective for you than others. Feel free to use your intuition and modify the images—for example, adding color, temperature, or other senses. On days you feel particularly tense or anxious, invite a calming energy to fill you. On days when you are tired, you might imagine a more vibrant, perky energy to flow through you. Similarly, if you feel hot or cold, choose an energy quality that brings you into a more comfortable balance.

- If visualization does not feel right for you, or is distracting or too cerebral, simply try to relax the various parts of your body progressively as you pay attention to them.

- In guiding negative energy out of your body, don't analyze, judge, process, or try to understand the source of this imbalance. Simply trust letting it go.

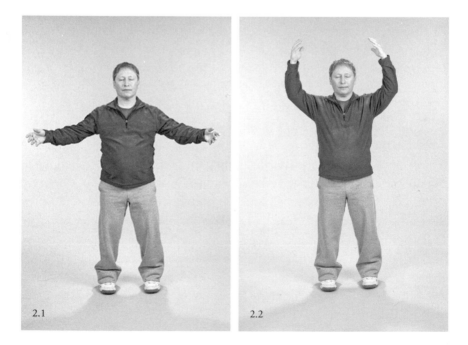

2.1

2.2

TAI CHI AND ITS ESSENTIAL ELEMENTS

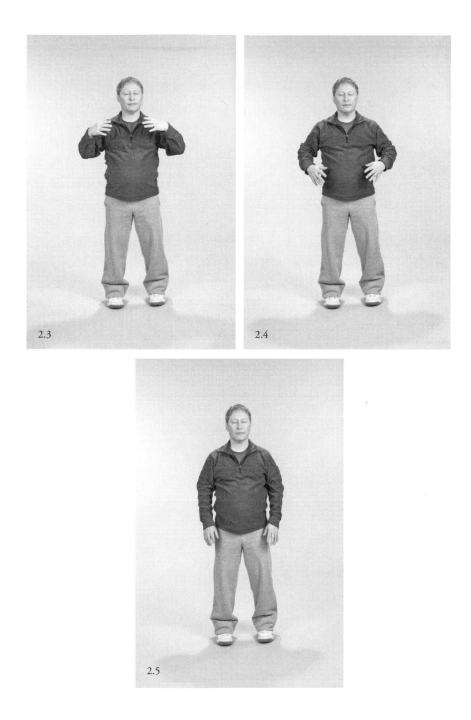

2.3

2.4

2.5

TAI CHI EXERCISES

Tai Chi Exercise 1: Raising the Power

This exercise integrates the upper and lower body by coordinating simple arm and leg movements, and strengthens and improves the flexibility of the ankles, knees, hips, and back. In addition, it challenges balance by continuously altering the position of arms relative to the torso and brings awareness to differences in energy between the left and right sides of the body. See photos 3.1–3.6 on pages 85–86.

Begin by standing with your feet shoulder-width apart. Gently, slowly bend your knees, no more than 10 percent, and at the same time, let your hands float upward in front of your body with the wrists bent and relaxed, about shoulder-width apart, and the hands and fingers hanging down. When your wrists reach shoulder height, allow your palms and then fingers to open slowly; your fingertips should feel perky, but the hands and arms relaxed. Then let your elbows feel heavy and sink, and as they descend, allow your relaxed wrists to float down the front of your body with the palms initially facing outward. As your arms move down, slowly straighten your legs. Do this again, and try to coordinate your arms and the legs. As you bend the knees slowly, without force or strain, let your arms float away from your body with relaxed wrists and fingers. Let your hands open when the wrists reach shoulder height, and straighten (but don't lock) your legs as your elbows sink and as your palms float down, with your fingertips trailing just a little bit.

As your hands rise, play with the image of them being almost like paintbrushes, with the backs of your hands painting on a wall. And, as your hands come down, the front of your palms are painting the wall. Coordinate the flexing of your legs with the floating of your hands away from your body. Keep your shoulders and elbows relaxed, and as your legs straighten, let your elbows and wrists sink and fingers trail as your arms come down.

Do this exercise 9 to 36 times, moving at your own pace. Each time you go up and down, sense a little more smoothness and evenness in the motion. Keep your spine upright, long, and relaxed, and feel your feet on the ground; the whole body is moving as one. As you finish, let your body settle and rest. If you like, rest in a chair before you start the next exercise.

Key Points to Keep in Mind

- Don't sink too deeply; there should be no strain in the knees.
- Don't lock the knee or elbow joints when you extend your legs or arms; don't let the wrists go higher than your shoulders. If you have shoulder discomfort, explore raising the arms to 50 percent or 75 percent of your shoulder height.
- Coordinate the timing of the arm and leg movements.
- Keep the spine upright. Don't lean back as your arms go up.

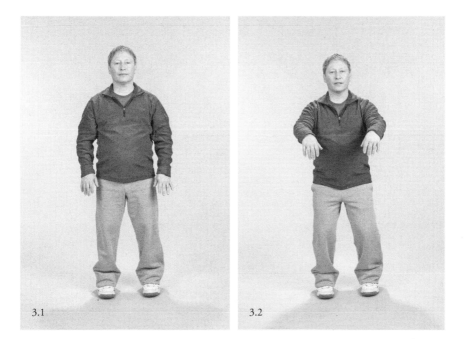

3.1

3.2

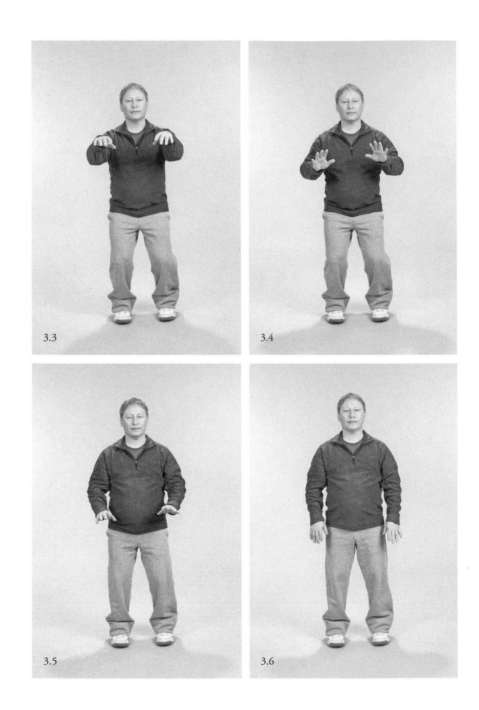

3.3

3.4

3.5

3.6

TAI CHI AND ITS ESSENTIAL ELEMENTS

Tai Chi Exercise 2: Withdraw and Push

This exercise adds the challenge of learning to rely on one leg (the rear one) for support and balance and then smoothly shift weight from one leg to the other, from front to back. It coordinates simple leg and torso movements with continuous changes in arm positions, develops dynamic balance, adds strength and flexibility to the legs and arms, and offers moderate aerobic activity. See photos 4.1–4.6 on pages 89–90.

Begin the same way as Raising the Power, with your feet roughly shoulder-width apart. Now you are going to change the stance to what's called the bow stance. To get into the bow stance, shift your weight to your left leg, and, as you leave your right heel down, turn the toes of the right foot out slightly, about 30 degrees, and shift your weight comfortably back onto the right leg. Now step forward with the left foot. Imagine that the left foot is on a railroad track, and place the heel directly in front of the left toes. Maintain the original width between your heels.

Then move your left knee over the center of your left foot, not going beyond the base of the toes, with about 60–70 percent of your weight forward. Square your hips so that your belly button, nose, and the toes of your left foot all point in the same direction. Now raise your hands to about chest height in front of you in a gesture as if you have just pushed something. The V-shaped angle of your elbow should not exceed 90 degrees. Keep your hands open and your shoulders and arms relaxed.

Begin a circular pattern of motion with your upper and lower body. Shift 100 percent of your weight back onto your right leg, and allow your arms to relax forward and downward in a circular movement. The angle your elbow joint makes will get much larger. Then, following the circular, falling movement of the arms, raise them in front of your body as you shift your weight forward again until your arms reach the original forward, pushing position. Do this series 9 times.

The weight shift should have the same quality as the warm-up exercises, with the feeling of pouring your weight. As you shift back and forth, feel your inner ocean bathing your feet and connecting them to your ankles, knees, hips, torso, and hands. Relax a little more deeply each time you release your arms. Relax your shoulders, and hang your elbows as you move into the active pushing phase. Throughout the exercise, your spine should strive toward the quality of a necklace of pearls hanging, with your neck relaxed. Be aware of your breathing, and keep it deep, slow, and comfortable, without forcing any rhythm or pattern. If a breathing pattern emerges with the movement, that is fine; just go with it. As you rock, feel your whole body, feet relaxed on the ground, spine long, breathing deeply, and arms and legs coordinated and integrated.

Finish by letting your arms fall to the sides, your weight shifting back, and the front foot sliding back to shoulder width. Adjust your feet to where you started, with feet parallel, shoulder-width apart.

Repeat this series, doing the mirror image of these movements. Shift your weight to the right; leave the left heel down; turn your right toes out 30 degrees; shift your weight to the left; move your right foot forward, putting the heel just in front of the right toes; and maintain shoulder-width distance between your feet. Shift your weight forward 60–70 percent, again making sure not to let your right knee pass the base of your right toes. Keep your palms up, neck long, and back straight as you push with your arms forward. Then let your arms relax and fall, making a circle down in front of your hips as you shift your weight onto the back leg. Do 9 cycles on this second leg.

As you finish, allow your arms to fall to your side and shift your weight back, sliding your right foot back to shoulder width, adjusting your feet to parallel. Again, as you stand here resting, just let your whole body and mind relax. If you want, sit and rest between the movements.

Key Points to Keep in Mind

- Make sure your bow stance has sufficient width (that is, it's shoulder width), but do not take too long a stance.
- If your knees feel strained, check the proportions of your stance. Also, try bending less deeply, and do not shift your weight as far forward or back. The forward knee should never extend past the base of the toes.
- The movements should become more continuous and smooth, what the Tai Chi classics say is seamless, with no obvious beginning, middle, or end.

- Maintain deep, unforced, natural breathing.
- Be aware of your whole body, feeling your feet on the ground, the spine hanging from the top, and the connection of the legs and arms throughout.
- After you learn these movements, think very little as you do them. It's more about feeling and listening to how your body is moving.

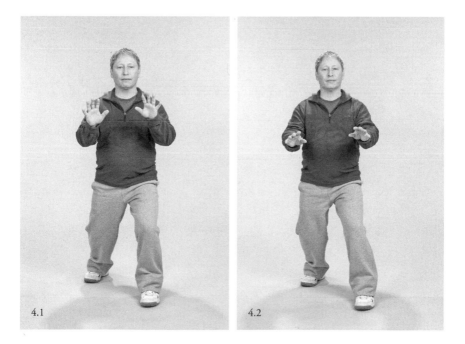

4.1

4.2

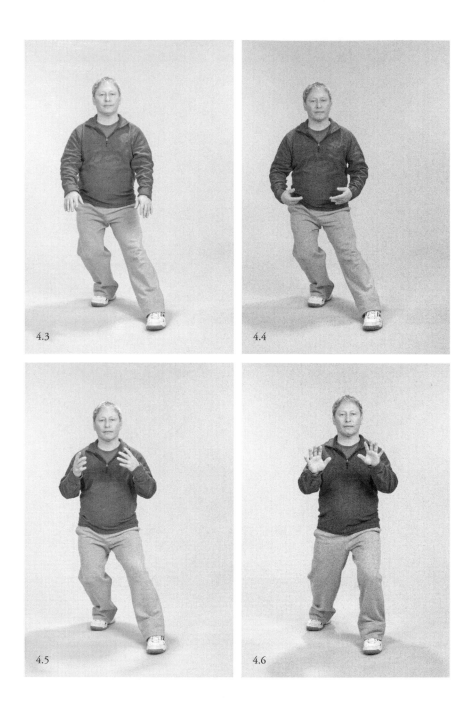

4.3

4.4

4.5

4.6

TAI CHI AND ITS ESSENTIAL ELEMENTS

Tai Chi Exercise 3: Wave Hands Like Clouds

This quintessential Tai Chi exercise integrates movements of the legs and waist with the arms, uses circular motion to improve blood and Qi flow to the extremities, and balances the left and right sides of the body. See photos 5.1–6.6 on pages 93–96.

First, get familiar with the movement of the legs and torso. Stand with your feet parallel, shoulder-width apart. Focusing first on the legs, hips, and torso, begin by shifting your weight to your right leg; turn your waist slightly to the right (knee stable and centered over the foot, no twisting of right knee or torso), and keep both feet flat. Your torso should rest into the kwah as a child harnessed and balanced in a Jolly Jumper; that is, hips and waist stay relaxed and elastic. While still oriented slightly to the right with your waist and head, shift your weight to the left leg so your weight is aligned over your left foot, and then close your left kwah (groin or inguinal fold) by turning the waist slightly to the left (again no twisting of knee or torso). Repeat this movement 9 to 36 times. Sense the movements gently massaging the feet, knees, and especially the hips and kwah, and feel the integration of these body parts.

Now add in arm movements. To help learn the choreography and experience key Tai Chi qualities, imagine your hands are soft, calligraphy paintbrushes. Picture your palm brushing against a surface—because it's pliable, it bends back slightly. If you made a brush stroke in the opposite direction with the back of your hand touching the surface, your wrist would bend gently toward the body. With this pliable quality of movement in mind, imagine your hand is filled with calligraphy Qi and begin to paint an oval with your right hand. Shift your weight from your right leg to your left leg and guide your right palm (facing slightly outward) from right to left around navel height making a smooth "brush stroke." Let the calligraphy Qi flow naturally out from the surface of your palm. As you complete the arm movement, turn your waist slightly to the left and then raise your right hand to chest height (without raising your right shoulder). As you shift your weight back to the right, make a smooth "brush stroke" with the back of your hand, letting the calligraphy Qi flow naturally from the back of your hand. Complete the oval by letting your right hand drop to navel height on your right side. Repeat 9 to 36 times with your right hand, and then repeat this series with your left hand.

All of these movements should feel very pleasant, as if you are internally massaging and making gentle waves throughout your body. Turn, float the hands, pour your weight, and complete the circular or oval motion. Throughout this movement, your body remains upright and comfortable; don't force or strain. Over time, the circle or oval that you are painting will feel more continuous and smooth, as all of your fingers become involved in the painting.

Throughout this movement, keep the breath deep, continuous, and relaxed. Feel a nice sense of integration from the hands all the way through the torso and legs, and in the other direction, from the legs all the way back up to the hands. To complete the movement, pause your hand in front of your shoulder, turn it to face down, and just let it float down lightly like a parachute. Feel the air under your hand. Also, feel your feet on the ground, and feel your whole body.

Again, think of the Tai Chi principle of seamlessness—continuous movement, with no stops or starts, no jerkiness in the movement. Someone watching you would have no sense of the beginning, middle, or end of the movement. The pouring is continuous; like waves washing through your body, your breathing is deep, natural, relaxed, and unforced. If some rhythms emerge for the breathing, that's fine. You want to feel as if your body is as light as a cloud and your hands are just floating through it.

Repeat the same movement with your left arm, completing 9–36 more cycles.

When you are comfortable performing this exercise with each arm, you can practice both arms together, working them in phase.

When you finish, feel free to take a few moments to rest, either sitting in a chair or standing, and notice changes in your body before you start the next movement.

Key Points to Keep in Mind

- Keep your spine upright, shoulders and neck relaxed throughout. Pay particular attention to relaxing your shoulders as your arms come up. Remain aware of how your feet stay in contact with the ground throughout the exercise.
- Remain aware of your breath, and keep it relaxed.
- Using the image of the hand as a paintbrush, notice whether some

fingers feel the flow of Qi more than others do, and try to even out the sensation. Similarly, balance out the sense of openness in the front and back of each hand.

- As you practice more, extend the concept of feeling like a brush to the length of your arm. Invite a freer flow of Qi though the entire body, integrating your legs, torso, and hands.
- Once you are comfortable with the choreography, feel free to explore a faster or slower pace of the "brush strokes," but always end with a short resting meditation.

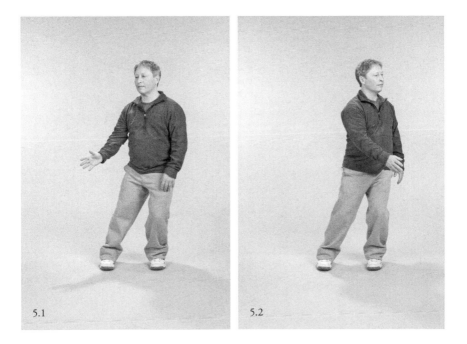

5.1

5.2

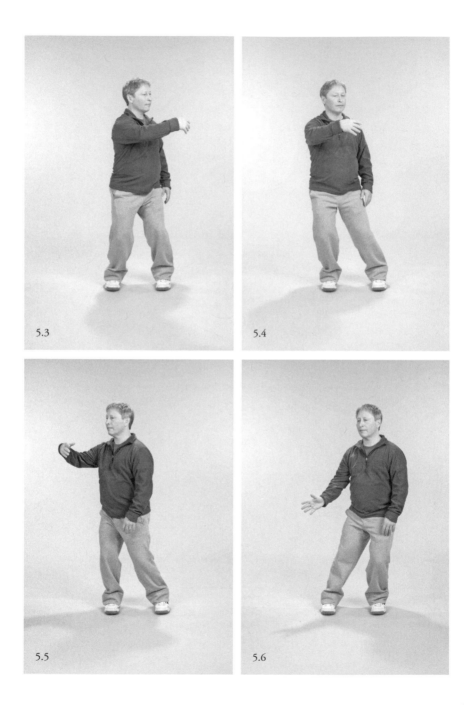

5.3

5.4

5.5

5.6

Tai Chi and Its Essential Elements

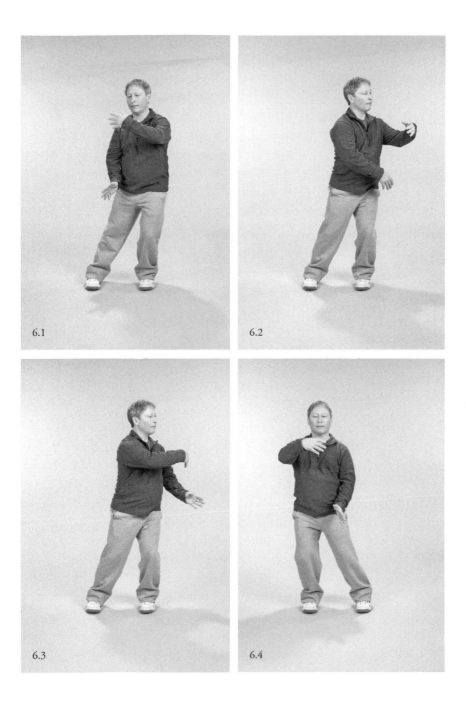

6.1

6.2

6.3

6.4

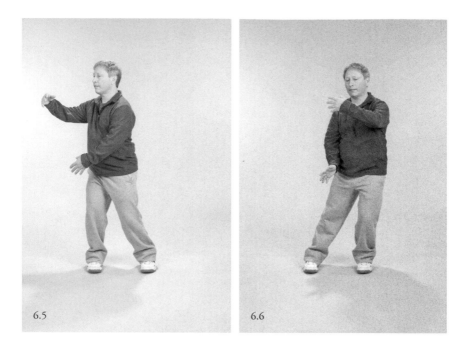

6.5

6.6

Tai Chi Exercise 4: Grasp the Sparrow's Tail

This exercise brings attention to the central role that the waist plays in integrated movement. Rotating the waist within a fixed stance develops flexibility in the hips and lower spine, massages the internal organs, and helps integrate the movements of the legs with the torso and arms. The large, circular movements of the arms improve your range of motion and the circulation to the upper extremities, develop dynamic balance, and provide moderate aerobic and strength training. See photos 7.1–7.8 on pages 99–100.

As with the other exercises, first you will learn the weight shifting and torso movements without the arm movements. Begin with your weight forward in a bow stance; your left knee is stable over the left foot with your torso facing forward (same direction as front toes), your right foot pointed 30 degrees to the right. Keep your weight forward, and slightly turn your navel and torso further to the left, closing or folding your left kwah. Then, still facing a little to the left, shift your weight back to 100 percent onto the right leg, and then turn your waist to the right, closing the right kwah.

Continuing to face slightly to the right, transfer your weight back to the left leg into the forward bow stance, and then turn your torso back to the original starting position (navel pointing forward in the same direction as your left toes).

Now you will integrate the arm movements, one arm at a time, with the lower body. Begin with your right arm by centering it in front of your chest, in a push gesture. Your right arm will follow the movement of your torso as it turns left; there should be no arm extension or change in your elbow angle during this small torso turn. Then release the right arm downward, creating a large, circular movement as your weight shifts backward. Now circle the right arm back up to shoulder height as your waist turns to the right. As your arm swings upward, the palm of your right hand faces the same direction as your navel. Then the shoulders and wrist relax, and the palm returns to the starting push gesture as your torso returns to the beginning of the bow stance.

For the left arm, begin with a round shape at chest height, as if you were cradling a large balloon or sphere against your chest. Maintain this "ward-off" gesture as your hips turn to the left. Shift your weight back as the left arm simply releases downward in a circular motion and sweeps across your groin area. The left arm swings back up to the same ward-off gesture. This gesture doesn't change throughout the remainder of the movement.

Finally, you move both arms together with the weight shifting. When you hold both palms in front of your chest, facing one another, this movement should resemble holding a small ball or bird, thus, "grasping a sparrow's tail." Do the coordinated movement 9 to 36 times.

When you are comfortable doing the movements with your left leg in the forward position, do the mirror image of the movement with the right side. Begin in a bow stance, right knee over the right foot, torso facing forward, left foot pointed 30 degrees to the left. With your weight forward, slightly turn your navel and torso further to the right, folding your right kwah, and while facing a little to the right, shift your weight fully back onto the left leg. Then turn your waist to the left, closing the left kwah. Still facing slightly to the left, transfer your weight back to the right leg into the forward bow stance, and then turn your torso back to the original starting position.

Move both arms together with the weight shifting. Begin with your left arm centered in front of your chest, ready to push. As your body turns, the arm follows your torso turn to the right, and as your weight shifts back to your left leg, your arm falls and circles back up to shoulder height, with palm facing the same direction as your navel. Meanwhile, the right arm begins in a round shape at chest height in the ward-off gesture as your hips turn to the right. During your weight shift to your back left leg, the right arm also releases downward and sweeps across your groin area, simply swinging back up to the same ward-off gesture. As you shift your weight again toward your front right leg, both your arms move to create the Grasp the Sparrow's Tail gesture, with one palm facing the other, in front of your chest. Turn your hips and torso to face straight forward, and begin a new cycle. Repeat 9 to 36 times.

Key Points to Keep in Mind

- When closing the kwah in the forward bow stance or when standing on the rear leg, be mindful not to twist the knee. If you feel any knee strain, bend your knees less, or explore a smaller stance.
- The head and shoulder should always point in the same direction as the navel. Be mindful not to twist the neck or spine.
- Don't get too hung up on details as you are first learning the movements. Try to feel the spirit of relaxed, flowing movements. The more you relax, the more likely your body will begin to flow in an integrated manner.

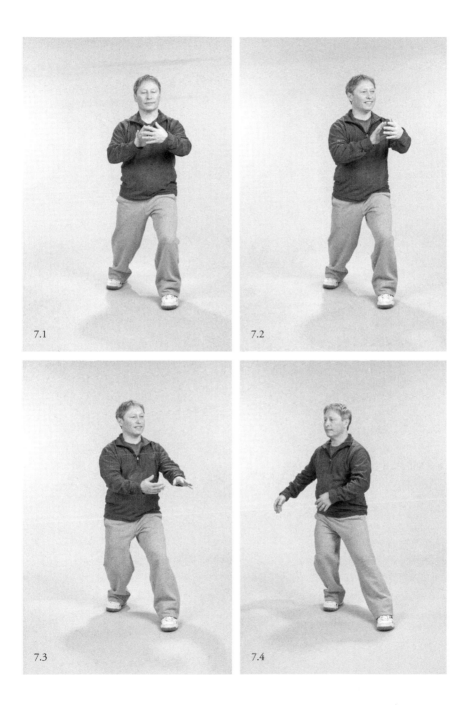

7.1

7.2

7.3

7.4

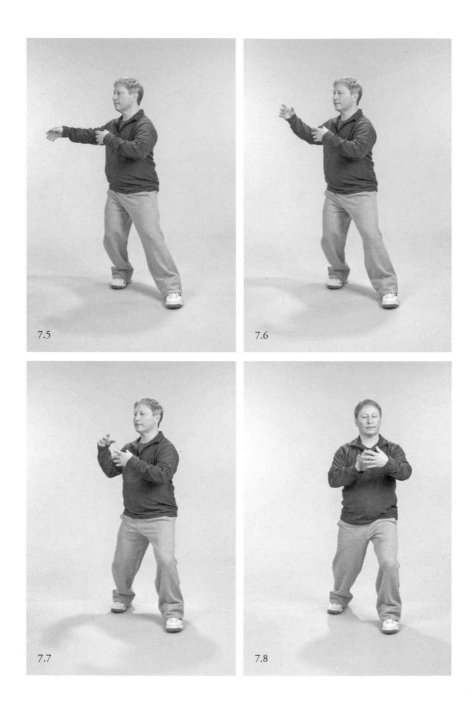

7.5

7.6

7.7

7.8

Tai Chi and Its Essential Elements

Tai Chi Exercise 5: Twist Step, Brush Knee

This exercise develops the ability to take slow, deliberate steps in a forward direction, while managing challenging balances imposed by constantly varying arm positions. Again, this exercise coordinates leg and arm movements, helping to integrate the upper and lower body. See photos 8.1–8.8 on pages 102–4.

Begin by standing with your right toes pointing 30 degrees to the right, your weight primarily on your right leg. Your left toes should be directly next to your right toes, touching the ground for balance, but without much weight on your left leg. While in this posture, hold your arms centered in front of your torso, as if you were holding a sphere, with your right hand on top of the left. Use this posture for balance.

Step out with your left foot to a bow stance, and while your torso faces the direction your right toes are pointing, shift your weight to your left leg. With 70 percent of your weight on your left leg, turn your hips and head to point forward, where your left toes are pointing. As you shift your weight, release your left hand so that it falls across your lower body and toward your left thigh. Let your right hand move slightly forward, fingers pointing up, to make the gesture of a push in front of your right shoulder. When you are in this forward bow stance, your right palm should be in a push position, with the palm facing out at about shoulder height. The left forearm and palm hang to the outside and slightly forward of the left thigh.

After making this shape, if possible, continue forward and balance on your left leg, bringing the right knee alongside the left knee and raising the toes of your right foot slightly off the ground. Then place your right foot back to where it originally was, and as you shift all of your weight back to the right leg, turn your waist to the right, draw your left toes alongside your right ones, release your arms, and guide the right one in a circular motion, first to an extended position with the palm facing out just below shoulder height, and then back to the beginning sphere position. Repeat this cycle 9 to 36 times on the right side.

Now practice the mirror image of this movement, beginning with your weight on your left leg, toes turned out 30 degrees, and right toes alongside the left foot and touching the ground for balance. Hold your arms as if you were holding a sphere in front of your body with your left hand on top of the right, step out to a right-footed bow stance, and shift your weight to your right leg; after your frame is in place and as you turn your torso to the right, allow your right hand to brush just above your right knee as your left hand pushes at shoulder height. Bring your knees next to each other, and then return first your left foot and then your right foot back to their original positions as you resume the beginning sphere position. Repeat this set 9 to 36 times on the left side.

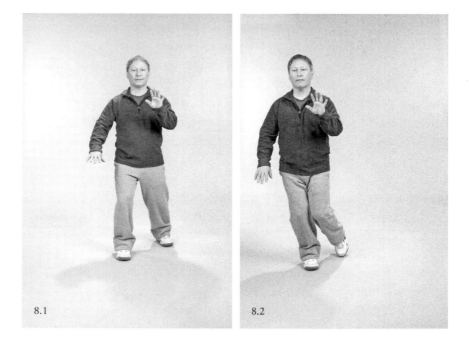

8.1

8.2

TAI CHI AND ITS ESSENTIAL ELEMENTS

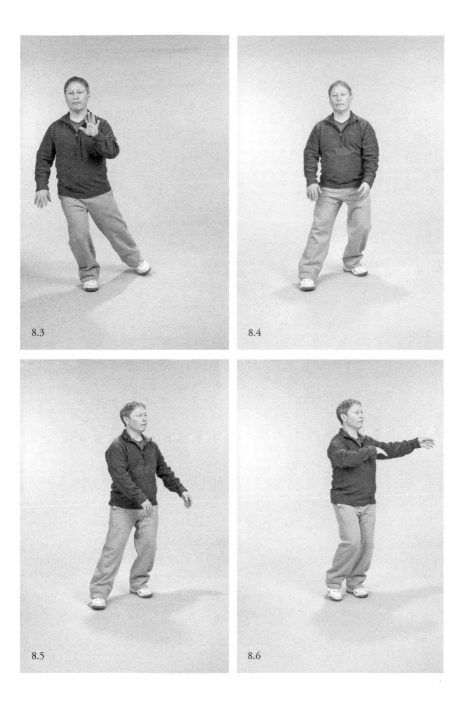

8.3

8.4

8.5

8.6

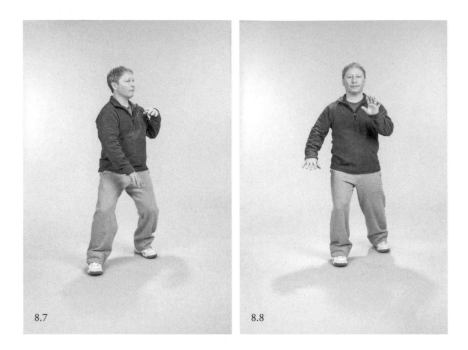

8.7

8.8

COOL-DOWN EXERCISES

Tai Chi Massage and Meridian Tapping

According to traditional Chinese medicine principles, these cool-down exercises assure that energy activated during the warm-up and Tai Chi exercises is evenly integrated within your body. These exercises help integrate the energy work by stimulating and balancing key acupuncture channels in the body that link the top and bottom, and left and right sides, of the body.

Begin by massaging your abdomen and then your lower back with the palms of both hands, each for about one minute. As you massage, feel as if you can move the Qi and juices deep beneath the skin surface. Follow this massage by gently tapping with your palms and fingers pathways that correspond with energy pathways or (acupuncture) meridians of traditional Chinese medicine. Start tapping the flank (kidney region) in the lower back, moving down the outside of your legs, knees, and calves to the outside of your ankles. Then move up from the inside of your ankles to the inner surface of your knees, thighs, and kwah back up to the navel and then around to your kidneys. Repeat this loop three times.

Continue tapping up your back, going as high as you can reach from the bottom to the top. Then reach over your shoulders and continue tapping upward toward the cervical spine. Use your fingers to tap lightly on your skull, forehead, throat, and down to your chest. Extend your left arm out to the side with the palm facing forward, and, using your right hand, tap from the chest outward along the inside surface of your left arm to your fingers. Then return by tapping the outside surfaces of your fingers to your shoulders and chest. Next, extend your right arm and tap from the chest to the fingers, and back to the chest. Repeat this loop three times on each side.

Complete the tapping massage from your chest down to the abdomen, ending by rubbing the abdomen again. Rest your palms on your abdomen as you rest for a minute and feel your breath.

Key Points to Keep in Mind

- Gently, lightly tap the various parts of your body without creating any pain.
- As you tap, relax the body so you can feel the vibrations deep into the tissues and organs.
- When tapping the lower legs, be careful to maintain your balance and not strain the lower back. Do not reach lower than is comfortable or safe for you.

PART TWO

Proof of the Promise:
Tai Chi through the Lens of Modern Science

4

Improve Your Balance and Bones

Losing any of the five traditional senses isn't necessarily life threatening. But to lose one's orientation to the earth, one's sense of up and down, one's position on the planet, is to undergo one of the most profound disturbances a human can experience.

—SCOTT McCREDIE, *In Search of the Lost Sense*

Balance is key to a healthy, full life. In older people, balance prevents falls and provides confidence to sustain physical and social activities. For younger people, better balance often translates into better performance in sports. For everyone, balance contributes to a grounded sense of well-being.

Balance and your relationship to gravity involve many interacting factors, including strength and flexibility, sensory perception, neuromuscular coordination or synergy, and cognitive processes. Understanding these components, including how they degrade with age or disease, and understanding how Tai Chi affects them will help you appreciate why Tai Chi is often so effective at improving balance.

One of the primary reasons you should be concerned about balance is fall-related fractures. Some 50 million Americans over age 50 have low bone density, and fractures in this group often result in great suffering and medical expense. Tai Chi offers a twofold effect of reducing fracture risk—not only does it improve balance and reduce falls, but also, preliminary studies, including our own research, suggest Tai Chi may also reduce rates of bone mineral density (BMD) decline, particularly in post-menopausal women.

In addition, elderly, frail, and deconditioned people who often have poor balance have found Tai Chi to be very safe. That makes Tai Chi an excellent response to the US Surgeon General's recent call for novel exercise programs for older adults diagnosed with low bone density. In fact, the Surgeon General's report specifically recommends Tai Chi as a good exercise for fall prevention.[1] Not surprisingly, community programs increasingly are adopting Tai Chi for balance rehabilitation and fall prevention.

SHADOWING IN A BALANCE REHABILITATION CLINIC IN PREPARATION FOR MY FIRST TAI CHI TRIAL

In preparation for my first Tai Chi trial with chronic inner-ear balance-disorder (vestibulopathic) patients, I arranged to shadow at the Massachusetts General Hospital Physical Therapy Clinic. There I met my first such patient, Charlene, a 53-year-old retired librarian. I was amazed at the level of Charlene's impairment and dysfunction. She was unable to do the simplest things, such as turn her head and look over her shoulder without losing her balance, steadily walk beyond a short distance, or close her eyes without nearly falling—tasks we normally take for granted.

Over time, as I met more patients and through the Tai Chi clinical trial we ran, I learned more about how debilitating balance impairments can be and how negatively they affect quality of life; activities of daily living, such as driving a car, playing with children or grandchildren, or shopping; as well as engaging in any type of exercise, work, finances, and family relationships.

Over the course of our first trial with dozens of balance-disorder patients, and now with years of studies of balance and Tai Chi, I realize how valuable Tai Chi can be to enhance stability and overall balance for nearly everyone from young athletes to normally aging people, as well as for rehabilitation and prevention of balance loss, falling, and subsequent fractures in those diagnosed with more severe balance disorders, people like Charlene.

What Is Balance?

The technical definition of balance, or postural stability, is the ability to maintain and control the position and motion of the center of mass of the body relative to the base of support. Humans' ability to balance, walk, and run on two legs, in comparison to our four-legged ancestors, represents quite an evolutionary feat (pun intended). When you stand or walk, your body is inherently unstable because two-thirds of your body's mass is located two-thirds of your body's height above the ground. Even the normal act of walking could be described as a continuous process of losing and regaining your balance. Master Morihei Ueshiba, founder of the martial art Aikido, stood less than five feet tall and weighed well under 100 pounds. Yet, he could remain centered, calm, and apparently stable, even while evading the attack of multiple opponents. He was fond of telling his students, however, that he was not as stable and balanced as they believed: "It is not that I stay balanced all the time. I just recover so fast, nobody notices the imbalance."

Balance is a feat that requires many systems interacting and coordinating in precise and complex ways. The elements involved in balance depend on the specific task—whether you are standing still or hopping on one leg—and also the environment where you are—whether you are standing on dark, slippery ice or a flat surface on a sunny day. Generally, four body systems must work together to keep you from falling over: musculoskeletal (muscle strength, flexibility), sensory, neuromuscular, and cognitive.[2]

- Musculoskeletal: Your muscle strength and flexibility, as well as the range of motion of your joints, all help keep you upright and affect your balance.

   Significant muscle weakness, especially in the hips, legs, and feet, is one of the primary factors in falls, particularly among the elderly.

Muscle strength decreases from 20–40 percent between the ages of 20 and 70. A correlation also exists between knee and ankle weakness and the risk of falls. Ankle flexibility, which is critical for postural control, declines by 50 percent in women and 35 percent in men between age 55 and 85. In addition, as we age, spinal flexibility is often the first thing to go, especially spinal extension (the ability to stand up straight). In fact, on average, we have 50 percent less spinal extension after age 70 than we had in our twenties.[3]

- Sensory: Your brain receives a combination of balance-related sensory inputs from your eyes; from pressure sensors in the skin, muscles, and joints; and from the vestibular system located in the inner ear.

Vision, in addition to allowing us to detect hazards in the environment, plays a direct and important role in balance; it provides the nervous system with continually updated information about the position and movements of body parts in relation to each other and the environment. For example, when people stand with their eyes closed, the amount the body sways increases between 20 percent and 70 percent.[4]

Proprioception, which relies on nerve cells throughout the body that are sensitive to mechanical pressures, provides additional information about the body's position and the limbs' movements. Pressure receptors located in the soles of your feet sense how the body makes contact with the ground and detect which way your weight is shifting or leaning. Feedback from these pressure sensors is essential to maintaining balance. For example, if someone bumps into you from one side, your body reacts by shifting weight rapidly to the other side. The change in pressure beneath your feet signals the movements your hips, knees, and ankles need to make to recover your balance.[5]

The vestibular system inside the inner ear plays an important role in balance. The inner ear continuously sends impulses that adjust your eyes to coordinate with the body's smallest movement. The vestibular system organizes the motion of your head and stabilizes your eyes relative to the surrounding environment. It also sends signals to the skeletal muscles that keep you upright.

Through experience, your body learns to evaluate the accuracy of this information and rely on it more or less. This process of selecting and integrating appropriate sensory information is called sensory organization. Several studies have shown that elderly people perform less well in maintaining a standing position than younger ones when under conditions of reduced or conflicting sensory inputs.[6]

As we age, the quality of inputs from all three systems declines. For vision, studies show that our ability to adapt to the dark, perceive differences between an object and its background, and perceive depth decreases starting at age 40; general visual acuity steadily declines starting at age 50. Try this: stand up and close your eyes—you will appreciate quickly the role vision plays in balance. Many studies support that impaired vision directly affects balance and predisposes older people to falls.[7]

The mechanical sensors throughout the body tend to lose their sensitivity as we age, causing a lag in communication with the brain. Sensory losses cause disruptions in the quantity, quality, and timing of sensory feedback. For example, sensory "alertness" in the feet remains stable until about age 40, and then it decreases by about 20 percent in our fifties and by a staggering 75 percent by age 80. This sensory loss is also associated with diseases such as peripheral neuropathy due to diabetes. Studies show that the more the soles of the feet experience loss of sensory input, the higher is the impairment in postural control.[8]

Finally, multiple aspects of the vestibular system decline with age or disease. Sensors located in the inner ear degenerate by 40 percent after age 70, and practical neuromuscular reactions associated with these vestibular sensors also have been reported to decline with age; these reactions affect head and neck movements. In addition, vestibular losses can be related to ear infection, head trauma, cancers, and toxicity to medications.[9]

- Neuromuscular: Groups of muscles often act together as a functional unit; this process is called neuromuscular synergy. This synergy helps you, for example, put one step in front of the other and makes walking more efficient. For you to start walking, numerous muscles throughout your body must contract in a coordinated fashion, from those in your spine to those in your feet. You commonly use neuromuscular synergies to recover from a perturbation in balance, such as when you slip on a wet sidewalk. You also use them when you get up from a chair. Again, as you age, the coordination of these processes may break down, which may put you at more risk for falls.[10]

- Cognition: Multiple thought processes interact with the other intrinsic factors to affect your balance. These processes include the fear of falling, planning or anticipating tricky situations (walking in the dark or across ice), and your ability to pay attention to postural control, especially while multitasking (for example, talking on a cell phone and walking at the same time).

The fear of falling is an increasing problem as we age, and is particularly prevalent in those who have balance disorders or a history of falling. Studies show that the tentative, physically tense, and mentally distracting behaviors associated with the fear of falling actually can increase the probability that you will fall. From a traditional Chinese medicine perspective, the anxiety associated with fear of falling creates an energetic imbalance in the body, drawing excessive Qi into the chest and head and weakening the energetic root in the legs, and therefore disturbing your sense of feeling grounded. Elderly people who have a fear of falling are more likely to be depressed and to restrict their activities, and these factors seem to feed on each other. Fearful people are also less active, which leads to muscle deconditioning and a loss of strength and balance.[11]

Many aspects of cognitive function decline with age, and one very relevant to balance is executive function. Executive function refers to your ability to organize thoughts and activities, prioritize tasks, and make decisions. A growing body of research suggests that poor executive function can affect balance and gait. You may have noticed that, for example, distracting thoughts affect your balance and walking speed. In addition, executive function seems to decline with age, studies show. Brain researchers believe that age-related decline in executive function may underlie some of the age-related loss of balance.[12]

The Burden of Balance Impairments

Deterioration of these four elements of balance control often leads to falls in older adults. Some 25–35 percent of the elderly over age 65 fall once or more each year. The likelihood of falling increases with age from 34 percent at ages 65–74 to 51 percent at age 85 and older.[13]

Tai Chi for Balance: Why It Makes Sense

The good news about balance problems is that most are fixable, and many falls are preventable. One of the key solutions to balance problems is exercise. Whether it's strength training, balance training, or Tai Chi, all have been shown to improve balance and reduce the number of falls.[14] Based on systematic reviews of exercise and falls prevention, Tai Chi may be one of the better exercises you can do. The diverse, multiple active ingredients inherent in Tai Chi allow you to compensate for deficiencies in the four body systems (musculoskeletal, sensory, neuromuscular, and cognitive) that underlie balance loss. Tai Chi's gentle, gradual approach also makes it accessible for people of all ages and stages of fitness.

FALLS AND FRACTURES: BOOMERS BEWARE

A primary reason we care about balance is to prevent falls and fractures. Older people have thinner bones and therefore have an increased risk of fracture. Every year, about 30 percent of people aged 65 and up who live in communities experience a fall; this figure translates into about 10 million falls per year. From 55–70 percent of these falls result in physical injury, and 30 percent of those who fall sustain serious injuries, such as hip fractures or head traumas, that reduce mobility and independence, and increase the likelihood of premature death. About half of those who suffer hip fractures will not return home or live independently. Only one in four fully recover, and about one in five will die within the first year due to complications. The estimated cost of falls in the United States in 2000 was $19.2 billion.[15]

All of these age-related fall/fracture issues will be exacerbated among the baby boomers, the 73 million Americans born between 1946 and 1964. By 2040, the numbers of people over age 65 are expected to double to 77 million. This statistic means that up to 25 million people are likely to fall and incur 8 million injuries, and 25,000 fall-related deaths will occur each year among this group.

Tai Chi and Reduced Falls

Systematic reviews and meta-analyses of clinical trials have studied the impact of Tai Chi on falls in the elderly. When viewed as a whole, the data suggest Tai Chi can significantly reduce the probability of falling, even when compared in randomized trials to other active exercise or balance-training interventions.[16]

One large randomized, controlled trial conducted at the Oregon Research Institute evaluated the impact of six months of Tai Chi, compared to a seated exercise control group. The study reported a 45 percent reduction in falls and increases in associated clinical benefits. A follow-up study by the same research team, evaluating a simplified Tai Chi intervention in community centers, found that the results from clinical trials successfully translate into practical community programs.[17]

Emory University researchers similarly reported a 46 percent reduction in falls following 15 weeks of Tai Chi training for community-dwelling adults age 70 and older.[18] In general, other studies also suggest a beneficial impact on fall risk and other clinical measures of balance, although some results are mixed.[19] Drawing on falls data such as these, cost-benefit analyses show that Tai Chi could significantly reduce costs associated with fall-related hip fractures. One recent systematic study in Australia concluded that Tai Chi was the most cost-effective falls prevention strategy.[20]

It's also noteworthy that the majority of these studies have focused on older, often frail and deconditioned adults, and few adverse effects have been reported.

How Tai Chi Helps Balance

"I had danced a lot as kid, but after a head injury in a car accident, I had balance problems and couldn't do that anymore," says Sandy, a 64-year-old teacher. "My doctor suggested I do Tai Chi exercises, and after six months, I felt my balance was somewhat better and I had more vitality. My Tai Chi instructor moved, but I continued to do Tai Chi on my own."

Sandy had a flare-up of balance problems a few years later and missed several months of work and her practice. "My doctor put me on medication for vertigo, which helped, and I started taking Tai Chi classes again," she says. "The classes help with my focus. I feel physically stronger and can concentrate better. I can stand with my eyes closed during a meditative relaxation without wavering. When I do the form, I feel connected to what I can do, and more graceful. I really enjoy the way it feels to be inside of me as I do the form."

The effectiveness of Tai Chi is due to its multiple active ingredients and subcomponents. Many studies have explored how the characteristics of Tai Chi might explain its effectiveness for postural control, which may underlie positive effects on fall rates. Here's how Tai Chi helps influence the four elements of balance:

Musculoskeletal

Tai Chi is a weight-bearing exercise. It involves a constant shifting of weight from one leg to the other, which facilitates improved dynamic standing balance and strength of the lower extremities (legs, ankles, feet). Laboratory studies support the idea that when practicing Tai Chi, you spend much more time on one leg compared to when you walk. Multiple longitudinal and cross-sectional studies show improved lower-extremity strength—in particular, knee strength, following Tai Chi training. Tai Chi also improves torso and limb flexibility and range of motion, which is an essential component for postural control.[21]

Tai Chi is widely believed to encourage better posture through body alignment and an emphasis on maintaining a vertical posture with an extended head and trunk position. Good alignment and appropriate use of the core muscles and spine allow you to stand more erect, and standing erect promotes a more stable, grounded, less rigid, and less top-heavy posture.

Sensory and Perceptual

Tai Chi's continuous, slow even tempo facilitates sensory awareness of the speed, force, trajectory, and execution of movements, as well as awareness of the external environment. With Tai Chi, your sensory systems become highly sensitized, which leads to better balance and function.

One Hong Kong study compared older Tai Chi practitioners to age-matched nonpractitioners and found that those who practiced Tai Chi scored higher on an instrument measuring overall body awareness. What's more, the Tai Chi practitioners had significantly better ability to lean further in most directions without losing their stability.[22] Tai Chi is also associated with improved joint proprioception. One study compared long-term Tai Chi practitioners to age-matched swimmers, runners, and sedentary controls. The Tai Chi practitioners had a better sense of the position of their ankle and knee joints in space, and were more sensitive to small movements of their joints.[23] So, Tai Chi may give you more accurate, quicker feedback for balance and posture, which could help prevent falling.

Some studies show that Tai Chi positively affects people who have peripheral neuropathy and experience little sensation in their hands and feet. Reduced sensation in the feet, for example, greatly affects balance.[24] This condition is common among those who have diabetes or people who are undergoing chemotherapy, among others. One promising noncontrolled pilot study by researchers at Louisiana State University showed the impact of Tai Chi on people who had plantar peripheral neuropathy due to diabetes. Tai Chi classes for 24 weeks led to an increase in sensitivity of the soles of the feet, greater balance, and faster walking speed.[25] Another nonrandomized trial reported that a 12-week Tai Chi program in diabetic patients who had peripheral neuropathy increased nerve conduction velocities.[26]

It's not just legs, but the hands as well that become more sensitive through Tai Chi. My colleague Dr. Cathy Kerr has studied sensitivity to touch, called tactile acuity in the fingertips, in a group of Tai Chi practitioners versus those who didn't do Tai Chi. Those who did Tai Chi, most notably older people, had the equivalent increase in sensitivity seen among blind people who read Braille.[27]

Our Harvard group, led by Dr. David Krebs, also has shown that Tai Chi can help patients who have vestibular-related balance problems. In a randomized trial, we compared 10 weeks of Tai Chi training to traditional vestibular rehabilitation exercises. While both interventions improved dynamic balance control, overall, Tai Chi was more effective. However, traditional rehabilitation exercises helped improve patients' eye gaze stability, which is related to vestibular function and overall balance, more so than Tai Chi. It appears that Tai Chi may affect different mechanisms of balance than traditional rehabilitation in patients who have vestibular problems. We hypothesized that Tai Chi may have led to changes in proprioception, leg strength, and flexibility, in addition to balance confidence, which together, may have helped compensate for a weaker vestibular systems. Thus, Tai Chi may provide an excellent adjunct, synergistic therapy for patients who have medical vestibular disorders.[28]

More generally, studies support that Tai Chi improves the ability to compensate when balance-related sensory input is limited or conflicting, what is called improved sensory organization. Studies have shown that during balance testing, if vestibular, visual, or proprioceptive inputs are experimentally reduced or purposefully made confusing, Tai Chi practitioners are better equipped to maintain their balance. In fact, some studies show that elderly Tai Chi practitioners attain the same level of balance control as young, healthy subjects during these experimental challenges. Since most falls occur when a person is in a difficult situation, such as when experiencing sensory conflict, Tai Chi's ability to compensate under these circumstances is noteworthy.[29]

Neuromuscular Synergy

The rich diversity of Tai Chi's movements—the sequencing, timing, and combinations of different muscle groups—provides excellent training for the coordination of neuromuscular patterns. Research supports that Tai Chi can improve your dynamic balance as you move and help you recover from perturbations in balance, for example, when you slip on a wet sidewalk.

One randomized trial of older adults studied reactions to experimentally induced slips during walking. Compared to a conventional balance-training program, those who were assigned to intensive Tai Chi training exhibited improved ankle neuromuscular reaction, better coordination of muscle groups, and better overall maintenance of balance.[30] Another randomized trial showed that Tai Chi improved coordination during the very initial stage of walking (gait initiation), a phase that is more likely to create a stumble or trip compared to when walking is under way.[31] Finally, our study with vestibular patients showed that Tai Chi improved organization of lower extremity neuromuscular synergies, leading to faster and more stable gait.[32]

Cognitive

It's highly likely that one of the primary ways that Tai Chi improves balance and reduces falls is by reducing the fear of falling and associated anxiety. Ironically, fear of falling is one of the biggest predictors of falls. Those who have a history of prior falls or who have impaired balance tend to walk in a guarded, tentative, "ungrounded" manner. They also stand a little more rigidly, breathe shallowly, are top-heavy, and their minds are anxious and preoccupied with not falling. All of these behaviors lead them to being less grounded and less aware of themselves and their surrounding environment.

Using Tai Chi lingo, fear of falling is the opposite of Sung, which is relaxed, sinking energy (see the end of this chapter for a Sung exercise). One of the participants in our vestibular study reported that she used to experience vertigo every time she stepped off a train onto the platform. But since doing Tai Chi, the second she begins to feel unbalanced and anxious, she feels her feet on the earth, imagines growing roots like a tree deep into the ground, and takes a number of slow, deep breathes. While she still experiences some instability, she feels less anxious or fearful about falling, and this confidence allows her postural control systems to work more efficiently.

Good evidence indicates that Tai Chi reduces the fear of falling, probably because this holistic intervention enhances relaxed, body awareness and provides more confidence from better strength and coordination. One randomized trial by Emory University researchers found that 48 weeks of Tai Chi reduced the fear of falling significantly compared to a wellness education program. An earlier study by the same group also reported a significantly greater reduction in fear of falling following Tai Chi compared to computerized balance training; improvements in fear of falling were correlated with a nearly 50 percent reduction in the fall rate.[33] Another trial reported that the combination of cognitive behavioral therapy (CBT) plus Tai Chi improved fear of falling, as well as measures of mobility, social support satisfaction, and quality of life, more than CBT alone.[34]

Researchers are just beginning to study how coordinating and managing the multiple mind-body components during Tai Chi training—that is, integrated arm and leg moves, continuously changing direction, memorizing sequences, breathing, and postural awareness and inner sensations—may further enhance the handling of concurrent mental tasks during physical activities, such as walking down a flight of steps. One creative cross-sectional study conducted in Hong Kong studied how older women who were experienced Tai Chi practitioners contracted their lower leg muscles in anticipation of bearing weight on one leg while descending stairs. These older women's muscle-firing patterns were compared to those of both older and younger people who had no Tai Chi experience. The participants repeated the experiment with and without a distracting mental task. The older women without Tai Chi experience braced their lower leg muscles inefficiently and much earlier when descending a step compared to the Tai Chi practitioners, whose muscle activation was indistinguishable from the more youthful controls. What's more, when distracted by a mental task, the leg contractions of the Tai Chi participants were not as affected as the other groups. The authors concluded that Tai Chi might help improve older adults' capacity to shift attention between mental and physical tasks.[35]

TAI CHI IMPROVES BALANCE AND MOTOR CONTROL IN PARKINSON'S DISEASE

Tai Chi appears to help Parkinson's disease patients improve their balance and motor control. Parkinson's disease, which affects more than 1 million Americans, is a brain disorder that affects muscle control, causing trembling and stiffness, slowness in walking, and difficulties with balance. These impairments greatly hinder everyday function and quality of life.

Some Parkinson's disease symptoms, such as tremors, respond to drug therapy. But others, like overall balance, do not respond well to medication, and the role of different types of exercise is still not well understood. A study published in the *New England Journal of Medicine* shows that Tai Chi can improve both balance and movement control for people who have Parkinson's disease. The study at the Oregon Research Institute included 195 people who had mild-to-moderate Parkinson's disease; they were randomly assigned to twice-weekly sessions of Tai Chi, strength-building exercises, or stretching. After six months, those who did Tai Chi were stronger and had much better balance than those in the other two groups. In fact, their balance was four times better than those in the stretching group and about two times better than those in the resistance-training group. The Tai Chi group also had significantly fewer falls and slower rates of decline in overall motor control.[36]

In addition, Tai Chi appears to be very safe, with little risk of Parkinson's disease patients coming to harm. Other smaller studies suggest that Tai Chi improves the quality of life for both Parkinson's disease patients and their support partners.[37]

These results are significant because they suggest that Tai Chi may be used as an add-on to current physical and pharmacological therapies to address some of the key problems patients with Parkinson's disease face.

Another small, uncontrolled study including 20 older adults reported improvements in executive function after 10 weeks of Tai Chi training.[38] However, another small, randomized trial that evaluated executive function using a "dual task paradigm"—having to maintain balance while simultaneously doing a challenging mental task—found no apparent benefits following Tai Chi training.[39]

While we need more research, current data indicate that Tai Chi has great potential as a safe, effective intervention to help prevent or rehabilitate balance problems, even in severely de-conditioned people, who are the most susceptible to falling.

Tai Chi and Bone Density

"In my mid-thirties, I developed a neurological problem, and my neurologist put me on mega-doses of intravenous steroids," says Kathleen, now age 45. "I was having problems with my leg strength and stability when my husband's friend suggested I try Tai Chi to help my balance and coordination."

Kathleen has been doing Tai Chi in group classes and on her own for five years now. "From the very first class, I enjoyed it," says the television executive. "It really calms my mind, and my body feels great, even after class."

When she started doing Tai Chi, yearly scans showed she had low levels of bone density. "After doing Tai Chi, despite the high levels of steroids, my bone density is now totally normal," says Kathleen, who also takes calcium and vitamin D to protect her bones. She attributes this improvement to her Tai Chi training.

Tai Chi classics say the body should feel like "steel wrapped in cotton," highlighting the image of how strong bones support relaxed muscles and connective tissues.

Most people commonly believe that to have an impact on bone, you need to do a significant amount of high-intensity resistance and strength training. What's more, many older adults just don't do conventional exercises, either due to health factors or a lack of sustained interest, among other reasons. However, research suggests that lower-impact exercises, such as Tai Chi, may possibly reduce rates of bone loss, especially in women with moderately low bone density (osteopenia) or osteoporosis.

Bone is a dynamic organ that undergoes remodeling throughout life. Bone density in women generally increases during the first three decades of life. At around age 40 years, BMD typically begins to decline, with more rapid changes following menopause, paralleling decreases in estrogen levels. However, continued bone loss in later life may also be related to other factors, including decreased calcium and vitamin D intake, decreased physical activity, and age-related impairment in bone formation.[40]

Osteoporosis is a disabling condition predisposing to fractures in both women and men. Osteoporosis means *porous bone*. If you have osteoporosis, typically you have low BMD, poor bone quality, and fragile bones. This combination, together with the increased risk of falling among older people, leads to painful fractures and other health problems.

About 10 million Americans (about 8 million women and 2 million men) have osteoporosis. More than one-third of Americans are now age 50 or older, so osteoporosis is becoming an increasingly greater health problem.[41]

Tai Chi and the Prevention of Fractures

The absolute risk of fracture is higher in women who have more advanced osteoporotic bone loss, but the far greater prevalence of osteopenia results in more fractures in women who have only moderate bone loss. Osteopenic women have a 1.7-fold higher risk of fracture than do women who have normal bone density. Left untreated, osteopenia puts women at high risk of losing additional bone and developing osteoporosis. Low BMD-related fractures are associated with significant long-term impairment, high morbidity rates, and high medical costs.[42]

Developing approaches to preventing bone loss and future fractures among those who have osteopenia, especially women, is one way to address these costly issues. Since lifelong drug therapy is an expensive option with uncertain consequences and fraught with potential side effects, non-pharmacologic therapy offers an attractive alternative for many women. For this reason, guidelines for the treatment of osteopenia include exercise. However, currently no consensus exists regarding the optimal types and regimens of exercise for treating low BMD, or for addressing other fracture-related risk factors relevant to women who have osteopenia.

Tai Chi and BMD Research

Our group's systematic review of the effects of Tai Chi on BMD in postmenopausal women suggests that Tai Chi may positively affect low BMD, but research results are not yet conclusive.[43]

One important source of information comes from studies of long-term Tai Chi practitioners. These studies are important because bone changes slowly; it's difficult to do experimental studies for long periods. One such study in Taiwan compared people who practiced Tai Chi for at least seven years to age-matched controls in the same community. Those who did Tai Chi had greater bone density at the hip and spine. Another study also showed that the rate of decline in bone density among Tai Chi practitioners was slower than among age-matched controls.[44]

The most rigorous support for the positive effects of Tai Chi on BMD comes from randomized trials. One trial observed that BMD at the lumbar spine significantly increased following 10 months of Tai Chi, while in sedentary controls, the BMD decreased.[45] A second randomized trial observed that for older women (but not men), 12 months of Tai Chi resulted in maintenance of total hip BMD levels when compared to non-exercise controls, who lost bone in their hips.[46] Also noteworthy in this study is that the beneficial effects of Tai Chi on hip BMD were equivalent to 12 months of resistance training.

Our group recently completed a small, randomized trial with 86 post-menopausal women diagnosed with osteopenia. Women randomly assigned to Tai Chi could pick from one of seven pre-screened Tai Chi schools in the Boston area; they received the full package of training typical Tai Chi students received. This approach differs from most other Tai Chi trials that test one specific training regimen. Over a period of nine months, women in the control group lost about 1 percent bone mass in their femur, which was about the amount we expected in this population. In contrast, those who attended Tai Chi classes regularly and practiced at home were able to maintain the BMD in their femur with no bone loss over the nine-month period. Tai Chi also improved multiple measures of balance that are known to reduce the risk of falls.[47] Another series of studies of osteopenic women conducted at Texas Tech University reported that a six-month course of Tai Chi had favorable effects of multiple markers of bone dynamics and quality of life, but little change in balance parameters.[48] Collectively, these studies suggest that Tai Chi may reduce multiple fall-related fracture risks, especially in post-menopausal women, but we still need results from larger, longer-term studies to make more-definitive recommendations.

TAI CHI EXERCISES FOR BALANCE AND BONES

Add the following exercises into your regular Tai Chi practice to have an additional impact on balance and bones.

SWINGING TO CENTER ("SUNG" TRAINING)

"Sung" training can help you center your body, breath, and mind. Stand comfortably with your feet parallel, shoulder-width apart. Gently swing both arms together slightly forward, no more than a few inches, and then together, a few inches behind your body. Notice the subtle shifts in weight as your arms swing gently. Allow your upper body to relax deeply. Feel as if you are one of those inflatable clown toys that rock forward and backward but maintain a stable base.

As you swing your arms, melt any tension in your shoulders. You might imagine squirting some natural lubricant into the shoulder joint to dissolve any friction. Melt any tension in your face, neck, chest, and upper back, as much as possible. Feel the weight and energy sink down through your body, like honey that settles to the bottom of a jar that's been held upside down and then turned up again. Let this sinking-of-weight sensation contribute to your sense of being more bottom-heavy, centered, and grounded. Dissolve as much upper-body resistance as possible to the swinging of your arms; sense how your movement, and the slight shift in weight it generates, helps you find and rest into your center.

After a minute or two of focusing on this physical centering, begin to center your breathing. Continue to allow your arms to swing together. As you breathe in, sense how each breath wave gently massages your belly and lower back, creating a slight expansion. As you exhale, relax your abdomen deeply; with each exhalation, relax just a bit deeper. Continue with this awareness of your breath being centered in your abdomen for another minute or two.

The third level is to center your mind and heart, and to shift the center of your cognitive awareness, thinking and emotions to the abdomen, or the "gut brain." Continue to swing your arms. Imagine the energy of your thinking and heart center settling down to rest and nourish your belly. You might even imagine your brain and heart sliding down the core of your body to reside temporarily in your abdomen. In Chinese medicine, this is referred to as the "merging of the three tan tiens." As you swing your arms, explore how having your brain's Qi centered in your belly can enhance your gut feelings, minimizing or temporarily shutting down the typical energetic and emotional chatter. Continue for a minute or two.

The entire exercise should take three to five minutes. This one is particularly good while you are waiting for a bus or when you need a short break from work to center yourself.

Lift Hands Standing Meditation

This exercise, based on a traditional Tai Chi posture, enhances the mind-body connection, develops awareness of postural alignment, and strengthens the lower and upper extremities. It also brings awareness to what the Chinese call "letting the Qi permeate your bones."

Take a comfortable shoulder-width stance, feet parallel. Gently shift your weight over your right leg, keeping the right knee aligned over the center of the right foot. Leaving the left heel on ground, turn the left toes out 45–90 degrees (depending on the range of motion in your hips) without twisting or straining your right knee. Have most, if not all, of your weight on your back foot. Raise your left wrist to shoulder height, and align it over the left ankle, palm facing to the right. Point the fingers in your left hand in the same direction as your left toes. Now raise your right hand in front of the chest, palm facing left, and point the fingers to the right to correspond with the left fingers—pinkie to pinkie, etc. Your upper body should take a triangular shape with both arms outstretched, but with your elbows relaxed and hanging between the shoulders and wrists.

Hold this shape for 15 to 30 seconds. Then repeat a mirror image of this posture standing on the other leg. Work your way up in 30-second increments to three to five minutes per leg. As you stand, keep your head lined up over the shoulders and hips. Practice the process of Sung, relaxing and letting go of any tensions that may arise in the shoulders, neck, and chest. Allow any tensions to release from the upper body, and let your abdomen (or tan tien) relax. As in the Swinging to Center exercise, let your mind, heart, and breath also rest in your tan tien. Stay connected to your roots.

You will feel energy building up as your muscles and connective tissues are "worked." As this buildup happens, try not to resist the sensation of building energy in your tissues by bracing against it. Instead, almost counter-intuitively, relax further and imagine energy permeating deeper into the muscles and bones themselves.

SHAKE EVERYTHING

This exercise for your bones takes you to a deeper level of awareness of your skeleton, using the vibrations of gentle shaking.[49]

Stand with feet shoulder-width apart, and let your arms hang straight down at your sides as you gently shake them. Notice the jiggling, and let the waves of energy pass through the arm muscles up into the shoulders. Now shake your whole body to loosen up the chest, back, and abdomen. Let the muscles around the pelvis shake—your hips and legs. Then feel the jiggle in your lower legs and feet so the muscles relax. Feel your neck and face relax. Let the internal organs gently shake—the heart, kidneys, and lungs. Take a few deep breathes, and as you exhale, shake off any tension.

Shake for two to three minutes. Then stand still and feel the vibrations you have generated throughout your body. Bring your attention to your skeleton, and let the vibrations permeate into your bones. Start with your feet. Feel the muscles around them relax, and invite the vibrations to seep into all of the bones of your feet. Remind yourself that bones are living tissue, rich in calcium crystals and collagen, and highly conductive of bioelectrical charges. Move up your body, and feel the vibrations and energy penetrate the bones of your legs, hips, spine, shoulders, arms, and even your head. Feel the capacity your bones have to absorb and hold the energy.

5

Ease Your Aches and Pains

"After my first Tai Chi class, I was gratified by the ease of movement; I knew it was something I could do easily," says Elaine, age 67, a freelance book editor. "After about two months of classes, I mentioned to my instructor that I felt so much more energy. Later on, I noticed that I did every chore I had to do for the week after I finished my class on Wednesdays. Also, when I came down the stairs for the first time each morning, I no longer had to place two feet on each stair before I proceeded because I ached from arthritis and general muscle fatigue." Now Elaine says she doesn't even think about it anymore: "I just come down the stairs like a fit 40-year-old."

A further benefit is the absence of back problems, she says. "I have four severely degenerated discs and used to 'throw my back out' at the slightest provocation. That hasn't happened once since I started doing Tai Chi. I am now in the process of cleaning out old magazines and files, and have moved at least a dozen heavy boxes without mishap. That is amazing."

Broadly speaking, traditional Chinese medicine considers pain to be associated with "stagnation" or "blockages" in the body's flow of Qi.

Healing occurs through remobilizing this flow and addressing longer-term structural or constitutional imbalances leading to the blockages. Traditional methods employed to treat pain and mobilize Qi include acupuncture, massage, topical balms and ingested herbs, and exercises like Tai Chi and Qigong. Underlying all these practices is the goal of "moving" Qi.

Until recent years, Western physicians widely believed that bed rest, and not movement, was the best prescription for many pain conditions like lower back pain. However, evidence from clinical trials has changed this view to one more in line with traditional Eastern approaches that emphasize keeping things moving.[1] Movement and simple exercises such as stretching, range-of-motion joint movements, and deep breathing now are prescribed increasingly as effective ways to help decrease pain and integrated into typical rehabilitation programs. Physicians now recommend regular exercise to improve function in people who have chronic ailments, including arthritis and back pain. The most optimal forms and regimens of exercise for different conditions, however, have yet to be determined.

Mind-body therapies such as Tai Chi, Qigong, and yoga are widely used by people who have back pain, as well as those who have osteoarthritis, fibromyalgia, and rheumatoid arthritis. A growing body of studies suggests Tai Chi may be effective for easing pain and improving quality of life for these and other pain conditions. This research also is beginning to show how Tai Chi may positively affect musculoskeletal pain conditions, such as by improving strength, flexibility, postural alignment, neuromuscular movement patterns, breathing, and psychological well-being.

This chapter reviews how great a role pain plays in some people's lives, maybe even yours, and how the many therapeutic components of Tai Chi may help relieve pain.

THE PREVALENCE OF PAIN

Pain is one of the most prevalent and costly medical conditions, and is a key reason why people go to the doctor and take medication. In fact, second only to the common cold, back pain is the most frequent problem that brings people to a doctor's office.

A staggering number of people experience acute and chronic pain and are diagnosed with pain syndromes. Data extrapolated from the 2005 National Health Interview Survey suggest that nearly one-third of Americans, that is, about 100 million people, experience some type of pain over any three-month period. Not surprisingly, a striking number of people seek help for their pain. Nearly half of all Americans see a doctor each year complaining of some kind of pain. Pain medications are the second-most prescribed drugs (after heart and kidney drugs) during visits to doctors' offices and emergency rooms. As a result, the costs of pain, including medical care for patients as well as the costs associated with disability, lost time from work, and reduced productivity, are an astronomical $150 billion per year, according to the US Census Bureau.[2]

Pain and Complementary and Alternative Medical Treatments

Conventional therapies and medications often do not treat pain adequately, so many people choose to use complementary alternative medicine (CAM), including mind-body exercises. National surveys have found that treating pain is one of the primary reasons people seek CAM. Approximately one out of five American adults with pain-related conditions specifically reports the use of mind-body therapies.[3] These mind-body therapies include relaxation techniques (deep-breathing exercises, guided imagery, meditation, and progressive muscle relaxation), yoga, Tai Chi, and Qigong.

Musculoskeletal conditions—in particular, low-back pain—are consistently among the top reasons patients seek CAM therapies. Researchers estimate that nearly one-third of all CAM provider visits in the United States between 1997 and 1998 were made specifically for the treatment of back or neck pain. Among individuals reporting low-back and/or neck pain over the prior 12 months, 54 percent used CAM to treat their condition. Mind-body approaches were among the most commonly used (13 percent) and were rated as "very helpful" in 43 percent of those sampled.[4]

My colleague Gloria Yeh and I conducted a small, unpublished pilot study in which we anonymously surveyed 144 practitioners, average age 53, two-thirds of them women, at Boston area Tai Chi schools. More than half of these Tai Chi practitioners said they had used Tai Chi for back or neck pain, and nearly all reported Tai Chi was "helpful" or "very helpful."

This high use of CAM and mind-body therapies for pain, and the large amounts of money spent on CAM therapies to treat and manage pain—

more than $4 billion each year for just mind-body therapies—has led medical researchers to evaluate rigorously which mind-body exercises are the most safe, promising, and cost-effective for treating painful conditions, and equally important, which are not safe or effective.[5] Because of its widespread use and potential promise, studying mind-body therapies for musculoskeletal pain is a stated priority of the National Center for Complementary and Alternative Medicine at the National Institutes of Health.[6] Emerging promising results regarding Tai Chi for musculoskeletal pain are summarized below.

DEFINING PAIN

Despite the high prevalence of pain, treatment is not that straightforward. In large part, this difficulty with treatment is because pain is not just a physiological phenomenon, but also has a large subjective component to it. Pain is really a mind-body phenomenon. Pain is a sensation that has both physical and psychological dimensions.

According to the International Association for the Study of Pain, the definition of pain is "an unpleasant sensory and emotional experience associated with actual or potential tissue damage, or described in terms of such damage." This definition means that pain is a perception, in the same way that what we see and hear are perceptions. The brain's perception of pain involves sensitivity to chemical changes in tissue, which the brain then interprets as changes that are, or may be, harmful. The perception is real, whether any harm has been done. The formulation of this perception involves thoughts, as well as the emotional consequences and behavioral responses to the cognitive and emotional aspects of pain. These psychological dimensions can become significant in managing chronic pain. They may have a long-term impact on your everyday activities and the quality of your life.

Acute Pain

Everyone has experienced acute pain—you jam or burn a finger, bang a shin, stub a toe, or pull a back muscle. Here's a simplified version of what typically happens when you feel acute pain. A stimulus (you touch a sharp or hot object) disturbs tissues, and the tissues release chemicals that the peripheral nerves sense. The nerves send signals that travel to the spinal cord and up to the brain. The brain "registers" the stimulus as pain. Over time, local inflammation and wound healing typically resolve the tissue trauma, and you return to normal.

Acute pain is important. It is an evolutionary "gift," that is, it serves to bring attention to a situation or guard against further injury. Acute pain motivates you to withdraw from potentially dangerous situations, protects a damaged part of the body while it heals, and teaches you to avoid those situations in the future.

Chronic Pain

Sometimes, and for reasons researchers do not fully understand, acute pain does not resolve and becomes chronic. Back pain is a good example. You may have experienced an episode of acute back pain that did not improve with treatment and progressed to become recurrent or chronic back pain. Despite a great deal of study, researchers cannot provide a reliable explanation of, or way to predict, chronic back pain. Medical studies using X-rays and imaging tools, such as computed tomography and magnetic resonance imaging, can help identify spinal abnormalities, such as a herniated disc or degeneration in a facet joint. However, the association between back pain symptoms and the results of imaging studies is weak, and up to 85 percent of patients who have chronic low-back pain do not receive a precise diagnosis.[7]

Psychological components of the mind-body system also contribute to understanding chronic back pain. Some researchers hypothesize that the development of chronic back pain is associated with psychological factors, such as depression, anxiety, catastrophizing, anger, fear/avoidance, and job problems, among other behaviors. In fact, some research suggests that psychosocial factors may be as important, or more important, than physical findings or imaging studies for the prognosis of low-back pain.[8] Screening for early identification of these factors has become a key element in occupational low-back pain research. Further evidence for the role of psychological factors in pain comes from motor imagery studies, which demonstrate that simply imagining certain movements can cause pain and swelling.[9] However, as with imaging studies, rigorous large-scale trials have not identified consistent relationships between psychosocial factors and the prognosis of chronic low-back pain.

The complex nature of pain may explain the lack of success in identifying specific factors that cause pain. Similarly, chronic back pain's complexity may be a reason for the limited success of most therapies. Even for so-called noncomplicated back pain, many different types of back-pain patients may each have unique, sometimes multiple, underlying causes, which require a slightly different therapeutic approach.[10]

My colleagues Drs. Helene Langevin and Karen Sherman, based at the University of Vermont School of Medicine and Group Health in Seattle, respectively, have advanced an innovative multifactorial model of chronic low-back pain that captures the complexity underlying some forms of back pain. The model also highlights how multicomponent interventions, like Tai Chi, may break the cycle of chronic pain and bring the body back to a more balanced state of health. A unique contribution of this model, particularly relevant to Tai Chi, is its inclusion of connective tissue/fascia—the sinews of traditional Chinese medicine.[11]

In brief, the model hypothesizes that in acute low-back pain that does not resolve quickly, in addition to local inflammation and pain, the fear of pain may lead to altered movement patterns. That is, you may favor one side of the body to avoid inducing pain by moving a certain way—a phenomenon call kinesiophobia. Chronic pain may also lead to pain sensitization, with some regions of the back remaining hypersensitive to pain well after injured tissues have healed. These changes may remodel connective tissue, making the tissue stiffer and less elastic, and lead to less efficient neuromuscular patterns—for example, how well you walk or maintain your balance.

What's more, this favoring and sensitization may set up a vicious cycle that leads to worse pain: If you feel pain, especially when you move, you may tend to avoid doing the things that provoke your pain. You rest, but unfortunately, resting does not help much, since it leads to further stiffness and weakness, and the symptoms you are trying to avoid just become worse. You may not be able to function at a high level––for example, go to work, play with your children, or participate in group activities, such as your weekly bridge game. This lack of functioning, in turn, leads to a loss of self-esteem and possibly other problems, such as financial hardship and strained relationships with family and friends. Your doctor may prescribe pain medication for your chronic pain, but these medications often have side effects, and, along with your pain, may interrupt your sleep and contribute to your mood disorders, again, worsening the situation. Obviously, chronic low-back pain, like many other chronic conditions, is a complex issue that is best viewed from a systems biology perspective.

Importantly, holistic and mind-body treatments such as Tai Chi may prevent, and possibly reverse, the development of these pathophysiological abnormalities; these treatments have the potential to influence multiple processes. For example, the gentle movements of Tai Chi might help begin to stretch and strengthen tissues and improve local circulation in the back. Because Tai Chi is done slowly and mindfully, it is less likely to cause more trauma to injured regions of the back. The reduction in what are often guarded movements and unconscious pain can lead to more efficient gait and posture, putting less biomechanical strain on tissues, including connective tissues. Mindful breathing might help you sense and even "massage" regions of the lower back, and the meditative, stress-reducing aspects of Tai Chi might improve your anxiety, mood, and sleep pattern. In addition, being in a group Tai Chi class, often with other people managing and recovering from various aches and pains, might provide the social support you need to stay upbeat and proactive about your rehabilitation.

CONNECTIVE TISSUE AND MUSCULOSKELETAL HEALTH

One of the strengths of the comprehensive Langevin-Sherman model lies in its recognition of the importance of connective tissue in the pathogenesis of chronic low-back pain. Many hands-on manipulative and mind-body therapies target connective tissue, specifically the fascia; however, the role of connective tissue in the physiology and biomechanics of low-back pain is generally underappreciated. Connective tissue adapts to the body's biomechanical and biochemical forces. The collagen and elastic fibers that provide fasciae their tensile strength are constantly being produced and remodeled. You might say that connective tissue senses and responds to your posture, movement, and activities. So, there is good reason to believe that Tai

Chi, with its emphasis on steady balance and dynamic, integrated movements, will substantially influence the body's network of connective tissue and modify its structure and function.

Recent studies by Dr. Langevin highlight the key role connective tissue may play in the pathology of musculoskeletal disease and the promising role that mind-body movements may play in prevention and rehabilitation.

In one study, Langevin's team used high-resolution ultrasound to compare the mobility and thickness of fascia around the spine of adults who had low-back pain for at least 12 months, along with a matched group who had no history of low-back pain. The researchers found that, on average, those with chronic low-back pain experienced impaired gliding motion of tissues during trunk motion. Interestingly, in males but not females, this impairment was associated with thicker connective tissue and overall reduced range of motion in the trunk.[12]

To better understand these results, and to test her back pain model further, she has conducted a series of innovative animal studies. One current set of studies is exploring if experimentally impaired movement, achieved by restraining the movement of one hind leg, leads to changes in connective tissue similar to that seen in chronic low-back pain patients. Even more striking, she has conducted a series of brilliant studies on how movement affects tissues and related symptoms of chronic back pain. In one study, she raised a group of rats to have connective-tissue inflammation; she then played with half of the group in a way that stretched and lengthened their spines. Specifically, she took advantage of a stretching reflex that occurs when a rat's tail is gently tugged, which results in a whole body stretch that looks just like a baby on its belly doing an "airplane" stretch (also similar to many Tai Chi and yoga stretches). She also played with the other half of the group, but without eliciting the same stretch reflex. She found that the more active stretching led to less inflammation in the fascia, as well as lower levels of inflammatory markers and improved gait.[13]

Taken together, Dr. Langevin's study and other studies support the central role that connective tissues may play in musculoskeletal health and the impact Tai Chi may have on the health of connective tissue. Researchers hypothesize that connective tissue is the central fabric of energy pathways (meridians) of Chinese medicine, and it is increasingly becoming appreciated as a communication system in many forms of integrative therapies. The impact of Tai Chi on connective tissue health may extend well beyond musculoskeletal health.[14]

Tai Chi for Chronic Pain Conditions

Two years ago, Anastasia, a 33-year-old linguist, felt a sharp pain in her hip. The constant pain became so severe that she had to stop jogging and jazz dancing. Even short walks became a challenge. "Overnight, I turned from an active young woman into a teetering old lady," says Anastasia. "I was a lost soul wandering from doctor to doctor, with no solution in sight. Some recommended pain medication; others alluded to cortisone injections. I wasn't thrilled with the idea of simply masking the pain; I wanted a real improvement."

An acupuncturist suggested that she take Tai Chi classes. "These classes are a place where I feel safe. I know I can move without hurting myself," says Anastasia, who now regularly goes to two or three classes a week. "Tai Chi seems to reorganize my internal structure and make my muscles less tense. I am encouraged to listen to my body instead of trying to copy someone else's movement. Over several years of class, my pain has steadily decreased. I can walk for hours, I can sleep comfortably, and I even go out dancing on occasion. Imagine my happiness when the other day I was able to run—run!—and catch a bus."

"I feel as if I am being healed not just by the movements we do in class, but also by the energy and humor of my classmates and by the feeling of community," she continues. "Tai Chi class is a place where it's OK to have a physical limitation, it's OK to make a mistake, and it's OK to crack a joke. It feels good to have companions on this journey."

Multiple Tai Chi principles and active ingredients may contribute to understanding and help explain how and why Tai Chi helps manage, resolve, and prevent musculoskeletal pain and pain-related symptoms. Research supports some of these purported mechanisms, although not always in the context of Tai Chi studies. Others include obvious mechanisms the Tai Chi community takes for granted, but they have yet to be substantiated with scientific research.

Postural Alignment and Control

All Tai Chi practitioners accept as a truism the notion that Tai Chi leads to a more efficient posture. Better structure and postural control is an explicit goal of Tai Chi and underlies its martial and health applications. As a teacher, one of my primary goals is to encourage students to carry themselves consciously in a more-upright posture, centering the head over the torso, the torso over the hips, and the feet so that key joints are aligned to maximize balance and minimize strain. It is very satisfying to watch a student's posture change over time, seeing the student move with more ease, efficiency, and awareness, both in and outside of classes.

From the perspective of traditional Chinese medicine, improved structure and posture frees and facilitates the flow of Qi, leading to higher levels of function and health. From a Western medicine perspective, better posture and biomechanics reduce strain and wear and tear on joints and tissues. Improved posture can also improve physiological processes that are more conducive to healing—improved blood and lymph circulation and reduced levels of stress markers associated with inflammation. Yet, surprisingly little data are available to characterize Tai Chi's impact on posture, and even less on how it impacts physiological processes related to pain.

The previous chapter summarized research suggesting that Tai Chi may improve dynamic postural control. Evidence also exists of improved gait biomechanics and improved balance during quiet standing, as well as during dynamic tasks. Interestingly, few, if any, studies to date have simply described basic postural changes following Tai Chi. Very few studies have explicitly explored the relationship between the characteristics of postural control and pain and function in those who suffer with musculoskeletal pain.

Here is a sample of a few key postural features of how Tai Chi training may contribute to better neuromusculoskeletal control and health.

Vertical Spine

The Tai Chi classics say: "The spine should be like a necklace of pearls hanging from heaven." This highlights how Tai Chi can improve the vertical stance by elongating the spine, including the neck, as well as reduce wear and tear on your discs. Verticality is also likely to lead to fewer unnecessary muscle contractions throughout the musculoskeletal system.[15]

Keen Attention to the Hips and Waist

In the Tai Chi classics, the waist, or more broadly, the segments of the body that connect the lower extremities with the trunk and upper extremities, is called the "commander." Physically and energetically, this region is prioritized as a central, coordinating hub. A key Tai Chi concept is "sitting into" or folding the kwa. The kwah generally corresponds with the inguinal fold, the fold or hollow on either side of the front of the body where the thigh joins the abdomen. So, being able to sit into the kwa means you have good flexibility and range of motion in the hip and pelvic area (the hip flexors and especially the psoas and the iliacus muscles), and symmetry on both sides of the body. A sedentary lifestyle and traumas to the pelvic area, even genetic issues such as a difference in leg lengths, may lead to imbalanced muscles. Some literature shows that imbalances in the psoas and related core muscles may be associated with back, knee, and neck problems, and they also may affect your gait and balance.[16]

Alignment of the Feet

The feet are the foundation of the body. If the foundation is askew, everything above it will be, too. Alignment can be off due to dropped arches or pronated feet (in which your feet and ankles turn inward), among other reasons. The very precise foot alignment in Tai Chi may help correct foot imbalances. Some studies in older adults who have arthritis show that Tai Chi improves ankle range of motion, and cross-sectional studies show that the plantar pressure distribution during standing and walking in experienced Tai Chi practitioners is more efficient than that of age-matched nonpractitioners.[17]

Tai Chi Master Bruce Kumar Frantzis has written extensively about the importance of proper alignment and described a vicious cycle leading to worsening pain and dysfunction. For example, the lack of support due to poor foot and knee alignment causes strain in the hip and back muscles. This strain can lead to muscle stiffness that eventually moves the vertebrae out of alignment, impinging the spinal cord. This poor alignment may then impair nerve impulses, weaken nerve signals to the legs, and cause pain. What's more, weak legs put more strain on the back, and the pain cycle continues.[18]

Through improving awareness of alignment and the range of motion and flexibility of the musculoskeletal system, and by training practitioners to move more efficiently, Tai Chi can help break cycles of dysfunction and reorganize negative patterns that underlie pain conditions.

Principle of the 70-Percent Rule

No pain, no gain? Just because it rhymes doesn't mean it makes sense!
—TAI CHI MASTER ROBERT MORNINGSTAR

Part of doing Tai Chi is learning how to move your body safely. One of the key principles and active ingredients of Tai Chi is moderation in effort, often called the 70-percent rule. Like the small amount of yin on the yang side of the Tai Chi symbol (the dark circle on the light side), the 70-percent rule supports never moving your joints or exerting effort in a stretch or stance more than 70 percent of your maximum potential. By avoiding the extremes of any movement or activity, you are less likely to cause trauma to tissues or to put yourself in a vulnerable position that might increase the likelihood of an injury. For example, if you lock your elbow during a Tai Chi push or punch, you could damage ligaments and tendons in the joint and make yourself more vulnerable to your opponent's control. Similarly, if you lock your elbow in reaction to a fall, you may increase the likelihood of a fracture. Leaving some flexibility or play in your elbow, or any other joint, affords a resiliency that may allow you to adapt your movements and prevent injury.

Not going to the extreme also minimizes an unconscious fear of movement (kinesiophobia).[19] Using the elbow as an example again, if you have tennis elbow and start to feel pain as you extend your elbow past a certain angle, the second you feel pain, and perhaps even just before that point, you naturally will guard against further injury and stop extending the elbow. That guarded movement may cause other tissues to compensate for your elbow weakness, possibly leading to shoulder or neck problems. From a Chinese medicine perspective, fear and guarding will limit the flow of Qi and blood to this area and slow down the healing process. Gentle movements, along with mindfulness and good intention, minimize the fear of pain and injury and create an environment for tissues to function safely at a higher level. For all joints, and especially injured ones, the intention is not to force healing, but to gently, gradually, nurture and nourish them.

Meditation and Psychological Components

The perception and experience of pain includes both physical and psychological components; thus, the meditative and cognitive aspects of Tai Chi are quite likely to affect positively any pain conditions. Chapters 8 and 9 discuss in more depth how the psychological, meditative aspects of Tai Chi might impact the perception of pain in many ways.

Numerous clinical trials of multiple meditative systems, including mindfulness-based stress reduction, loving-kindness meditation, and transcendental meditation, have shown them to reduce pain symptoms and improve function among those who have chronic pain conditions.[20] These meditative practices encompass a broad range of techniques, and so it's likely they impact pain and function via different physiological mechanisms.

One pathway might be through the immune system. Some meditation studies report reduced levels of inflammatory compounds that are known to exacerbate pain.[21] A handful of Tai Chi and Qigong studies in diverse populations, including cancer survivors and osteoporotic women, suggest that Tai Chi may have a positive impact on markers of inflammation.[22] Other experimental studies, including some with Zen monks, have shown that experienced meditators have higher pain thresholds, both while meditating and not meditating.[23] These higher thresholds may be due to meditators' ability to not dwell on or exaggerate pain sensations, but rather simply to just experience what is happening. Studies employing neuroimaging have reported meditation-related decreased pain sensation and decreased activation in regions of the brain associated with executive functioning, evaluations, and emotions.[24]

Placebos, Intention, and Pain Relief

Further evidence of the mind's power in pain perception comes from placebo research. A large, exponentially growing body of research unequivocally demonstrates that the manipulation of expectation and belief can markedly alter the levels of pain people may experience. This outcome is regardless of whether it happens in the context of receiving a real or placebo pill, an intervention, or even surgery.[25]

One of my favorite placebo-pain studies, due to its elegance and (unintentional) use of primary energy centers focused on in Tai Chi (the centers of the palms and soles of the feet), was conducted by Fabrizio Benedetti and colleagues in Turin, Italy. In this study with healthy volunteers, researchers used a small needle to squirt capsaicin (the chemical component of hot peppers) to produce a painful burning sensation just under the skin of the left palm, right palm, left foot, and right foot, simultaneously. The subjects' expectations of pain relief were raised by applying on only one of these body parts a cream researchers told them was a powerful local anesthetic. In actuality, the cream was a placebo and did not contain any anesthetic. Benedetti and colleagues induced a placebo response only in the treated body part; in other words, the subjects felt less pain in the treated part, but experienced no variation in pain sensitivity in the untreated parts.

Even more fascinating, if the researchers repeated the same experiment after giving the subjects the drug naloxone, which blocks the effect of the body's natural opium-like painkiller, they could totally abolish this highly specific placebo response. This outcome proves that the body's own natural pain-killing system completely mediated the placebo effect. These studies show that raising expectations of pain relief can induce a very specific effect to specific body parts.[26]

This concept of inducing a mind-body placebo effect may underlie some of the fundamental concepts of Tai Chi. Chinese medicine states that the mind leads Qi, and Qi moves and influences the body. In Chapter 2, you learned how imagination can become reality. This notion may be particularly true for pain. Imagining healing energy flowing to arthritic hands, knees, or the spine may actually elicit measurable neurochemical changes that relieve the pain.

Breathing

The breathing component of Tai Chi can lead to many changes, including enhanced relaxation, blood flow, and tissue massage. In addition, with a little practice, you can use breathing as an internal awareness tool. Some evidence also suggests that breathing, in and of itself, can affect pain.

Breath therapy is a mind-body therapy that integrates body awareness, breathing, meditation, and movement. A small study at the University of California at San Francisco found that six to eight weeks of breath therapy relieved chronic low-back pain better than standard physical therapy.[27] Slowed-down breathing used in Tai Chi, yoga, and Zen meditation also has been shown to reduce the intensity and unpleasantness of pain for fibromyalgia patients.[28]

Social Support

How much social support you receive can make a difference in how much pain you can tolerate. Being in a Tai Chi class, studying with a like-minded group, gives you the added impetus to continue to come to class, even on days when you feel achy. Many studies show that people who receive social support experience less cancer pain, take less pain medication, are less likely to suffer from chest pains after coronary artery bypass surgery, feel less pain during labor, and are less likely to use epidural medication during delivery of a baby.[29]

As discussed in Chapter 2, and later in Chapter 9, Tai Chi classes are a rich social environment. Rituals, like going to Tai Chi class regularly, can give you a feeling of community and companionship, and provide you with an outlet to share with others, which can be particularly important when you are in pain.

In conclusion, the multimodal approach of Tai Chi can lead to pain relief in many ways. Clinical studies bear out this belief.

CLINICAL EVIDENCE OF TAI CHI FOR PAIN

Despite the widespread use of Tai Chi for pain conditions, only a few large-scale clinical trials, to date, have evaluated Tai Chi's effectiveness and safety for chronic pain conditions. Nevertheless, numerous preliminary studies have evaluated Tai Chi for back pain, arthritis, and fibromyalgia with promising findings.

Back Pain

Given the prevalence and burden of back pain, as well as the widespread use of Tai Chi for back pain, it is surprising that so few Western studies have evaluated Tai Chi for back pain. In 2011, the first larger-scale clinical trial studying the effect of Tai Chi on persistent low-back pain was published by an Australian team led by Dr. Amanda Hall. This randomized trial assigned 160 adults (average age 44) to either 10 weeks of Tai Chi training based on a simplified form, called "Tai Chi for Back Pain" developed by Dr. Paul Lam, or to a control group. The results showed that Tai Chi significantly improved bothersome back-pain symptoms, which was the study's primary outcome. The participants also said they experienced lower pain intensities, less pain-related disability, and felt their health-related quality of life had improved, and, in general, felt better for having done Tai Chi.[30]

In another smaller trial conducted in Korea, patients suffering from ankylosing spondylitis (a form of chronic inflammation that causes pain and stiffness in and around the spine) were randomly assigned to eight weeks of Tai Chi plus usual care or to usual care with no additional treatment (the control group). Compared to the control group, those who performed Tai Chi exhibited significant improvements in fatigue, pain, stiffness, flexibility, and depression.[31]

Additional research based in China adds further support for the potential benefits of Tai Chi for those who have back pain. My colleagues and I conducted an unpublished review of Chinese-language literature between 1990 and 2007, using the keywords "taiji," "taijiquan," and "back pain." We found six studies specifically evaluating Tai Chi for back pain or neck pain. Two of the studies were randomized controlled trials and reported increases in flexibility and decreases in pain with Tai Chi.[32] The other studies suggest that adding Tai Chi to other therapies such as acupuncture is beneficial and that Tai Chi has the potential to improve quality of life, pain, emotional stability, and sleep in patients having back conditions.[33] However, these studies were generally small and suffered from methodological problems, so the results must be interpreted cautiously.

Finally, additional indirect support for Tai Chi for back pain comes from recent high-quality, large-scale trials of relatively dynamic forms of yoga. These trials show that a 12-week course of yoga improves function and pain in patients who have chronic low-back pain, is markedly superior to usual care, and may be equal to or better than some forms of comprehensive conventional back pain exercises.[34]

Osteoarthritis

Osteoarthritis, sometimes called degenerative arthritis or degenerative joint disease, is a condition involving the wearing away of protective tissues in the joints (cartilage) that cushion the bones and allow bones to glide over one another. While osteoarthritis can damage any joint in your body, the disorder most commonly affects joints in your knees, hips, hands, neck, and lower back. Symptoms commonly include joint pain, tenderness, stiffness, locking, and swelling. These symptoms can lead to reduced exercise and social activities, which in turn can affect the overall quality of your physical and mental health. For example, patients who have osteoarthritis of the knee and hip have a 15–20 percent reduction in their aerobic capacity and an increased risk for cardiovascular disease, obesity, and other inactivity-related conditions.[35]

Osteoarthritis is one of the leading causes of chronic disability in the United States. According to the Centers for Disease Control, in 2011, osteoarthritis was estimated to affect more than 26 million people. Not surprisingly, osteoarthritis is associated with high medical costs: in 1997, an estimated $7.9 billion was spent on osteoarthritis-related knee and hip replacements alone.

Over time, osteoarthritis gradually worsens; no cure exists. But physicians now consider nonpharmacological treatments, including exercise and physical therapy, first-line interventions that can slow the progression of the disease, relieve pain, and improve joint function.[36]

A growing number of studies, including more than a half-dozen randomized controlled trials, suggest that Tai Chi may be a safe, effective way to delay progression and manage osteoarthritis symptoms. However, most of these studies are smaller pilot studies, and some have significant design issues, which limits the conclusions we can draw from them.[37]

Dr. Chenchen Wang, a rheumatologist based at Tufts Medical Center, has conducted some rigorous, although small, randomized trials. One trial included 40 people (average age 65) with symptomatic knee osteoarthritis. These osteoarthritis patients were randomly assigned to either 60 minutes of a 10-forms version of Tai Chi, modified from the classic Yang style, or to wellness education and stretching twice weekly for 12 weeks. Importantly, these studies include a long follow-up period to assess how stable or transient any observed changes were. Those in the Tai Chi group exhibited significantly greater improvements in pain and physical function. They also reported they felt less depressed and had a better quality of life, compared to the control group. Tai Chi was also deemed to be safe.[38]

Several studies have evaluated the benefits of a simplified Sun-style form of Tai Chi developed by Dr. Lam specifically for arthritis patients. A randomized clinical trial of older patients who had chronic symptomatic hip and knee osteoarthritis found that both 12 weeks of Tai Chi and hydrotherapy classes provided large, sustained improvements in physical function when compared with a control group. Interestingly, hydrotherapy, but not Tai Chi, also led to sustained improvements in pain and psychological well-being.[39] Two other studies of older women who had osteoarthritis compared 12 weeks of Tai Chi to routine care. In one study, those in the Tai Chi group said they felt significantly less pain and stiffness, and they also exhibited improvements in balance, physical function, and abdominal strength. In the second study, those who practiced Tai Chi had greater knee extensor endurance, greater bone density in the hip, and a reduced fear of falling. Since osteoarthritis impairs balance, leads to joint weakness, and markedly increases the risk of falling, Tai Chi's improvement in balance and bone strength suggests it may help prevent fall-related fractures in older adults with osteoarthritis.[40]

Finally, studies conducted by researchers at Texas Tech University shed some light on how important it is for osteoarthritis patients who want to maintain the benefits of Tai Chi to continue practice. One study found that a six-week Yang-style group Tai Chi program, followed by six weeks of home Tai Chi training, significantly improved knee pain, physical function, and gait characteristics (walking speed and stride length) compared to a non-exercise control group. However, six weeks after their formal training ended, all of the Tai Chi–derived improvements disappeared.[41]

In summary, these and additional studies suggest that Tai Chi is a promising, safe, effective treatment for osteoarthritis symptoms, especially for the knee and hip, and can help improve quality of life. However, we need larger-scale trials to draw more-definitive conclusions. Even so, the Arthritis Foundation does advocate Tai Chi as a good choice for those who suffer from joint discomfort.[42]

RHEUMATOID ARTHRITIS

Rheumatoid arthritis is a chronic inflammatory disorder that typically affects the small joints in the hands and feet. Unlike the wear-and-tear damage of osteoarthritis, rheumatoid arthritis affects the lining of the joints, causing a painful swelling that can result eventually in bone erosion and joint deformity. Weakened muscles, ligaments, and tendons can also lead to joint instability.

An autoimmune disorder, rheumatoid arthritis occurs when your immune system mistakenly attacks your body's tissues. In addition to affecting the joints, it commonly causes fatigue. And, as with osteoarthritis, rheumatoid arthritis leads to symptoms that can make it difficult to exercise and perform daily activities, such as climbing stairs or carrying groceries, or to participate in social activities, leading to overall decreased quality of life and reduced psychological well-being.

Although rheumatoid arthritis has no cure, medications can reduce joint inflammation to relieve pain and prevent or slow joint damage. Gentle exercise has also been shown to help strengthen the muscles around the joints, as well as to help fight any fatigue. Tai Chi's gentle, adaptable approach, and its positive effect on muscle and bone strength, postural control, stress reduction, and cardiovascular health, has led researchers to evaluate its safety and effectiveness for those who suffer with rheumatoid arthritis.[43]

To date, only a handful of small, randomized trials and observational studies have evaluated Tai Chi for rheumatoid arthritis. Dr. Wang from Tufts University has conducted a small, pilot randomized controlled trial, mostly with women who were long-term sufferers from rheumatoid arthritis. The patients were randomly assigned either to 12 weeks of Tai Chi based on the Yang style or to a control group that did modest stretching exercises and received education regarding rheumatoid arthritis self-care. After 12 weeks, half of those in the Tai Chi group experienced a clinically relevant improvement in their rheumatoid arthritis symptoms; none in the control group showed improvement in their symptoms. The Tai Chi group also had greater reductions in disability and depression, but had no reported reductions in pain. Importantly, no patients withdrew from the study and no adverse events were observed, which suggests that Tai Chi is enjoyable, safe, and may well be beneficial for rheumatoid arthritis patients.[44]

Results of other studies are mixed, but generally supportive. They all suggest that Tai Chi is safe for rheumatoid arthritis patients.[45]

FIBROMYALGIA

Fibromyalgia is a disorder characterized by widespread musculoskeletal pain accompanied by fatigue, sleep, memory problems, and mood issues. Researchers believe that fibromyalgia amplifies painful sensations by affecting the way the brain processes pain signals. Unlike osteoarthritis and rheumatoid arthritis, the pain of fibromyalgia is not due to joint degeneration but rather to a more diffuse set of tender points, most commonly in the soft tissue on the back of the neck, shoulders, chest, lower back, hips, shins, elbows, and knees. Many people who have fibromyalgia also have tension headaches, temporomandibular joint (TMJ) disorders, irritable bowel syndrome, anxiety, and depression. As with other musculoskeletal conditions, fibromyalgia affects one's ability to exercise and overall quality of life.

While no cure exists for fibromyalgia, a variety of medications can control symptoms. These medications, however, are associated with multiple side effects. Exercise, relaxation, and stress-reduction measures may also help with symptoms.

Recent research suggests Tai Chi may offer significant symptom relief for fibromyalgia. A recent study published by Dr. Wang in the *New England Journal of Medicine* reported the results of the first randomized controlled trial to evaluate Tai Chi for fibromyalgia patients. Using a protocol similar to her osteoarthritis and rheumatoid arthritis studies, 66 patients were randomized to either 12 weeks of Tai Chi training or to a control group. Again, Tai Chi was successful. In this trial, Tai Chi led to large improvements in symptoms listed on a clinically validated questionnaire about fibromyalgia symptoms, as well as separate measures related to pain, sleep quality, depression, and quality of life. What's more, these improvements were maintained for six months, more Tai Chi subjects cut back on their use of medication compared to controls, and, again, there were no Tai Chi–related adverse events.[46]

Additional support for using Tai Chi to treat fibromyalgia comes from smaller noncontrolled studies and case series,[47] as well as from studies reporting positive effects on fibromyalgia following mind-body therapies, including Qigong[48] and mindfulness-based stress reduction.[49]

In summary, although a paucity of large-scale definitive trials evaluating Tai Chi for pain conditions still exists, growing evidence suggests that Tai Chi, when taught by experienced teachers, is safe and potentially an effective adjunct therapy for people who suffer with back pain, osteoarthritis, rheumatoid arthritis, and fibromyalgia. By treating the whole person, Tai Chi targets not only pain but also many of the secondary factors associated with pain, and it sets up behaviors that may slow down disease progression.

TAI CHI EXERCISES FOR PAIN

A good way to experience the interactions between gentle, pulsing movements, relaxation, imagery, and intention and their potential to alleviate pain is by practicing a simple exercise I developed called "Hand Tai Chi." As a Tai Chi teacher, I have found that this exercise is often therapeutic for those who have arthritis or repetitive-stress injury. More generally, I have found that this exercise helps students experience a number of the core principles of Tai Chi. Once they experience therapeutic Tai Chi qualities in the hand, it's easier for them to experience and begin integrating these principles into the rest of the body.

HAND TAI CHI

Hold your right hand in front of your body in a relaxed way, palm up. If it's tiring to hold it up, rest it on your thigh. Slowly and mindfully, extend all your fingers and separate them, and then relax them. Don't try too hard, no more than 70 percent effort. As you stretch, take time to notice which knuckles and surrounding tissues feel as if they are opening and which ones are not. It's more important at first to just feel and notice without trying to affect any change. Feel the network of elastic fascia in and around each joint, and notice how the gentle stretching and resting begins to allow the surrounding inner ocean or living matrix to rehydrate and nourish the tissues. Compare the front and back of your hand. Invite the warm, inner ocean to spread more deeply and freely into all tissues, with each cycle of the palm stretching and relaxing back to neutral.

Now add a bit of imagery or intention. Imagine warm, healing energy, perhaps a miniature radiant yellow sun, in the palm of your hand, relaxing and nourishing the tissues.[50] As you open and gently stretch the palm, allow the healing energy to radiate out into every cell of the hand, adding a gentle, charged quality to the inner ocean. As you relax your hand, feel the energy become more focused in the heart of the palm.

Each time you open the hand, the movement of the joints and the flow of the energy should be a just a little easier. Do this for three to five minutes with your right hand, and then compare it with how your left hand feels. Sometimes, the right hand feels warmer, sometimes more tingly, sometimes a little "bigger." It's different for each person. Switch to the left hand, and do Hand Tai Chi for three to five minutes. Now feel how the left hand feels compared to your right hand.

The principles of Hand Tai Chi are the same as those you use to practice the essential Tai Chi forms. For example, as you move forward in the "Push," the palms open to strengthen the connection between the joints and to express energy. Once you "Push," your palm returns to a more neutral, relaxed (or yin) phase. During the same movement, more experienced Tai Chi practitioners may sense the opening and closing of many more body joints—the spine, ribs, and lower extremity joints. And, during certain stages of Tai Chi training, the whole body feels like a hand, opening and closing, and being bathed with awareness and energy.

6

Strengthen Your Heart

Worry affects the circulation, the heart, the glands, the whole nervous system, and profoundly affects heart action.
  —Dr. Charles Mayo (1865–1939), founder of Mayo Clinic

When the Heart is at ease, the body is healthy.
  —Chinese proverb

Whether viewed from Western or Eastern medicine, the heart is considered a central, integrating hub for health and well-being. In the West, the heart is viewed as the body's primary pump, beating 100,000 times per day to circulate blood through its 60,000 miles of vascular plumbing. The heart and its vascular system play an integral role in connecting all of the body's physiological systems. The cardiovascular system delivers oxygen and nutrient-rich blood to every tissue of the body, including muscles and bones, nerves, and every internal organ; it also carries away waste from these tissues, to remove them from the body. Blood also serves as a delivery system for the endocrine and immune systems, transporting chemical messages that help regulate hormonal balance and fight off infections.

Like Eastern medicine, Western medicine increasingly appreciates how the heart interconnects with the nervous, endocrine, and immune systems and how the interactions between these systems may explain everyday phrases like "worried to death" and "heart broken."[1] Extending a little beyond the edges of science and medicine, we poetically attribute some of the most fundamental human behaviors, such as love, courage, wisdom, honesty, and even memories to the heart. This holistic perspective of the heart aligns with the Eastern medicine belief that Qi from the heart simultaneously governs a person's physical, emotional, and spiritual characteristics.[2]

Given the integral role the heart plays in supporting physical and emotional well-being, it is not surprising that an unhealthy cardiovascular system is one of the most prevalent causes of illness and death worldwide. Despite great breakthroughs in medications and surgical procedures for preventing and managing cardiovascular disease (CVD), it remains the number-one killer of Americans, claiming more lives than the next five leading causes of death combined.[3] This fact is particularly disturbing since most people can prevent CVD by living a healthy lifestyle and managing known cardiovascular risk factors, such as uncontrolled hypertension (high blood pressure), high cholesterol levels, physical inactivity, high levels of stress and anger, uncontrolled diabetes, and being overweight.

Tai Chi may be one of the more effective, versatile nonpharmacological interventions to prevent and rehabilitate CVD. The multicomponent approach of Tai Chi that combines physical exercise, stress reduction, emotional regulation, improved breathing efficiency, and social support targets many of the modifiable CVD risk factors. The gentle, adaptable nature of Tai Chi makes it safe and accessible for people of all fitness and health levels, including those who have CVD.

This chapter provides the rationale for using Tai Chi to improve heart health and summarizes a growing body of research that supports Tai Chi's positive effects on CVD risk factors. Tai Chi also has a promising track record as an effective adjunct therapy in the rehabilitation and management of multiple CVDs, including heart failure, coronary heart disease, and stroke.

CVD Prevalence and Risk Factors

Cardiovascular disease, including heart disease, stroke, atherosclerosis (or blocked arteries), and high blood pressure, is a major cause of morbidity and the leading killer of US men and women. Experts estimate the economic cost of CVD in the United States to be $431.8 billion per year, including both direct health-care costs and indirect costs from lost productivity caused by illness and death.[4]

Some CVD risk factors are controllable, while others are not. Uncontrollable risk factors include your gender (being a male), being older (age 50 and up), a family history of heart disease, and race (African Americans, American Indians, and Mexican Americans are more likely to have heart disease than Caucasians). However, if you control modifiable risk factors, you can reduce your chances of CVD: don't smoke; maintain low levels of low-density lipoprotein cholesterol (LDL), or "bad" cholesterol, and high levels of high-density lipoprotein cholesterol (HDL), or "good" cholesterol; maintain healthy blood pressure; be physically active; achieve good body weight; control blood sugar; and manage stress and anger. New research suggests that lower levels of inflammation, as reflected by blood markers such as C-reactive protein, are also associated with lower risks of cardiovascular events.

If you use preventive strategies, you may avoid the ravages of CVD. Even if you already have established CVD, complementary and adjunct therapies may help to reduce the dosage and number of medications you need, and therefore, reduce your risk of side effects and delay or prevent additional surgical procedures. For these reasons, conventional health-care providers and heart patients have a growing interest in holistic, lifestyle modification programs targeting CVD. These include mind-body exercises such as Tai Chi, meditation, and yoga, often along with special (usually low-fat) diets, and group support. Members of the medical community are beginning to adopt what is being called a "TLC" (Therapeutic Lifestyle Changes) approach for heart disease, which shows promise based on preliminary clinical research.[5]

Heart patients want more mind-body therapies. US surveys suggest that heart patients are particularly attracted to mind-body therapies like Tai Chi, yoga, and relaxation techniques. These surveys also reveal that 95 percent of those who use mind-body therapies for cardiovascular conditions perceive the therapies to be helpful.[6]

TAI CHI: A MULTICOMPONENT MIND-BODY EXERCISE

"Tai Chi, to me, is like a leaf that slowly floats down from a tree and then a cool breeze comes by," says Bonnie, a heart-failure patient in her eighties who participated in a Harvard Medical School heart failure study. "It is loosening me up. I am standing straighter, and I sleep better. I find myself 'pouring' from side to side when I am peeling potatoes in the kitchen or doing the dishes."

A number of the active ingredients of Tai Chi are highly relevant to cardiovascular health.

Tai Chi Is a Safe, Adaptable Form of Aerobic Exercise

Physical activity, without a doubt, strengthens the heart. Multiple large-scale, prospective epidemiological studies show that even moderate aerobic exercise and a physically active lifestyle improve heart health compared with a sedentary lifestyle.[7] It is also never too late to take advantage of the benefits of exercise for heart health—even light activity later in life can reduce your risk of dying of heart disease, compared to remaining sedentary.[8]

If you watch people practice Tai Chi, it might not seem as if they are getting any aerobic benefit. But they are. Numerous studies have shown that Tai Chi can be considered an aerobic activity of low-to-moderate intensity, depending on your training style, how deep you sink into the postures, how fast you move from one posture to the next, and the duration of your practice. The physical activity of Tai Chi ranges between 1.6 and 4.6 metabolic equivalents (METS). To put this measurement in perspective, your resting metabolic rate while sitting quietly is equal to 1 MET. The majority of studies report the intensity of Tai Chi at about 3.5 METS, which is about the same intensity as walking at a moderate pace (about three miles per hour) on level ground. Tai Chi can get your heart rate up to between 50 and 74 percent of maximum, depending on the type and intensity of Tai Chi and your age.[9] Importantly, Tai Chi is highly adaptable to your heart's capacity for exercise because you can modulate the intensity.

Tai Chi Can Reduce Stress and Improve Psychological Well-Being

A strong body of research demonstrates the relationship between psychological factors and the risk of CVD.[10] Sustained periods of depression lasting from weeks to years have been associated with an increased CVD risk, and a history of depression can raise the risk of a heart attack.[11] Mental stress and outbursts of anger have also been associated with acute coronary events.[12] In addition, heart attack rates are 20 percent higher on Monday mornings, an indication of the influence of increased work stress.[13]

Tai Chi can help you manage and reduce stress, improve your mood, including depression and anxiety, and may help you soften unhealthy, overly aggressive behaviors by increasing your self-awareness and promoting a balanced lifestyle. (Chapter 9 discusses more about how Tai Chi affects psychological well-being.)

Tai Chi Improves Breathing Efficiency

The heart and lungs work in concert to assure oxygen-rich blood is available to every cell in your body through the exchange of two gases, oxygen and carbon dioxide.

The emphasis on diaphragmatic breathing in Tai Chi (see Chapter 7) may result in greater efficiency in gas exchange, and this efficiency may lessen the heart's workload. The slow, deep meditative breathing associated with Tai Chi has also been shown to reduce blood pressure, dilate blood vessels, improve circulation, and calm the nervous system.[14] Collectively, these potential benefits of Tai Chi breathing may underlie some of its clinical effects on CVD.

Tai Chi May Improve the Confidence to Exercise and Motivate Healthy Behavior

Another way Tai Chi enhances fitness and heart health is by giving you the confidence to exercise and motivating you to seek out other healthy behaviors. Studies show that Tai Chi enhances what is called exercise self-efficacy, that is, the belief and conviction that you can successfully engage in exercise. Enhanced exercise self-efficacy translates into greater physical activity.[15]

Tai Chi's meditative, self-reflective components, as well as its connection to Eastern philosophy, which espouses a balanced lifestyle, may also foster your awareness of unhealthy behaviors and motivate you to make more healthy behavior changes. These changes may include an improved diet and overall lifestyle, which can only help your heart health.

Tai Chi Leads to Social Support

Tai Chi is a social activity. As a Tai Chi student, you interact with your instructors and other students. You may also feel as if you are broadly connected to a larger community of those who practice Tai Chi regularly. A strong body of research suggests that this form of social support and a sense of connection can positively affect your health, including prevention of and rehabilitation from cardiovascular events, such as heart attacks.[16] The underlying mechanisms of social support are not fully clear, but they may be related to reducing stress and depression. As you have read above, both chronic and acute psychological stress can increase the risks of heart disease.

TAI CHI FOR HEART HEALTH

Several systematic reviews have summarized the clinical and basic research evidence for Tai Chi as an intervention for heart health. This research suggests that Tai Chi is a safe, promising intervention for the prevention and rehabilitation of multiple CVDs. However, more-definitive conclusions are not yet possible because only a few large-scale trials are studying Tai Chi and the heart.[17]

Tai Chi impacts key cardiovascular risk factors, including blood pressure, cholesterol levels, blood sugar metabolism, and inflammation. (For Tai Chi's impact on stress and mood, see Chapter 9). Tai Chi also affects specific cardiovascular conditions, including heart failure, coronary artery disease, and stroke.

High Blood Pressure

High blood pressure, or hypertension, is a serious condition in itself as well as a risk factor for other cardiovascular conditions. "Blood pressure" is the force of blood pushing against the walls of the arteries as the heart pumps blood. If this pressure rises and stays high over time, it can damage the body in many ways. Blood pressure is measured as systolic and diastolic pressures. "Systolic" refers to blood pressure when the heart beats while pumping blood. "Diastolic" refers to blood pressure when the heart is at rest between beats. You most often will see blood pressure numbers written with the systolic number above or before the diastolic number, such as 120/80 mmHg. The mmHg is millimeters of mercury—the units used to measure blood pressure. All levels above 120/80 mmHg raise your CVD risk, and the risk grows as blood pressure numbers rise.

Many studies have shown that Tai Chi will lower high blood pressure. In a 2008 systematic review conducted by our group, we identified 26 studies that assessed the impact of Tai Chi on blood pressure. We found that in 85 percent of trials, Tai Chi lowered blood pressure, with improvements ranging from 3 to 32 mmHg in systolic pressure and from 2 to 18 mmHg in diastolic pressure. Some of these studies were of poor quality, so we should interpret the results cautiously, but collectively, these data suggest that Tai Chi may be as effective in controlling blood pressure as other lifestyle approaches, including weight loss, a low-sodium diet, and moderating alcohol use.[18]

In one of the smaller but higher-quality randomized trials in our review, researchers at Johns Hopkins Medical Institutions recruited 62 older sedentary adults with pre-hypertension and compared the impact of a moderate-intensity aerobic exercise program to a light-intensity Tai Chi program. Both programs held group classes that met for one hour, twice weekly, and instructed participants to practice at home. The results show comparable and clinically significant blood pressure changes in both groups (–8.4 and –7.0 mmHg systolic blood pressure; –3.2 and -2.4 mmHg diastolic blood pressure for the aerobic and Tai Chi groups, respectively). Notably, the Tai Chi group was more likely to continue home exercises than the aerobics group.[19]

A number of other randomized controlled trials (RCTs) including hypertensive patients have also reported a positive effect of Tai Chi on blood pressure.[20]

High Blood Cholesterol Levels

Cholesterol is a fat (also called a lipid) that your body needs to work properly. Overly high cholesterol levels can increase your chance of getting heart disease, stroke, and other problems.

A handful of studies, including multiple RCTs, have examined the effects of Tai Chi on cholesterol and related lipids. Some have found that Tai Chi leads to favorable changes as compared to no significant changes in nonintervention (control) groups.[21] Other trials, both randomized and nonrandomized, among people who were obese, diabetic, or had lipid disorders—and also among healthy people—have reported positive effects of Tai Chi on cholesterol and blood lipid levels.[22] However, other studies report no effects of Tai Chi on blood lipids.[23]

Impaired Blood Sugar (Glucose) Metabolism

Most of the food you eat is broken down into glucose, the form of sugar in the blood. Glucose is the body's main source of fuel. After digestion, glucose enters the bloodstream, and then goes to the cells throughout the body where it is used for energy. A hormone called insulin, produced by the pancreas, must be available to allow glucose to enter the cells.

However, in people with diabetes or pre-diabetes symptoms, the pancreas does not make enough insulin, or the cells in the muscles, liver, and fat do not use insulin properly, or both. As a result, the amount of glucose in the blood increases, while the cells are starved of energy. Over time, high blood-glucose levels damage blood vessels, leading to increased risks for heart attack and stroke.[24]

A few studies, including one randomized trial, have reported improvements in blood sugar control following Tai Chi training.[25] However, most of the more rigorous RCTs have not reported any apparent benefit of Tai Chi on glucose metabolism.[26]

Inflammation and CRP

Inflammation, the process by which your body fights off infection and heals itself, is now widely believed to be associated with the development of cardiovascular disease. Although we don't yet understand the precise mechanisms between inflammation and cardiovascular disease, increased inflammation is associated with narrowing and clotting of the arteries, both key processes associated with heart disease and stroke.[27]

One key marker of inflammation is the protein CRP. High levels of

CRP in the blood indicate an increased risk of heart disease and low levels of CRP, a low risk. This marker is independent of cholesterol levels.[28]

A few small studies suggest that Tai Chi may positively affect inflammation and CRP levels. One recent RCT including Taiwanese obese patients who had Type 2 diabetes found that 12 weeks of Tai Chi reduced CRP levels, but conventional exercise did not.[29]

Another small Australian RCT designed to study the effects of Kung Fu on metabolic health in obese adolescents used Tai Chi as a "placebo control." After six months of training, CRP decreased significantly in both groups, and a trend toward decreased markers of blood sugar control existed. No apparent advantage appeared in the more physically demanding Kung Fu versus the "placebo" of Tai Chi![30]

Exercise Capacity and Fitness

Good evidence suggests that Tai Chi can improve aerobic capacity and overall fitness in both healthy people, as well as in those with CVD.

A recent RCT of more than 370 relatively healthy community-dwelling adults conducted in Hong Kong compared the effects of a 12-week Tai Chi program to both brisk walking and non-exercising controls. At 12 weeks, exercise capacity increased in both the Tai Chi and walking groups about equally. In addition, Tai Chi led to improved weight and general physical fitness. Interestingly, the Tai Chi group did this with 33 percent less increase in heart rate. These results support the idea that when exercise intensity is a concern, as it is in many heart conditions, Tai Chi may be the preferred form of exercise since it puts less demand on the heart.[31]

Another longer, nonrandomized study at the National Taiwan University Hospital monitored the health of 35 older Tai Chi practitioners, average age 69, over five years and compared them with a matched group of sedentary elderly people from the same community. As expected in this older age group, exercise capacity declined over time. However, Tai Chi helped both men and women substantially slow down this age-related decline compared to the sedentary controls. Those who practiced Tai Chi also showed smaller increases in body fat and less decrease in flexibility compared to the controls.[32]

Many other randomized and nonrandomized trials also support that

Tai Chi may improve exercise capacity and fitness among those who have CVD risk factors.[33]

Tai Chi for Rehabilitation and Management of CVD

If you have heart disease, then Tai Chi may be one of the better ways to help you rehabilitate and manage the effects of such conditions as heart failure, coronary heart disease, and stroke.

Tai Chi for Heart Failure

Jackie, age 58, the owner of a food market, had had congestive heart failure for 10 years when her doctor suggested that she enroll in the Tai Chi study at Beth Israel Deaconess Medical Center in Boston. "My doctor told me I was almost ready for a pacemaker. I was tired and couldn't endure much," says Jackie, the mother of two teenagers. Jackie received educational materials and did aerobic exercises for 12 weeks as part of the study's control group, and then accepted the researcher's offer to take the Tai Chi classes for another 12 weeks. She learned Tai Chi breathing, strength, and flexibility exercises and a simplified Tai Chi protocol she could practice on her own.

After three months of the Tai Chi classes, as well as an hour of aerobics twice a week, Jackie's doctor told her she didn't need a pacemaker after all. "My heart was more stable, and I felt stronger," she says. "I had more energy to run my business and to keep up with my kids."

To learn more about Tai Chi, she began taking a class at a community Tai Chi center in Boston. "I always feel more energized after a Tai Chi class. I have no problem doing two hours of Tai Chi, whereas I'm counting the minutes during aerobic exercise," says Jackie, who drives one hour each way from her home outside Boston to do the Tai Chi classes. "I can easily incorporate Tai Chi into my life. I take breaks at work to do Tai Chi, and when my kids start to get to me, I do some Tai Chi breathing to help calm me down."

Chronic heart failure is a condition in which the heart cannot pump enough blood to the rest of the body. Heart failure includes problems due to the heart muscle's inability to pump blood out of the heart efficiently.

This condition is called systolic heart failure. Heart failure also includes problems due to stiffness in the heart muscles that make it difficult for the heart to fill up with blood easily. This condition is called diastolic heart failure. Our study team at Harvard Medical School, led by Dr. Gloria Yeh, has reported that Tai Chi has positive health benefits for both systolic and diastolic heart failure patients.

We began our research on Tai Chi for heart failure with a pilot study of systolic heart failure patients. Thirty patients were randomized to either 12 weeks of Tai Chi training or usual care (the control group). For this study, we first developed a simplified, tailored twice-weekly protocol of traditional warm-up exercises and five Tai Chi forms adapted from Cheng Man Ching's Yang-style Tai Chi, which we have subsequently used in all our heart failure clinical trials. At 12 weeks, the patients in the Tai Chi group demonstrated a significantly improved heart failure–related quality of life, walked farther on a six-minute test, and had greater decreases in blood levels of B-type natriuretic protein (a marker for heart failure) when compared to the control group. We also saw trends toward improvement in increased aerobic capacity in the Tai Chi group. And those in the Tai Chi group also experienced more stable sleep.[34]

Based on these promising preliminary results, we conducted a larger follow-up study of 100 systolic heart failure patients. In this study, the comparison group was a heart-health education program. As in our pilot study, participants in the Tai Chi group experienced clinically significant improvements in quality of life, as well as improvements in exercise self-efficacy and mood. However, unlike the pilot study, improvements in six-minute walking distance and exercise capacity were small and not statistically different from in the education group.[35]

Our group recently completed a smaller pilot study with diastolic heart failure patients. We were specifically interested in learning if the benefits of Tai Chi were simply due to moderate aerobic training or to mind-body components, such as meditation and controlled breathing. In this study, 16 patients with diastolic heart failure were randomized to either Tai Chi or a low-impact aerobics class twice a week for 12 weeks. We found that Tai Chi provided significantly less-intense exercise than the aerobic exercise group. However, at the end of 12 weeks, those who had participated in Tai Chi increased their six-minute walk distance more than those in the aerobic group, and patients in both groups had equal improvements in quality of life. So, it appears that Tai Chi's success is due to other mechanisms than just aerobic training in improving exercise capacity and quality of life among heart failure patients.[36]

Importantly, about 90 percent of the participants across all of our heart-failure studies regularly came to the Tai Chi classes and practiced Tai Chi at home as well. This result means that Tai Chi is enjoyable and can be safely incorporated into regular activities, even for patients who have chronic heart disease.

Researchers in Italy have reported results of an RCT that demonstrated that adding Tai Chi to endurance training for heart-failure patients resulted in greater improvements in the distance walked in six minutes, systolic blood pressure, quality of life, and lower-extremity strength, as compared to a control group.[37] Other researchers have also shown positive improvements among heart failure patients who practiced Tai Chi.[38]

Tai Chi for Coronary Heart Disease (CHD)

Coronary heart disease (CHD) is a narrowing of the small blood vessels that supply blood and oxygen to the heart. Also called coronary artery disease (CAD), this is the leading cause of death in the United States for both men and women. CHD is caused by the buildup of plaque in the arteries to the heart. It can result in angina, a type of chest pain and discomfort due to poor blood flow through the blood vessels of the heart muscle, or a heart attack (myocardial infarction) when blood flow to a part of the heart is blocked for a long enough time that some heart muscle is damaged or dies.

A handful of studies have evaluated specifically the potential benefits of Tai Chi for patients diagnosed with CHD.[39] One RCT in England, using patients recovering from a heart attack, found improvements in systolic blood pressure in both Tai Chi and aerobic exercise groups, but only the Tai Chi group showed improvements in diastolic blood pressure. In addition, those who did Tai Chi were more likely to stick with exercise compared to the aerobic exercisers or a control group.[40]

Other studies show that Tai Chi may lead to a better prognosis for cardiac events in patients who have CAD, increase the rate of return to a resting heart rate following exercise, and help to balance out the autonomic nervous system.[41]

Tai Chi also may aid recovery from bypass surgery. A small, nonrandomized study at National Taiwan University looked at 20 men, average age 57, who were recovering from bypass surgery. Over one year, about half of the men practiced Tai Chi, while the other half participated in a home-based cardiac rehabilitation program. After one year, the men who did Tai Chi showed a 10 percent increase in aerobic fitness, while those who walked briskly showed little change in their fitness levels. Again, the Tai Chi group was more likely to adhere to their exercise regimen than those in the traditional rehabilitation group.[42]

These and other recent studies have found that exercise at a lower intensity can provide benefits to those recovering from heart disease. That's why Tai Chi is being increasingly accepted as an alternate exercise program, particularly for unfit or elderly people with heart problems.

Recovery following Stroke

A stroke happens when blood flow to a part of the brain stops. If blood flow stops for longer than a few seconds, the brain cannot get blood and oxygen. Brain cells can die, causing permanent damage. Stroke is the third leading cause of death in the United States and is the leading single cause of disability. More than 4 million Americans have had a stroke, or brain attack, and are living with the aftereffects.[43]

A handful of studies have evaluated Tai Chi as a rehabilitation exercise for stroke survivors. The largest published study to date investigated whether Tai Chi could improve standing balance. Researchers in Hong Kong randomly assigned 136 subjects who had suffered a stroke at least six months prior either to 12 weeks of Tai Chi or to a control group who practiced general exercises for 12 weeks. The Tai Chi group showed greater ability to maintain balance, to reach and lean both forward and backward, and also demonstrated faster reaction times. These benefits persisted through a second assessment at 18 weeks.[44]

Israeli researchers conducted another smaller RCT in which they compared a Tai Chi program to balance training for stroke survivors. After 12 weeks, those attending the Tai Chi classes showed improvements in general functioning and social functioning, but they did not exhibit changes in balance or walking speed. The balance training led to improvements in balance and walking speed, but not in general functioning. Tai Chi appears to have potential benefits for stroke survivors, but we need additional and longer-term studies to evaluate its full benefits.[45]

CLINICAL IMPLICATIONS AND ADVANTAGES OF TAI CHI FOR CVD

If you have heart disease, you need to find an appropriate, nonthreatening, easy-to-perform physical activity that you will maintain. Tai Chi may be just what the doctor ordered. Based on the existing evidence, Tai Chi is a promising adjunct to conventional heart care.

Cardiac rehabilitation programs, unfortunately, are underutilized. Tai Chi may be appropriate if you are unable or unwilling to engage in other forms of physical activity, or as a bridge to more rigorous exercise programs, particularly if you are frail or deconditioned.

If your doctor says you have borderline hypertension, and you are not certain you want to begin drug therapy, a nonpharmacological approach such as Tai Chi may be a way to keep your blood pressure in check. If you have established hypertension and find it difficult to engage in regular exercise, again, think about using Tai Chi to aid the treatment program your doctor has designed for you. Tai Chi may also help you improve your aerobic fitness and manage your cholesterol; its effects on blood sugar control are less clear.

Importantly, all studies to date suggest that Tai Chi may be safe for heart patients. Tai Chi may offer you additional options, whether as an adjunct to formal cardiac rehabilitation, as a part of maintenance therapy, or as an exercise alternative.

Deepen and Enrich Your Breathing

"I feel like my breathing has freed up quite a bit since I started taking Tai Chi classes two years ago," says Lois, 65, a retired real estate broker who has asthma episodes after allergy attacks. "I live at the top of a steep hill above where my Tai Chi class meets. It's hard to contemplate walking up that hill, but after Tai Chi class I kind of sail up the hill."

Now that her husband has been diagnosed with Parkinson's disease, Lois has to complete daily tasks by herself. "I carry the grocery bags, bring boxes to the basement, and do all the laundry," she says. "I used to be wary about doing those things. Now I do them without thinking about it. I have a lot more energy, stamina, flexibility, and strength. Tai Chi has really helped me cope physically and emotionally.

"And I can take long walks every day and spend hours working in the garden without resting," says Lois, who also has enough energy to take her two grandchildren to the aquarium and museums, and play with them in the playground and on the basketball court.

Strong lungs and efficient breathing are central to overall health, well-being, and living a long life. One of my Tai Chi teachers liked to remind us that while most of us could live for quite some time, even days, without food and water, no one could live for more than a few minutes without breathing air. On average, you breathe more than 20,000 times per day, so it naturally follows that efficient, mindful, and freer breathing patterns have the potential to significantly enhance and sustain your health. In fact, sound epidemiological data supports that less-restricted and higher-volume breathing may lead to a longer life.[1] On the other side of the coin, inefficient, constricted breathing may exacerbate, or contribute to, illness.

Breathing is great example of how the active ingredients of Tai Chi are interwoven and synergistic. A mindful breath brings attention into the deepest, most intimate places within ourselves. Breath is also a vehicle for intention, for good air and vibrant Qi going in and bad air and bad Qi going out. The breath helps integrate the body with the mind, and with the key Tai Chi concept of relaxing.

How you breathe is regulated and intertwined with nearly all core physiological systems, including the musculoskeletal, nervous, cardiovascular, and endocrine systems. Slow, deep, mindful, and rhythmic breathing developed in Tai Chi potentially affects breathing and lung health, as well as other multiple physiological systems that control cardiovascular processes (such as blood pressure), nervous system processes (such as involuntary control of blood flow to organs or muscle contraction in the intestines), and even perception and tolerance of pain.

> A Tai Chi joke:
> Student: "Master, what is the secret of a long life?"
> Master: "Keep breathing as long as you can!"

BREATHING CAPACITY AND LIFE SPAN

One indication that good breathing affects health is the strong association between breathing function and longer life span. Two studies illustrate this association nicely. The first is the landmark Framingham Heart Study, in which a cohort of 5,209 men and women, aged 30 to 62, was followed for more than 20 years.[2] At the beginning of the study, all participants underwent pulmonary testing and had an evaluation of a key index of healthy breathing called "forced vital capacity" (FVC), which is simply the amount of air you can forcibly exhale from the lungs after taking the deepest breath possible. Over the course of the study, FVC was a very strong predictor of cardiovascular-related death and disease. This relationship was robust, even when factors such as initial age, smoking status, and prior pulmonary and heart disease were taken into account.

A second, more recent, study at the University at Buffalo followed 1,195 men and women for 29 years and also reported a strong relationship between lung function and mortality using a measure called FEV1—a measure of the maximal amount of air you can forcefully exhale in one second.[3] In this study, lung function was a significant predictor of all-cause mortality, not just heart disease, as in the Framingham study. Again, this relationship was strong even after factors such as smoking, blood pressure, and age were considered. What's more, the risk of death was increased for participants who had only moderately impaired lung function, not only those with severe impairments.

In summary, long before you become diagnosed with a serious illness, the health of your breath may predict your life span. The good news not mentioned in these studies is that exercises like Tai Chi can improve the functional quality of your breathing and therefore potentially help you lead a longer life.

BREATHING BASICS

To appreciate how Tai Chi and Tai Chi breathing might affect pulmonary health, we need to know a bit more about breathing and how age and disease change it.

The anatomy and physiology of human breathing has evolved to enable us to harvest oxygen from the atmosphere to fuel our metabolism of energy-rich molecules, such as glucose, and to release carbon dioxide back to the atmosphere as one of the byproducts of this metabolism. Based on multiple sources of feedback from the body, including the chemistry of the blood and immediate physical demands, the brainstem sends signals that trigger the body to inhale or exhale.

Muscles, including the diaphragm and intercostals, play big roles in mechanically expanding and contracting the lungs, drawing in and expelling air. The diaphragm is a dome-shaped sheath of muscle sitting on top of the stomach and liver, and it is the primary muscle of healthy breathing. When the diaphragm is relaxed, it assumes a domed, upward shape. When it contracts, it pushes downward. Along with some help from the intercostal muscles (which pull the ribs upward), the downward movement of the diaphragm opens the rib cage, decreases pressure on the lungs, and creates a vacuum (negative pressure) that draws outside air in all the way to the bottom of the lungs. Upon exhaling, the diaphragm returns to its relaxed, upward dome-shape, compressing the lungs and squeezing air out.

The respiratory system is technically elegant and sophisticated; however, most of us do not use it anywhere near to its highest level of efficiency. In typical breathing, most adults only use the upper regions of their lungs. But, we can learn to use more of our lungs. For example, a highly trained athlete can develop a 50 percent greater lung capacity than the average adult.

AGE-RELATED CHANGES IN BREATHING AND LUNG FUNCTION

Just as with other bodily systems, the efficiency of breathing and lung function declines with age. For example, shortly after we reach the age of 20 years, our FVC decreases 200 to 250 cc every 10 years. Remember, vital capacity predicted cardiovascular death and disease in the famous Framingham study. In contrast, functional residual capacity—that is, the amount of air left in the lungs after normal expiration—increases slightly as we get older. This air in the lungs can be problematic as trapped carbon dioxide in the airsacs of the lungs is a primary symptom of chronic obstructive pulmonary disease (COPD).[4]

Several physical and physiological processes are believed to underlie these age-related changes; they include changes in muscles, lung elasticity, and lung structure, as well as stress.

Musculoskeletal Changes: Two of the most important age-related changes relate to the structure of the chest wall. First, the chest wall becomes stiffer due to changes in the shape, calcification, and health of the joints of the rib cage. Second, the strength of the respiratory muscles, including the intercostals and the diaphragm, decreases.[5]

Elasticity of the Lungs: Aging causes subtle changes in the connective tissues of the lungs, changes including a decrease in elastic fibers and an increase in more rigid type 3 collagen. Increases in cross links and fiber orientation also occur. All of these changes alter the elastic property or springiness of the lungs and the airways, with a loss of elastic recoil, and thus, the loss of an ability to squeeze air out during exhalation.[6]

Efficiency of Gas Exchange: Structural changes also reduce the number and surface area of the air sacs (alveoli) in the lungs.[7] This reduction is important because these air sacs are where gases (oxygen and carbon dioxide) are exchanged through tiny blood vessels (capillaries).

Emotions and Stress: Emotions can affect breathing and, over time, affect the quality of your breath. An obvious example of the effect of emotions on breathing is a frustrated young child crying. The plaintive crying makes it difficult for the child (and sometimes the accompanying adult!) to catch a breath.

One key factor is chronic stress. When our evolutionary ancestors perceived something as potentially threatening (for example, an encounter with a sabertooth tiger while hunting), their brains sent warning signals through their central nervous system. Their adrenal glands produced hormones (adrenalin and noradrenalin), which in turn caused the heart to beat faster. Muscles tensed and pupils dilated. Their lungs breathed faster to match the immediate demands of the heart, and the result was more shallow breathing.

Our bodies still maintain the same evolutionary sense to confront a threat and deal with it, even if it does not mean running away from the threat as quickly as possible. While shallow, rapid breathing is a good match for the short-term "fight-or-flight response," it's not efficient for everyday cardiorespiratory function. Unfortunately, in today's stressful society, high levels of anxiety resulting from real or simply imagined threats—the bombardment of stressful stories in the news, the possibility of losing a job, a dispute with a family member—can cause continual activation of elements of the "fight-or-flight response," leading to chronic shallow breathing. In fact, shallow, rapid breathing shares qualities with breathing patterns associated with chronic anxiety and panic disorder symptoms; it may even contribute to them becoming chronic.

LEARNING TAI CHI BREATHING

The Tai Chi way of breathing is to be gentle and gradual. Breathing potentially is connected to emotional and physical patterns, so being gentle allows you to experience breathing mindfully and gives your mind and body time to reorganize and stay balanced.

The first phase is simply to observe the breath, without any intention to change it. Notice where the breath goes and where it does not go; feel the sensation of breathing in your nose, throat, chest, and throughout your body.

Sometimes, I first teach breathing while students are sitting or lying down; this position allows them to focus on the richness of breathing, without becoming distracted by the choreography of movements in the Tai Chi form. As with any Tai Chi training, don't attempt to force the breath; you do not want to create new stresses over old ones. Over time, natural, deep breathing becomes part of the movements.

Imagery can also affect the breath. Generally, I'll suggest that students imagine breathing in air from nature with qualities that bring them to a greater sense of balance. For example, they might imagine breathing in vibrant sunshine-filled air (e.g., recalling a warm summer day near the ocean) if they are sleepy and a cold, or calming, cooler energy (e.g., recalling a walk around a placid lake) if they are stressed and a bit overheated. A substantial body of imagery research, as well as a burgeoning number of placebo studies, demonstrates that what people imagine and expect can affect how their body reacts. For example, multiple placebo studies have shown that people who are told they are breathing in a toxin (e.g., ragweed) when in actuality it's only saline will have an asthma attack, and when they are told they are breathing in rescue medicine (again only saline), the attack stops.[9] This knowledge helps Tai Chi students better understand, and legitimizes, the use of intention and breathing practices, such as when I ask students to imagine breathing in fresh, Qi-filled healing air from a mountaintop or a forest.

The Benefits of Tai Chi Breathing

Breathing in Tai Chi serves more than the function of bringing oxygen into and expelling carbon dioxide out of the body. Breathing provides an internal massage, serves as a tool for bodily awareness and focus, balances the nervous system and emotions, and regulates and enhances Qi flow. The quality of our breath, easy or labored, shallow or deep, also provides feedback that informs our posture and movement patterns.

During typical Tai Chi training, the air that is breathed in and out should have a soft, continuous flow. The idea is to attain a level of natural breath that flows regularly, lightly, slowly, and deeply. During some Tai Chi exercises, you may benefit from coordinating breathing with your movements. For example, when you expand your body and stretch your arms out, breathe in, and when you relax your body and allow the arms to move inward, breathe out. However, be careful in consciously coordinating breathing with movements—controlling a breathing pace that is too slow or too fast to match your movements can have unwanted physiological and energetic effects. While I occasionally explore breath-movement coordination, most of the time, I follow the advice of one of my teachers who emphasized the principle, "Let the body breathe you."[8]

DIAPHRAGMATIC OR TAN TIEN BREATHING

Diaphragmatic or tan tien breathing (sometimes called abdominal or belly breathing) is natural, deep breathing without any forceful effort (think of a sleeping baby). To get a sense of this type of breathing, I sometimes use the image of a balloon centered in the abdomen. During inhalation and exhalation, imagine that the balloon is expanding or stretching, and then deflating. The inhalation and exhalation is sometimes coordinated with an opening and closing movement of the hands and arms in front of the abdomen. The idea is to take unstrained, slow, deep, rhythmic breaths.

Here's how I introduce tan tien breathing during a seated resting meditation:

Sit comfortably, feet flat on the ground, palms resting on your thighs, eyes closed, and sitting upright. Relax your mouth, tongue, and jaw. Allow your whole body to relax . . . allow your thoughts to relax . . . allow your breath to relax. Now imagine that you have a balloon in your abdomen, and as you breathe in, the balloon gently inflates. As you exhale, the balloon naturally deflates. Imagine that the air you are breathing in is mist-like and filled with a vibrant, positive, or healing nourishing energy—whatever qualities you sense will best balance your body today. As you breathe in, simultaneously move your arms in front of your abdomen to mimic and encourage the expanding of the balloon. As you exhale, allow your arms to return to a more neutral position, with the palms facing inward toward the abdomen. Repeat this inhale-exhale cycle 9 to 36 times. As your body relaxes and your breath deepens, allow the volume of the expanding balloon to grow to include the middle and upper regions of the torso as well as your feet. When you are done, sit comfortably in an upright position. Return your hands to rest on your thighs and simply relax, especially the abdomen and feet, and observe changes throughout the whole of your body (without "thinking").

Better Breathing through Tai Chi

Studies have shown better respiratory function in Tai Chi practitioners compared to those who are sedentary. What's more, Tai Chi appears to slow the loss of respiratory function in older adults over time in studies up to five years long.[10]

Better breathing through Tai Chi may be due in part to increased torso flexibility.[11] This increase is likely due to stretching, a less-flexed posture, and the impact of deeper, more mindful breathing while practicing Tai Chi. You would expect that regular, deep breathing would keep your lung tissues more flexible and help them maintain their elasticity, but no long-term studies have proven this assumption yet.

Slow, diaphragmatic breathing may also improve lung efficiency, allowing more oxygen to reach the capillary-rich alveoli for better absorption of oxygen into the blood.[12]

Taking Control of Breathing

Breathing, like digestion of food, occurs naturally below the level of your consciousness. This automatic control is great—it allows you to go about your day, even while you sleep, without having to remember to breathe. However, breathing can also be voluntarily controlled. You can learn to breathe more deeply, slowly, smoothly and mindfully, and improve your respiration as well as bring it into greater balance.

Slow, deep breathing encouraged in Tai Chi positively affects the balance between the sympathetic (arousal) and parasympathetic (calming) aspects of the nervous system, which in turn, affects many other processes, including blood pressure regulation and immune function.[13] We now widely recognize that many chronic diseases, such as heart failure and COPD, are highly associated with overactive sympathetic nervous activity. This connection may partially explain why in our clinical trial of heart failure, as well as in other's heart trials, Tai Chi seems to affect heart-lung symptoms and quality of life positively.

Psychological Well-Being and Mood

The meditative movements and exercise components of Tai Chi can help you manage stress, both the psychological and physiological responses to stress. Tai Chi may even rehabilitate stress-related, inefficient breathing. Shallow breathing is associated with the physiological flight-or-flight response. Slow, deep, mindful breathing is associated with more relaxation and more-efficient gas exchange. In fact, healthy breathing patterns are associated with less hostile behavior and improved cognitive function as you age.[14] Chapter 9 summarizes research supporting the more general positive effects of Tai Chi on stress and mood.

Internal Physical Massage

In Tai Chi, one of the main functions of breathing is to massage the internal organs and body tissues. Diaphragmatic breathing is associated with internal pressure changes, so the idea of the internal organs being moved around and "massaged" during Tai Chi seems quite logical. One of my

Tai Chi teachers, Robert Morningstar, likened breathing to blowing up a balloon under water. Pressure changes caused by the expansion of the balloon-like lungs displace fluids and fluid-filled tissues surrounding the lungs and the diaphragm. This displacement, in turn, leads to what in effect are liquid pressure waves in surrounding tissues.

When coordinated with specific Tai Chi postures and movement patterns, these pressure waves can be directed throughout the body. A handful of studies on breathing physiology support the idea that deep breathing generates measurable changes in abdominal pressure—that is, breathing creates an internal massage.[15] Deep breathing is also associated with altered blood flow throughout the body.[16]

Cognitive Focus and Attention

Attention to the breath is central to Tai Chi, as well as many Eastern healing and meditative traditions. To achieve enlightenment, Buddha is said to have sat for an extended period to become aware of each breath, from moment to moment, feeling its flow through the nostrils, the rise and fall of the chest, its movement from the nose to the belly—not trying to control or fix it, just noticing it. In this sense, you can use the breath to develop focus. This idea of being mindful as the breath comes in and goes out is a way to practice living in the present moment without the unfocused, distracting thoughts of the "monkey mind." This idea is captured in a quote by one of the leading teachers of Buddhist meditation in the West, Thich Nhat Hanh: "Feelings come and go like clouds in a windy sky. Conscious breathing is my anchor."

Energy Flow

Western researchers are just beginning to examine the physiological and biophysical effects of bioelectricity within the body. For a Western scientist, breath-related internal pressure changes and autonomic system–mediated changes in blood flow may partially explain how breathing affects energy flow, just as, according to traditional Chinese medicine, blood and Qi flow are connected. Although studies are lacking, it is plausible that each breath induces electrical charges in the fascia, fluids, nerves, and blood. Your breath can direct the movement of energy and—

when combined with the intention and shape of Tai Chi—can lead to rich patterns of energy flow throughout your body, sometimes along very specific pathways relevant to healing as well as the martial applications of Tai Chi.

CLINICAL RESEARCH ON TAI CHI FOR RESPIRATORY CONDITIONS

A growing body of research suggests that the slow, rhythmic breathing during Tai Chi, along with its other active ingredients, may enhance the health of patients with COPD and asthma.

ON BREATH AND SPIRITUALITY

The link between breath and vital energy is not unique to Chinese medicine. The concept of "Pneuma," the root for pneumonia, pneumatics, and other lung and breath-related contemporary words, derives from the ancient Greek word for breath. In ancient Greek medicine, Pneuma was considered the "Breath of Life" or a form of kinetic energy responsible for all function and movement.

Breathing may have a spiritual connotation as well. From the perspective of energy exchange, breathing from the universe into the body and back out creates an exchange that makes us feel more "porous," less distinct, and more connected to, and integrated with, the larger environment around us. Many Tai Chi practitioners say they feel connected to part of some larger whole—perhaps, using Ted Kaptchuk's description of Chinese cosmology, part of what he calls the "Web that has no Weaver."

In Chinese, one of the characters for breath often is used synonymously with the character for Qi.[17] In Latin, the word for breathing is *spiritus,* which serves as the root for "inspiration" and "spirit." In the New Testament, the Holy Spirit is used interchangeably with Pneuma; it also includes references to the breath of God. In his book on Tai Chi imagery, Martin Mellish writes that if there were one translation of "Holy Spirit" into Chinese, it would simply be Qi.[18]

Clinical Research on COPD

"I think the thing that changed the most after going through the Tai Chi for COPD study at Harvard was understanding my breathing better, my breathing patterns, and breathing deeply," says James, age 55. "I'm one who is used to shallow breaths, but now I try to be much more aware of that. If I'm having a bad day, I try to give myself some time to rest and get my breathing back in sync.

"I like the pace of Tai Chi, the gracefulness of it, and that it's non-stressful," he says. "If you're doing other forms of exercise, you often have more on your mind. If you're on the treadmill or the bike, you're watching to see how long you're on, the speed you're going, whereas in Tai Chi it's nothing—it's just you."

Chronic obstructive pulmonary disease (COPD) is one of the most common lung diseases. The two main forms of COPD are chronic bronchitis, which is defined by a long-term cough with mucus, and emphysema, which is defined by destruction of lung tissue over time. Most people with COPD have a combination of both conditions.

COPD is projected to be the third leading cause of death in the United States by the year 2020, and it is the only major disease with an increasing death rate. An estimated 16 million Americans are currently diagnosed with COPD, and an additional 14 million or more still may be undiagnosed because they are in the beginning stages of the disease with minimal symptoms and therefore have not sought health care yet. The total estimated annual cost of COPD is more than $32 billion.[19]

The leading cause of COPD is cigarette smoking. The more a person smokes, the more likely it is that person will develop COPD, although some people smoke for years and never get COPD. The most common symptoms include cough with mucus, shortness of breath (dyspnea) that gets worse with mild activity, fatigue, frequent respiratory infections, and wheezing.

Conventional pulmonary rehabilitation programs focus on aerobic exercise and strength training to improve exercise capacity, quality of life, and symptoms in patients with COPD.[20] Tai Chi extends the breathing techniques taught in pulmonary rehabilitation by integrating novel elements, such as progressive relaxation, imagery/visualization, mindfulness of breathing and overall body sensations, postural training, and coordinated patterns of breathing and movement. These additional therapeutic elements make Tai Chi an effective adjunct to conventional rehabilitation. Mind-body exercises like Tai Chi may also allow patients with COPD to feel more confident about their ability to exercise and entice them to continue to exercise, which, of course, has the potential for lasting benefits.

COPD Study Results

Several studies have been completed or are under way to evaluate Tai Chi for COPD.

In our group, we have completed a small, pilot randomized controlled trial designed to determine the feasibility of administering a Tai Chi program to improve the quality of life and exercise capacity in COPD patients. We randomized 10 patients, average age 66, with moderate-to-severe COPD, to 12 weeks of Tai Chi plus usual care or usual care alone. The Tai Chi training consisted of a one-hour class, twice weekly, that emphasized gentle movement, relaxation, meditation, and breathing techniques.[21]

Our participants told us they enjoyed the Tai Chi program and said they could participate without experiencing any adverse reactions. After 12 weeks, the Tai Chi participants felt significant improvement in chronic respiratory symptoms compared to the usual-care group. The Tai Chi group also had slight improvements in their six-minute walking distance, depression, and shortness of breath. Our conclusion: Tai Chi as an exercise appears to be a safe, positive adjunct to standard care and warrants further investigation. Led by Drs. Gloria Yeh and Marilyn Moy, our group is now conducting a much larger trial sponsored by the National Institutes of Health; this trial compares Tai Chi to both meditative-breathing exercises (isolated out of the Tai Chi program) as well as to a non-exercise education program.

An already completed large, randomized controlled COPD trial conducted in Hong Kong compared a program of Tai Chi Qigong to walking plus breathing exercises or usual care for three months. The Tai Chi Qigong group improved key measures of respiratory function and participated in higher levels of activity. The group also reported greater improvements in respiratory health–related quality of life.[22]

After initial gains in lung function from a pulmonary rehabilitation program, COPD patients typically lose these benefits after about six months. One reason may be due to poor compliance with existing forms of home exercise, such as walking and weight training. Studies show that Tai Chi–like exercises, including Qigong, may help sustain the gains COPD patients make after they complete pulmonary rehabilitation.[23]

The Epidemic of Asthma

"I had asthma when I was little and 'outgrew' it, but I started to get winter colds that dragged on and on, so my doctor prescribed an inhaler," says Liz, 65, a retired musician. "I didn't want to get hooked on the inhaler. Instead, I really began to focus in on different kinds of breathing during Tai Chi classes."

Through Tai Chi, Liz learned how to tune in deeply to her breathing. "If I felt resistance in my breath, I visualized where the tightness was—a space in the left edge of my right lung—and I literally felt it let go," she says. "Sitting relaxed and breathing deeply, I paid attention to my breath. This allowed my mind to rest and my body to feel refreshed with each breath."

Tuning into her breathing at rest "has been a great discovery. I'm not always gasping for breath. I have a reference point that is more prevalent than I thought," she says. The good news is that even though she got a few short-lasting colds last winter, she didn't have any asthma attacks and didn't need to use her inhaler.

Asthma is characterized by inflammation of the air passages, resulting in the temporary narrowing of the airways that transport air from the nose and mouth to the lungs. Symptoms include difficulty breathing, wheezing, coughing, and tightness in the chest. In severe cases, asthma can be deadly.

About 23 million Americans, including almost 7 million children, have asthma. The numbers of people with asthma are increasing at an alarming rate. Experts estimate that the number of asthmatics will grow by more than 100 million by 2025. The overall prevalence of asthma increased 75 percent from 1980 to the mid-1990s, and among children under the age of five, it increased more than 160 percent. The annual economic cost of asthma is $19.7 billion, with adults missing more than 10 million workdays and children missing 13 million school days each year due to asthma.[24]

It is not clear what underlies this epidemic. Research suggests it's unlikely to be just one factor, but rather a mixture of factors, including sedentary lifestyles, static indoor microenvironments, poor diets predisposing to obesity, and stress, all of which may influence asthma.[25]

Asthma Clinical Studies

Some preliminary studies suggest that Tai Chi, as well as other mind-body exercises such as Qigong, may be helpful for asthmatics, both children and adults.

Twelve weeks of Tai Chi training improved the lung function of children with asthma in a small Taiwanese study. We need larger studies with longer periods of follow-up to show whether Tai Chi can also help reduce the severity of asthma symptoms in children.[26]

A small study from Thailand also suggests adult asthma sufferers may be able to better control their breathing and improve their exercise performance using Tai Chi training. After six weeks of Tai Chi training, the patients said they felt more comfortable during a six-minute walk and increased their maximum work rate and maximum oxygen consumption. We need further research to show whether Tai Chi can help control asthma.[27]

8

Sharpen Your Mind

"In my mid-30s, I began to experience neurological problems," says Taylor, a 44-year-old marketer. "Stress in my life triggered an autoimmune response. When I woke up, my limbs would be numb and they felt as if they weighed 100 pounds. I had been an athlete all my life, and now it was a chore just to get dressed in the morning." After neurologists ran a battery of tests, they told Taylor her condition was similar to multiple sclerosis.

She went on and off multiple medications over a dozen years, and then found Tai Chi. "From the first class, I enjoyed it and felt better," Taylor says. "The sitting meditation made my brain and body feel so calm and relaxed, even after class."

Now Taylor does a group Tai Chi class once a week and takes private lessons at home as well to help her learn the form. "I feel that I'm making good progress. I definitely think I will learn the entire form. I really believe that Tai Chi is helping me rewire my brain," she says.

The complexity of the human brain truly is amazing. Your brain is a liter and a half in volume and weighs an average of 2.8 pounds; it contains approximately 100 billion nerve cells (neurons)—more than the number of stars in Milky Way—with an average of 7,000 synaptic connections for each neuron. The cerebral cortex, the most recently evolved part of the brain, and the one centrally involved in "thinking," has about a trillion synapses per cubic centimeter, with a computational capacity that far exceeds any computer imaginable. To stay fed, your brain has 100,000 miles of tiny blood vessels and uses 20 percent of your body's total oxygen, despite weighing in as only 2 percent of your body's mass.

To take care of yourself, you need to take care of your brain. Your brain is a huge part of what makes you "you." Modern neuroscience supports that the brain is the home to your mind and personality; it houses cherished memories and future hopes. It orchestrates the symphony of consciousness that gives you meaning, passion, and emotion. The brain is perhaps the only organ we cannot replace with a transplant without changing our fundamental identity.

One of the biggest developments in neuroscience in the past 20 years has been our ability to understand the dynamic qualities of the brain. Until recently, scientists believed that the brain produced new cells only early in life; in adults, the fixed allotment of cells started to dwindle. Now research shows that new brain cells grow throughout all stages of life, replacing dying ones, and existing cells become connected to new communication networks within the brain.

Many aspects of the brain continuously remold, a process known as neuroplasticity. This brain remodeling helps you meet the ever-changing physical, cognitive, emotional, and environmental demands that you are exposed to over the course of your life. The brain is now viewed as an organ built to last, and change, even well into later life. In the words of Professor Richard Davidson, Director of the Waisman Laboratory for Brain Imaging and Behavior at the University of Wisconsin at Madison and a leader in field of meditation research, the brain is "a life-long learning machine."[1]

With the advent of sophisticated medical-imaging technology, researchers have gained insight into the brain's structure and function and how it regulates basic physiological functions, such as the pumping of the heart and breathing of the lungs. In addition, this unprecedented research has led to a better understanding of the connections between the body and the mind—for example, how exercise and emotional stress can affect memory, or how mental focus helps us sustain balance or learn new movements. This research is also beginning to elucidate the understanding of how mind-body therapies such as Tai Chi and meditation help to enrich physical and cognitive function as you age.

This chapter discusses how the multiple active ingredients of Tai Chi— including aerobic and mobility exercises, stress reduction, learning new skills, engaging in socially rich leisure activities, and focused attention— may contribute to brain health, which, in turn, may lead to optimal cognitive and physical function. You'll read about a brief comparison of Western and Eastern concepts of the relationship between the mind, brain, and body, and learn about the concept of plasticity and age-related changes in cognitive function and memory. This chapter also explores specific, subtle aspects of the mind-brain-body connection, including how Tai Chi's emphasis on mental attention and imagery may improve how you move, and how this is relevant to balance, the ability to learn sequences of movements, and sports performance. Finally, you will understand how the meditative, mindfulness aspects of Tai Chi lead to improved focus and attention, and possibly long-lasting changes in the brain's structure and function.

Body-Brain-Mind Connections: West vs. East

From antiquity, philosophers, scientists, and spiritual thinkers have proposed various theories regarding the origin of what we call the mind. The Greek physician Hippocrates, the father of Western medicine, wrote that the brain is the "organ of the mind." The idea that the mind is essentially a projection of the brain remains the predominant biomedical theory today. The American Heritage Stedman's Medical Dictionary defines "mind" as "the human consciousness that originates in the brain and is manifested especially in thought, perception, emotion, will, memory, and imagination." According to this framework, the mind has a material basis—that is, the brain.

Many Eastern traditions view the relationship between the mind-brain-body as a continuum, with less of an emphasis on one having responsibility for the others. In traditional Chinese medicine, no absolute distinctions exist between what the West classifies as the mind versus the activity of the brain versus the physiology of the physical body. The mind helps shape what we call the body, and the body influences what we call the mind.

This mind-body connection is referred to as the Shen-Jing continuum. *Shen* is generally used to characterize a person's less physical or tangible qualities, such as the thought, spirit, or emotion. A traditional Chinese medicine doctor may look at the vitality expressed in your eyes or face to gain insight into your Shen. *Jing* refers to tangible material qualities, such as the organs, flesh, and blood.

In this Chinese medical framework, you are a field of Qi, with Shen and Jing simply representing different vibrational or qualitative states of energy or information. This idea is somewhat analogous to the three different energy states of water (water, ice, and steam). Like the Tai Chi concept of yin and yang, Jing and Shen arise mutually and are interdependent. That is, the brain informs the mind and the rest of the body, including organs such as the heart and liver, as well as other tissues, including muscles, bones, and interconnecting fascia. What's more, the mind shapes the body and brain. This notion parallels more-contemporary ideas emerging in the field of cognitive science related to the principle of embodiment.[2]

The Shen-Jing framework is central to Tai Chi philosophy and training. In Tai Chi, the body and mind are inseparable—the body is considered a dynamic, organic site of meaningful experience, not just a physical object that is distinct from the self or the mind. Consequently, Tai Chi emphasizes simultaneous, integrated training of mind and body. In his provocative book, *Mind over Matter: Higher Martial Arts,* martial arts master and scholar Shi Ming states:

> When all is done and said, the origin, core, and highest level of the inner and outer work of martial arts are all in refinement of mind. The basic principle of the training, that inside and outside join, enables people to gradually attain intercourse and merging of the totality of body and mind.[3]

Shi Ming highlights how studying this interaction from a scientific perspective, as it manifests in Eastern practices like Tai Chi, offers researchers a unique opportunity to further the understanding of basic human health, physiology, and nature.

Brain Plasticity

In the past few decades, neuroscientists have come to appreciate that brain changes occur throughout life. Your neural networks continually reorganize and reinforce themselves in response to new stimuli and learning experiences. The brain's ability to change and shape itself according to experience is called plasticity—from the Greek word meaning "molded" or "formed."[4]

Your brain's plasticity is analogous to general physical training and conditioning. If you go to the gym several times a week, you will build muscle and become more physically fit over an extended period. Similarly, a wide variety of activities, such as learning a new language, playing a musical instrument, or doing meditative exercises like Tai Chi, can affect the brain's structure and function.

Brain plasticity in response to learning can manifest itself in many ways. Sometimes, new brain cells grow and replace dying ones. New cells form in the hippocampus—one of the key memory centers in the brain— well into the later years of life. Existing brain cells can also grow and connect with other brain cells, and extend the intricate branches of nerve fibers called dendrites (from the Latin word for "tree") to foster communication between nerve cells. Or, neurotransmitters (chemical substances that regulate cell-to-cell communications) and neuroreceptors (the docking point where chemical messages are received) can change and affect brain function. These changes can affect how individual parts of the brain work, as well as how these parts network together.[5]

A landmark study by (now) Harvard Professor Alvero Pascual-Leone was one of the first to demonstrate how both physical and mental practices can affect the brains of adults. People who had never studied piano were randomly assigned into three groups. One group learned one-handed, five-finger piano exercises over a five-day period, training for two hours a day. A second group sat in front of the piano for the same period and simply visualized their fingers performing the same exercise. They were to imagine the sound, but were not allowed to touch the piano keys or to rehearse the exercise by moving their fingers in the air. The third (control) group did not practice.

All three groups had their brains mapped before and after the experiment. The surprising results: five days of physically practicing these piano movements led to increased activity in the area of the brain that represents finger muscles, but, even more remarkably, five days of mental training also led to the same plastic changes in the brain. Mental training alone, however, resulted in less physical mastery of the sequences.[6] This study shows that mental training, like the mind components of Tai Chi practice, may play an important role in motor control and, along with physical practice, can help shape the brain.

How Tai Chi May Keep Your Mind Sharp

Starting around age 50, most people experience some brain changes that directly affect their working memory, as well as other cognitive functions, such as the ability to perform multiple tasks, pay attention to detail, and mentally process information quickly. Age-related decline results from several changes in the brain. These changes include decreases in the number of synapses, or connections, between neurons; reductions in the number and function of chemical receptors across synapses; and fewer bundles of fibers that transmit messages throughout the central nervous system.

As an unprecedented number of Americans approach old age, a growing concern exists about the loss of cognitive function that is often attributed to aging. Mayo Clinic researchers have found that by around age 70, one in six people have mild cognitive decline. Mild cognitive decline is considered an intermediate state between the cognitive changes of aging and the earliest clinical features of dementia, particularly Alzheimer's disease.[7]

The good news is that due to your brain's plasticity, you may be able to improve your cognitive function and offset age-related decline through exercise, stress reduction, learning new tasks, staying socially active, and learning how to focus better—all integral elements of Tai Chi training. A body of studies on Tai Chi and cognitive function lend support to the promise of Tai Chi for your brain and mind's health. Two randomized trials have evaluated Tai Chi in adults diagnosed with moderate levels of dementia. In one large Chinese trial, a group assigned to Tai Chi showed greater improvements in cognitive performance after one year than a group assigned to a stretching and toning program. In addition, fewer of those in the Tai Chi group progressed to dementia. The authors' conclusion: Tai Chi may offer specific benefits to cognition, but we need longer follow-up periods to make stronger conclusions.[8]

In a smaller study at the University of Illinois, a group of adults with dementia showed small increases in mental ability and self-esteem after 20 weeks of a combination of Tai Chi, cognitive behavioral therapies, and a support group as compared to an education group, who had slight losses of mental function.[9] Interestingly, a follow-up companion study reported benefits of Tai Chi training to the caregivers of people with dementia.[10]

A few randomized trials have evaluated the impact of Tai Chi on cognitive function in healthy older adults. A University of Arizona study found that Tai Chi led to greater improvements in cognitive function, including attention, concentration, and mental tracking, as well as balance, after six months compared to either education or exercise groups. These differences in cognitive function between the groups persisted for 12 months.[11] Another randomized trial reported that 40 weeks of Tai Chi training led to increased brain volume and greater performance in multiple aspects of cognitive function, when compared to walking, being part of a social group, or not receiving any intervention.[12]

Results are mixed on whether Tai Chi helps improve executive function—that is, cognitive skills related to multitasking, managing time efficiently, and making decisions or doing a challenging mental task while maintaining one's balance.[13] Some studies of longer-term Tai Chi practitioners add further support to the potential benefits of Tai Chi on cognitive function in older adults. Hong Kong researchers found that a group with an average of eight years of Tai Chi training outperformed an exercise group and a non-exercise group in evaluations of attention and memory.[14] In a Chinese study, older adults who practiced mind-body exercises, including Tai Chi and Qigong, or cardiovascular exercises, such as tennis or swimming, showed similar levels of memory. In addition, their learning capacity and memory was better than that of those who did not exercise regularly. It's not surprising that those who both practiced Tai Chi and did cardiovascular exercise performed the best on memory tests. But, the older adults who did no exercise showed signs of age-related decline, which was not seen among those who practiced mind-body exercises.[15]

The factors that attenuate age-related cognitive decline provide some additional insights into interpreting which of Tai Chi's active ingredients may contribute to better cognitive function.

Exercise

The impact of Tai Chi on cognitive function may be due, in part, to its effects on fitness. Physical activity and exercise, including moderate aerobic exercise (such as walking), can markedly slow or reverse age-related cognitive decline. However, of particular relevance to Tai Chi, recent studies suggest that the benefits of exercise on cognitive function are not solely due to cardiovascular fitness, but also to motor fitness, which includes balance, speed, coordination, agility, and power. Motor fitness is also called skill-related fitness.[16]

Numerous prospective, randomized trials support a positive effect of physical activity, especially aerobic exercise, on cognitive function. Exercise can lead to a 50 percent improvement in cognition—in particular, executive function, or planning, scheduling, working memory, and multitasking. This effect is greater when aerobics is combined with strength and flexibility training compared to just aerobics alone.[17] Older adults who have no cognitive impairment and who participate in exercise programs, including combinations of training, may have more brain changes and greater neuroprotective effects.[18]

Moderate aerobic exercise appears to be better for your brain than stretching and toning. A University of Pittsburgh study showed that a group who did toning exercises lost slightly more than 1 percent of the volume of the front part of the hippocampus—a normal amount of brain shrinkage that comes with aging—in one year. However, a group of walkers (who walked up to 40 minutes at a time three times a week) had about a 2 percent increase in this area of the brain. In addition, the walkers achieved higher scores on memory tests, a result that makes sense since the hippocampus is a key memory center in the brain. They also possessed more brain-derived neurotrophic factor (BDNF), which is a brain protein that helps neurons to grow and survive.[19] Other trials support that exercise may protect cognitive function due to plastic, structural, and physiological changes in the brain.[20]

Some studies in older adults show an association between more exercise and less cognitive decline. Seattle researchers followed more than 1,700 adults, ages 65 years and up, who had normal mental function. The incidence of Alzheimer's disease and other forms of dementia among those who exercised more than three times a week for six years was much less than those who exercised less often. Interestingly, the positive, protective impact of exercise was the same for those with and without genetic predispositions for Alzheimer's disease.[21] Studies have correlated greater cognitive function with routine walking and stair-climbing, with those who walk the most (17 miles per week) showing the least cognitive decline.[22]

The combined positive impact of Tai Chi on both aerobic and motor fitness (balance, agility) may underlie its impact on cognitive function. Studies show that the benefits of exercise on cognitive function are not solely due to aerobic capacity and general fitness; mental health may also be affected independently by agility and motor fitness. Brain imaging studies show that those with higher levels of physical versus motor fitness use different parts of the brain to perform executive function tasks.[23]

Some research suggests Tai Chi's lower-intensity form of exercise may be more beneficial than all-out effort. Moderate activity may be protective, but long-term, strenuous activity, particular in women before menopause, may actually lower cognitive performance later in life.[24]

STRESS

You've probably forgotten something during a stressful situation—where you left the car key as you rush out the door, forgot a simple answer during an exam, or forgot the first words of a speech. This forgetfulness is, in part, due to stress hormones, especially cortisol, that interfere with the function of neurotransmitters and, therefore, disrupt how brain cells communicate with each other. Long-term stress and chronically high cortisol levels can make it difficult to think of or retrieve long-term memories. Tai Chi's favorable impact on stress and stress hormones may be part of the reason for its positive effect on cognitive function.

Stress is normal. How much stress is too much is not easy to say. The real issue with stressful events is not the events themselves but how you perceive, and then react to, them. Typically, during a perceived threat, the adrenal glands immediately release the hormone adrenalin into the bloodstream. If the threat is severe or persists for a few minutes, the adrenal glands then release cortisol into the blood. Once cortisol goes through the bloodstream and gets into the brain, it remains there much longer than adrenalin and continues to affect brain cells.

Chronic oversecretion of stress hormones can adversely affect your brain function, especially memory. Too much cortisol can prevent the brain from laying down a new memory or accessing already existing memories. Sustained stress specifically can damage the hippocampus, which you may remember is the brain area central to learning and memory.

What's more, the effects of chronic stress result in a continual loop of stress hormones. The hippocampus is part of the feedback mechanism that signals the adrenal glands when to stop producing cortisol. The more stress on the brain, the smaller the size of the hippocampus. Therefore, a stressed person has poorer control of cortisol, which leads to more cortisol-related damage. This negative feedback cycle ends up keeping stress levels high.[25]

Stress has a well-documented impact on age-related cognitive function.[26] A now-famous epidemiological study of Catholic nuns, priests, and brothers shed important light on the relationship between stress-related personality types and cognitive function. The Religious Orders Study, which researchers at the Rush Institute for Healthy Aging in Chicago conducted, measured "distress proneness" to quantify a clergy member's tendency to experience events as psychologically distressing. Those prone to high distress had a much higher decline in memory compared to those who had a low tendency toward distress.[27]

A unique aspect of this study was that the clergymen and women donated their brains to science when they died, enabling the researchers to do a postmortem examination of those brains to evaluate any evidence of Alzheimer's disease. Among those who died, those prone to high distress had twice the risk of developing Alzheimer's disease than those prone to low stress, even though their brains did not show the typical physical markers of Alzheimer's disease (that is, plaques and tangles). Proneness to experience psychological distress may be a risk factor for Alzheimer's disease, independent of whether a person has other markers of Alzheimer's disease.

Managing stress can counteract stress-related cognitive decline, and, again, this may be one of the ways that Tai Chi aids cognitive function. Studies show that Tai Chi may reduce anxiety and perceived stress (for more details, see Chapter 9 on mood and psychological well-being).[28] Some small studies suggest that Tai Chi and Qigong can reduce anxiety and stress by reducing cortisol levels, although this result is not consistent.[29] More evidence that Tai Chi's effect on stress may impact cognitive function comes from interviews of clinical trial participants, including one study with HIV patients, who reported Tai Chi enhanced their psychological coping abilities.[30]

MEDITATION AND THE BRAIN

Meditation studies, especially studies of mindfulness meditation, provide additional support for the positive effects of mind-body practices on stress and cognitive function.

One of the most exciting frontiers in mind-body research is the neurophysiological basis of meditation.[31] Here are the highlights of a few emerging trends:

- Meditation may enhance multiple dimensions of cognitive function. Systematic reviews of prospective clinical trials have found that meditation boosts working memory (the ability to hold information that you need to do complex tasks, such as reasoning, comprehension, and learning) and some aspects of executive function, although these conclusions are not based on definitive large-scale trials.[32] US soldiers who regularly practice meditation increase their capacity for working memory.[33] Other meditation studies report decreases in stress and cortisol levels, suggesting that stress reduction and an ability to reappraise stressful situations may benefit cognitive function.[34]
- Meditation can change memory-related brain activity and structure. A study at Harvard-affiliated Massachusetts General Hospital showed greater activation in the brain area associated with memory, as well as in areas related to attention and autonomic nervous system control.[35] Mindfulness-based stress reduction also can lead to brain changes in the regions involved in learning and memory processing, regulation of emotions, and taking perspective.[36] Long-term meditators also have a larger size hippocampus, studies show.[37]
- Meditation enhances the ability to focus and alters brain networks that enhance cognitive skills. Meditation produces behavioral changes that correspond to changes in the insula of

the brain, a key center for processes related to awareness,[38] as well as to changes in the function of brain networks associated with focus, sensory processing, and awareness of sensory experiences.[39]

LEARNING NEW SKILLS, LEISURE ACTIVITY, AND SOCIAL INTERACTIONS

Learning new skills, participating in leisure activities, and maintaining strong social networks have all been associated with a lower risk of dementia. Each of these factors may contribute to Tai Chi's positive effect on delaying a decline of cognitive function with age.

Learning New Skills

Many studies support the notion that learning new motor skills leads to cognitive changes in healthy adults. Learning to juggle may increase brain white and gray matter, studies show, and improve connections in the parts of the brain involved in making the movements necessary to catch a ball.[40] Importantly, this research also supports that older adults have the potential for learning new motor skills.[41] Similar studies show that music training can enhance behavioral and anatomical responses in the brain.[42] In addition, dance activities, which, like Tai Chi, include sensory, motor, and cognitive learning, also may help preserve cognitive function as people age.[43]

A remarkable study of London taxi drivers shows that learning can positively affect memory and the adult brain. Scientists at the University College London compared the brains of taxi drivers with those of bus drivers. London cabbies have to learn the layout of streets and the locations of thousands of places of interest to get an operating license. Bus drivers, who must deal with daily stresses of driving in London, stick to regular routes and do not need to memorize complex maps. It turns out that the taxi drivers' brains had more grey matter, which is associated with memory, in the mid-posterior hippocampus, which is where they store a mental map of London.[44]

So it's possible that the memory training associated with Tai Chi, which uses spatial relations, kinesthetic movements, and sequential learning, may contribute to increased cognitive function.

Leisure Activities

Many people consider Tai Chi to be a leisure activity, and participation in leisure activities has been associated with enhanced cognitive function in the elderly. Studies show that those who participate in leisure activities that involve thinking, such as reading, playing board games, playing a musical instrument, or dancing, have reduced rates of memory decline.[45]

Social Support

One of the key ingredients of Tai Chi is psychosocial support. Not surprisingly, research supports that older adults who have greater social networks have lower risk for cognitive decline, even after controlling for education levels or amounts of physical activity.[46]

MINDING THE MOVEMENT OF THE BODY

Movement and self-defense were driving forces in the evolution of animal brains, so thinking about the brain in context of Tai Chi makes sense since it is a martial art. The evolution of the earliest nervous systems was driven largely by the need to coordinate movement to help an organism go out and find food. Jellyfish and their relatives, who were the first animals to develop nerve cells, had a tremendous advantage over sponges and other "brainless" sedentary organisms that simply waited for their dinner to come to them. As larger hunters learned to prey on smaller hunters, and one another, animal brains evolved further to coordinate movements for self-defense so they could fight back and escape being eaten.

Movement is a key feature of Tai Chi, which, legend has it, was based on the movements of animals in battle. This phenomenon is not solely physical, but reflects the connection of the body and the mind. In the early stages of Tai Chi training, the mind often is occupied with learning gross motor sequences and movement patterns, which, as you read above, can be helpful for memory. However, after practitioners learn the gross move-

TAI CHI IMAGERY: SWIMMING IN THICK AIR

Here's one way I explore imagery in my classes:

"Soften any tensions in your body, and feel as if your body is flowing through water. Feel the flow and continuity of your movements. Master Cheng Man Ching, and many of his students, including my teacher Robert Morningstar, used to suggest practicing Tai Chi as if you were swimming in thick air. Keep the image of moving through thick air in your mind and body. This imagery will help you generate a gentle, palpable sense of drag or resistance to the movements. Meet this resistance with an appropriate, moderate amount of relaxed strength, and you may experience connectedness among your body parts and increased internal energy."[47]

ment patterns and become comfortable with them, the "thinking" mind begins to relax during practice and shifts more to observing the body in motion. As you progress further in Tai Chi, your mind begins to feel at home in your body as you move from posture to posture. Over time, you can begin to add intention through imagery, which enhances the quality and characteristics of the movements.

At even higher levels of practice, movement and thoughts become one; no time lag occurs between an intention to move, act, or react. You don't "try" to move a certain way, you just "do" the movement. No distinction occurs between consciously "thinking" about the movement and the body physically fulfilling that request. Master Wang Xiang Zhai, founder of Yi Chuan, another internal martial art, said, "In a fight, if you have to think and then respond, you are too late."

If you play sports, you may have felt this hyper-merged mind-body state, often described as "being in the zone." I recall an interview with legendary Dallas Cowboys running back, Hall of Famer Emmitt Smith (later a *Dancing with the Stars* champion), who talked about those unique moments where time seemed to slow down. He could see plays unfold in ultra-slow motion, which gave him the time to choose the best direction to run the ball. (Think Keanu Reeves' character in the *Matrix*). Others have described similar mind-body states during meaningful religious or artistic experiences. For most athletes, these moments are atypical, occasional, and fleeting. In contrast, those who have attained higher levels of Tai Chi and related mind-body training apparently can shift into these states of "being in the zone" at will and sustain them for significant periods.[48] You might say that they can dissolve the hyphen in the phrase "mind-body."

One practical expression of the merging of mind and body in Tai Chi is the quality of strength or force used in movements, especially when doing interactive Tai Chi with a partner. Tai Chi classic and contemporary texts distinguish between strength that is primarily generated by physical force, called Li, and an internal strength that reflects a more conscious movement, called Jin. Robert Chuckrow, a physics professor and high-level Tai Chi teacher and scholar, translated Li as ordinary strength and Jin as "educated" strength. He speculates that the use of intention and mindfulness in movement may generate low-level nerve impulses to muscles and surrounding tissues. These impulses are below the threshold of generating observable movement, but they may add an energetic quality or liveliness—an intrinsic energy—to Tai Chi movements. This liveliness may also prime your body so that you are more prepared to respond, if need be (for example, react to an attack), in a more efficient, coordinated manner. This model of a highly sensitized neuromuscular system could explain how your body becomes attuned to react quickly.[49]

MOVE BEFORE HIM

Two of my Tai Chi teachers, Robert Morningstar and Arthur Goodridge, believed that a highly sensitive Tai Chi practitioner could take advantage of intention during two-person Tai Chi, such as Push Hands. They regularly reminded me not to telegraph my movements by revealing my physical or mental preparation before I attacked. "For most Tai Chi players, all movements are preceded by an intention or thought to move in a certain way," they said. With practice, they said, I could learn to sense this energy and preempt or redirect the attack. They said this mechanism explained the Tai Chi principle repeated in multiple classics: "Wait for your partner to move, and then move before him!"

Motor Imagery

A fascinating branch of Western mind-body research adds support to the idea that intention affects movement and neuromuscular physiology. Many studies show that simply imagining a movement can improve the actual performance of that movement. This research also suggests that mental training, even without physical training, can change brain structure and function, similar to physical training. Motor imagery, as this process is called, is commonly defined as the cognitive process in which motor acts are mentally rehearsed without any overt body movements. Motor imagery has been widely used as a tool for improving sports performance and is increasingly being explored as a promising tool for rehabilitation of neuromuscular conditions, such as stroke and Parkinson's disease.[50]

One study conducted by researchers at the Cleveland Clinic Foundation demonstrated that healthy young adults who mentally practiced simple muscle movements could increase strength and change brain activity. One group in this trial practiced only mental exercises to increase pinkie strength. Researchers asked group members to think as intently as they could about moving the pinkie sideways without actually moving the finger. A second group practiced actual physical finger exercises, and a third (control) group did no mental or physical exercises. The mental and physical exercise groups practiced for 12 weeks, five minutes a day, five days a week. Compared to the control group, those in the mental exercise group increased their pinkie muscle strength by 35 percent and those doing the actual physical exercises increased their pinkie strength by 53 percent. What's more, significant increases in a measure of the brain's ability to control voluntary muscle contractions accompanied the improvement in muscle strength for the motor imagery group.[51]

In other studies, as Chuckrow speculated, motor imagery or intention resulted in measureable changes in muscle activation. For example, in one study, participants imagined lifting heavy weights, which enervated electrical activity in their bicep muscles.[52] Many other motor imagery studies report improved physical performance of a task and measurable changes in the brain; however, these studies have not observed changes in muscles. This result has led some researchers to hypothesize that the impact of motor training occurs primarily in the brain.[53] The lack of electrical response in muscles may be too low to be detected by instruments. Just the idea that mindful movement can improve motor function and learning is quite remarkable.

How are these results relevant to Tai Chi? The majority of studies to date suggest that the best way to learn a new physical movement is to combine motor imagery with actual practice of the movement, which works better than either motor imagery or physical practice alone. Successful results with this combined approach suggest that Tai Chi may be an excellent choice to rehabilitate and manage neuromuscular diseases, such as stroke-related paralysis, Parkinson's disease, and multiple sclerosis, and may explain why Tai Chi shows promise in preliminary evaluations of these conditions.[54]

In summary, the cognitive components of Tai Chi—perhaps the most unique aspect of Tai Chi—may underlie its benefits to the health of the mind and the body. Chapter 9 continues the exploration of the mind-brain-body interactions to address how Tai Chi impacts mood, psychological well-being, and sleep.

9

Enhance Psychological Well-Being and Sleep Quality

"When I go to Tai Chi class, whatever frame of mind I'm in, it changes and shifts. If I feel down, once the class gets going, chances are good my energy level increases within a few minutes," says Monique, age 58, a teacher. "After class, I go home and feel better about myself, and I sleep better. And when I do a class with younger people, it's invigorating for me."

During the rest of the week, Monique is not free of sadness, depression, or anxiety, "but when they come in, I recognize the feelings and know they will go away quickly," she says. "I can be with them. By doing Tai Chi, I have more confidence that I will not lose my footing in the world."

The vast majority of people I know who practice Tai Chi, including me, do so in large part for greater peace of mind. Like many of my students in my community-based classes, I typically arrive at an evening class a little stressed, exhausted, and physically tense after a long day at my demanding academic "day job." As I jokingly, but honestly, share with my students, Tai Chi research can be stressful! As the class unfolds, and through the practice of Tai Chi, we begin to get our blood and Qi flowing. Then, as we relax and redirect our preoccupied minds back into our bodies and focus more on the sensations of the moment, we begin to let go of many of the psychological and physical stresses we brought with us. While many of us admit that it's often hard to drag ourselves to class on some days, it's extremely rare that anyone leaves feeling worse. Sometimes the relief is only temporary, just a couple of hours' break from the stress. But for most people, including those who suffer from chronic psychological illnesses, such as anxiety and depression, Tai Chi provides the practical tools to manage or restructure behaviors and to cultivate coping skills, self-awareness, insight, resiliency, and hopefulness.

This chapter explores in depth the psychological benefits of Tai Chi, highlighting how the recent growth in mind-body practices parallels a greater appreciation of the role of mental health and stress in overall health, and how mind-body interventions make good sense for managing and treating mental health issues and improving psychological well-being. You'll read about a growing body of evidence that suggests Tai Chi can positively affect multiple aspects of psychological well-being, including depression- and anxiety-related disorders. Finally, you'll learn about sleep, a topic integrally related to both psychological and physical well-being, and you'll learn how Tai Chi may help you get the critical rest you need at night.

Mental Health and Psychological Well-Being

Joy and Temperance and Repose
Slam the door on the doctor's nose.
—Henry Wadsworth Longfellow

Those who keep their minds unimpaired within,
externally, keep their bodies unimpaired.
—*Nei Ye* ("Inward Training"),
fourth century b.c.e., author anonymous

The Western approach to health looks for the physical, material, biological basis of disease. Not that long ago, people who had mental disorders were considered to be "possessed." Even today, phrases like "it's all in your head" have a judgmental connotation: if no material basis for the problem seems apparent, it's not real. However, great changes in the appreciation and understanding of mental health are reflected in the rapid growth of psychiatry and many branches of psychology. Paralleling these changes, and perhaps even influencing them, has been our look to the East for practices that hold a more holistic appreciation for the health of the mind and body. A practical tool like Tai Chi can help sustain and better integrate the connection between mind and body.

This more integrated view of health is reflected in the World Health Organization (WHO) constitution, which states: "Health is a state of complete physical, mental, and social well-being and not merely the absence of disease or infirmity." The WHO defines mental health itself, as "a state of well-being in which the individual realizes his or her own abilities, can cope with the normal stresses of life, can work productively and fruitfully, and is able to make a contribution to her community." As with overall health, mental health is not defined as the simple absence of a mental disorder.[1]

STRESS AND EMOTIONAL RESILIENCE

I try to take one day at a time,
but sometimes several days attack me at once.
　　　　　—JENNIFER YANE (CONTEMPORARY ARTIST AND AUTHOR)

Stress is a natural part of being human. According to the National Health Interview Survey, 75 percent of the US population experiences at least some stress every two weeks, and half of these respondents report experiencing moderate or high levels of stress. Stress can be caused by many factors, including family or personal illnesses, social relationships, and work, among others. Considering only work, surveys conducted in the 1990s suggest that 40 percent of interviewed American workers reported their job was very or extremely stressful.[2]

Stress contributes to most chronic medical conditions, including heart disease, strokes, diabetes, chronic obstructive pulmonary disease, and autoimmune diseases. Not surprisingly, chronic stress also affects mental health, increasing the risk of depression, anxiety disorders, suicide, substance abuse, and other harmful behaviors. Public health leaders around the world have made stress reduction a leading health priority.[3]

The Subjective Nature of Stress

You know stress when you feel it. Yet, defining stress is still problematic. The Merriam Webster dictionary defines stress both as a causal factor, that is, "a physical, chemical, or emotional factor that causes bodily or mental tension and may be a factor in disease causation," and also as a response to "bodily or mental tension resulting from factors that tend to alter an existent equilibrium."

Stress means different things to different people. If you asked 10 people to discuss how they experience stress, you would get 10 different answers. Stress is a very subjective thing—both in what causes stress and in how people perceive it. The American Institute for Stress uses an excellent example of a roller coaster ride to illustrate this point.[4] On any given ride, people in the last car are likely to be holding on with eyes closed, feeling highly stressed and truly fearing for their lives, praying the ride will end soon. Those in the front row are likely to appear very different—eyes wide open, not holding on, hands waving up in the air screaming with elation, thinking they want to get on line again as soon as the ride ends. Those in the middle might be bored; it's just another ride. On the same ride, we find three very different perceptions of, and reactions to, this potential cause of stress.

It's now clear that stress has more to do with how you judge a situation than the situation itself. Dr. Hans Selye, a pioneering endocrinologist and stress researcher, wrote, "It's not stress that kills us, it is our reaction to it." Sometimes you may even react to misinformation—getting angry because you assessed a situation incorrectly, misheard what someone said or misread their body language, or recalled a very different scenario than what actually happened. Mark Twain beautifully captured this subjective source of stress and suffering when he wrote: "I am an old man and have known a great many troubles, but most of them never happened."

The good news is that within this subjective nature of stress lie some of the solutions to managing it. A growing body of research suggests that mind-body practices like Tai Chi can improve the accuracy of your perceptions and can increase the gap between your observation of an event and your conditioned reaction, giving you a bit more time or emotional distance to more clearly appraise it and act accordingly. Mind-body therapies may improve your ability to bounce back or recover from emotional stress, or what is known as resiliency.[5]

Emotional Resilience

Even if you are emotionally and mentally healthy, that doesn't mean you never experience stress or emotional problems. Everyone suffers disappointments, losses, and changes. These are all normal parts of life and can lead you to feel sad, anxious, or stressed. People who have good mental health have an ability to bounce back from stress, adversity, and trauma. This ability is called *resilience*. Emotionally and mentally healthy individuals have the tools for coping with difficult situations and maintaining a positive outlook. As you will see, Tai Chi may enhance your emotional resiliency through its emphasis on physically and cognitively "letting go" and paying attention to the present moment, as well as through the development of coping strategies——including, for example, techniques for feeling grounded and centered, meditative breathing, and imagery leading to an enhanced sense of being connected to supportive healing energy from nature.[6]

COMMON MENTAL ILLNESSES

Few families are untouched by mental illness. According to the National Institute of Mental Health, in a given year, approximately 57.7 million Americans suffer from a mental disorder listed in the Diagnostic and Statistical Manual of Mental Disorders (DSM) published by the American Psychiatric Association. That figure represents more than one-quarter of all American adults. In the United States and much of the developed world, mental disorders are the leading cause of disability among people aged 15 to 44.[7]

In addition to personal suffering, mental illness has huge medical costs. For example, direct medical costs in the United States associated with mental health were estimated to be $69 billion in 1996, nearly 8 percent of all medical spending. These values did not even include the high costs associated with Alzheimer's disease and substance abuse treatment, and did not consider the indirect costs associated with lost productivity at work, schools, and the home due to mental illness, which is estimated to be even higher than the direct costs.

The most common forms of mental illnesses fall into two classes: anxiety disorders and mood disorders. Anxiety disorders are the most common mental illnesses. In 2000, estimate show that one in six Americans experiences some form of anxiety disorder in any given year. Examples of anxiety disorders include phobias, generalized anxiety disorder, post-traumatic stress disorder, and panic disorders.[8]

Mood disorders, also known as affective disorders, are also widespread. The Surgeon General's Report on Mental Health estimated that 7.1 percent of the US population experiences some kind of mood disorders in a given year. Those who suffer with these illnesses share disturbances or mood changes, generally involving either mania (elation) or depression. Examples of mood disorders include major depression, bipolar disorder, and seasonal affective disorder.

Causes and Treatments

The precise causes of most mental disorders, like many other health conditions, are likely shaped by the interaction of biological, psychological, social, and cultural factors. Many mental health disorders run in the family. Depression studies report that even when identical twins are raised apart, up to a 67 percent chance exists that if one twin is clinically depressed, so is the other. Genetic makeup also plays a role in schizophrenia and anxiety disorders.[9]

However, even in conditions where a significant genetic predisposition to having mental illness exists, other factors clearly play an important role, suggesting that environmental, behavioral, and social factors may help prevent you from developing a mental health condition. Physical exercise, stress reduction, cognitive restructuring, and social interactions may be important elements of maintaining sound mental health and psychological well-being. Evidence presented in this chapter suggests that using tools like Tai Chi and related mind-body exercises in combination with pharmacological and behavioral interventions may help reduce the severity of some mental health conditions.

OLYMPIANS OF MENTAL HEALTH

In 2003, I had the opportunity to hear the Dalai Lama facilitate a fabulous discussion between leading cognitive neuroscientists and Buddhist meditation practitioners at the Mind and Life Conference at the Massachusetts Institute of Technology. Topics discussed included how the study of meditation may contribute to understanding cognitive behavior and how our brain works.[10]

One specific exchange stood out for me. One Western scientist asked the monks if researchers had not yet considered any outstanding questions or issues. One of the monks very eloquently and humbly, and with no judgment whatsoever, stated something like this: "It is clear from research that you have learned a great deal about mental illness, and what the brains of people suffering from mental illness look like. I think it would be interesting to explore what the brains of very healthy, happy people look like. What would the brain of an Olympian of mental health look like?"

In fact, a growing field of positive psychology is dedicated to the impact and biological basis of positive emotions, such as happiness and joy. Obviously, happiness alone may not cure most illnesses, but it might protect you against becoming ill. One systematic review of 30 studies found a strong association between happiness and longevity in healthy people.[11]

In studies with Tibetan monks who have extensive meditation experience, researchers have found striking increases in brain regions associated with happiness.[12] For example, while practicing one form of compassion meditation, which involves wishing for happiness and relief from suffering in others, advanced Tibetan Buddhist practitioners are capable of strongly and reliably inducing brain patterns associated with positive emotions.[13] And recent research shows that even short periods of this kind of meditation training can lessen distress and, even more remarkably, positively affect the immune system.[14]

To sum up, a growing body of evidence suggests that positive psychological states, such as happiness, joy, and compassion, are not entirely hardwired. Meditation can lead to changes in the brain and behavior, which may in turn contribute to mental and physical well-being. These meditation-induced changes in cognitive function, which likely occur during Tai Chi's "meditation in motion," may underlie some of the clinical benefits of Tai Chi on mental health.

TAI CHI AND PSYCHOLOGICAL WELL-BEING

"I have just gone through a provoking chapter in my life with my father dying and my mother being hospitalized," says Sandy, age 55, who is a high-powered executive. "Moods bubble up when I'm grieving, or just in general. With Tai Chi, I'm more cognizant of the moods, and I feel I have inner strength to deal with them. There is no 'mood manual.' Tai Chi helps replace the manual to help me navigate my emotions.

"When I go to the Tai Chi studio, I know I will feel better, more relaxed, my body at ease with the flow of emotions. It's like a vibrant, comfortable massage, and validation that my body responds to the flow."

Tai Chi's connection between mental and physical health is an essential tenet that links to its roots in traditional Chinese medicine. For example, in the first chapter of *The Yellow Emperor's Inner Classic* (*Huangdi Neijing*, approximately 111 C.E.), perhaps the most important ancient text in Chinese medicine, it was written: "If one is calm, peaceful . . . then true Qi follows. If essence and spirit are protected inside, from where can illness come?"[15]

More contemporary traditional Chinese medicine has a well-formulated, systematic correspondence between emotions and physical health. For example, excessive anger is believed to both negatively affect and reflect an imbalance in liver Qi, and excessive grief is similarly associated with imbalanced lung Qi. In balancing the flow of Qi, Tai Chi positively affects both mood and physical health.

Many people are attracted to Tai Chi explicitly because of its emphasis of integrating body, mind, and spirit. Yet, some classic Chinese texts tend toward emotional reserve, avoiding or even repressing emotional extremes. In some ways, this view contrasts with the more outgoing American culture, which values going more deeply into feeling and fully experiencing and expressing emotions.

Peter Deadman, a world authority on Chinese medicine and long-term practitioner of Tai Chi and related arts, wrote thoughtfully about this issue in the forward to Giovanni Maciocia's contemporary textbook, entitled *The Psyche in Chinese Medicine*. Deadman and Maciocia argue that one interpretation of this cultural difference may be that emotional self-discovery and expression was not as pervasive in China, perhaps due to Confucianism, where the self is often viewed as less important than society.[16]

Deadman and Maciocia were writing to acupuncturists treating patients with mental illnesses, but I think clear parallels with Tai Chi are apparent. We are currently experiencing a new stage in the evolution of Tai Chi in which emotional self-defense is more important for most practitioners than physical self-defense. Not surprisingly, many Westerners attracted to Tai Chi also undergo psychotherapy, and many use Tai Chi in combination with pharmacological treatments for mood disorders. Appreciating the apparent differences between traditional Eastern and contemporary Western cultures, Deadman offers a Tai Chi–like balance between reserved introspection and honest emotional exploration: "Quieting the mind, and dwelling in the present allows us to connect with what is universal and withdraw from the peripheral debilitating noise of what is emotionally unnecessary. At the same time, cultivating this deeper awareness allows us to feel and explore the truer currents of our emotional life. Perhaps in that way, we can hold a vision of emotional health that is neither repressive nor self-indulgent."[17]

As you will see, some evidence supports Tai Chi and this integrative approach to mental health.

CLINICAL EVIDENCE OF HOW TAI CHI IMPROVES PSYCHOLOGICAL WELL-BEING

A growing number of studies support the positive impact of Tai Chi on many aspects of psychological well-being. A comprehensive systematic review and meta-analysis published in 2010 by my colleague Dr. Chenchen

Wang based at Tufts University School of Medicine identified 40 studies conducted both in the West and in China that included an evaluation of Tai Chi for psychological outcomes. These studies primarily evaluated Tai Chi for psychological outcomes in people being studied for other health conditions, such as heart failure or arthritis. Also included were a small number of trials specifically designed to study the effects of Tai Chi for psychological disorders—that is, patients were recruited based on a clinical diagnosis of depression or anxiety.

The review concluded that Tai Chi appears to be associated with improvements in stress, anxiety, depression, mood, and increased self-esteem. More definitive conclusions were not possible due to methodological limitations of many of the studies. You'll read summaries of some of the studies below, as well as more recent findings that highlight a few other significant studies.[18]

DEPRESSION

> "I like everything about Tai Chi, particularly that I can go at my own pace. It has boosted my energy level to a point where I never thought I'd be," says Janice, a 59-year-old participant in one of our heart failure trials. "I was severely depressed before, crying almost every day. I can't take depression medication because of my heart. Now my outlook on life is so much higher. I can only attribute it to Tai Chi."

More than 20 Tai Chi studies identified in Dr. Wang's review suggest that Tai Chi tends to reduce depression. Nearly all of these studies included people diagnosed with other health conditions or relatively healthy, older adults. Dr. Wang has led three separate randomized trials of Tai Chi in patients with fibromyalgia, rheumatoid arthritis, and knee osteoarthritis. Her results show these patients experience significant reductions in depression, as well as changes in pain and musculoskeletal function.[19] Similarly, in our own recent trials with heart failure patients, we saw reductions in depression that paralleled overall improvement in quality of life and exercise capacity.[20] These studies show that chronic diseases and diminished psychological well-being are often intertwined. Shifts in one dimension of illness often lead to shifts in emotional health as well.

Well-designed randomized trials also show that Tai Chi can improve the quality of life of older adults whose symptoms of depression are not fully relieved through drug therapy. Those who do Tai Chi also make significantly greater improvements in physical function and do better on cognitive tests.[21] We have seen similar results in a small, exploratory randomized study of Chinese Americans with major depressive disorder, the majority of whom were also taking antidepressants. Working in collaboration with Dr. Albert Yeung and colleagues at the Massachusetts General Hospital Depression Unit, we found that 12 weeks of Tai Chi training led to trends in lessening of depression symptoms.[22] These studies nicely illustrate the potential of Tai Chi for treating depression in older adults and show how to combine Tai Chi with other therapies.

Anxiety and Psychological Stress

A number of studies report that Tai Chi improves anxiety-related symptoms. As with depression, the majority of studies primarily focus on relatively healthy adults or people who have other medical issues, such as HIV infections, balance disorders, or cardiovascular conditions.

In one representative study conducted in Taiwan, researchers randomly assigned 76 subjects who had high blood pressure to 12 weeks of Tai Chi or a control where they remained sedentary. Tai Chi led to marked improvements in blood pressure as well as anxiety levels as compared to controls.[23]

Dr. Wang also identified 11 studies (including five randomized controlled trials) that evaluated Tai Chi for stress. A meta-analysis of a subset of these studies showed significant improvements in stress management and psychological distress.[24]

How Tai Chi Impacts Mood

Tai Chi can affect your mood through exercise and stress reduction.

Exercise

Exercise is a powerful antidote to stress, anxiety, and depression. Paralleling the effects of exercise on cognitive function discussed in Chapter 5, multiple large-scale epidemiological studies have shown associations between increased physical activity and psychological well-being. Conversely, physical inactivity appears to be associated with the development of psychological disorders.[25]

Randomized trials show that exercise can elevate mood,[26] and may be as effective as medication in treating major depression in women who are over age 50[27] and also augment the beneficial effects of antidepressants.[28]

Exercise also seems to improve anxiety symptoms, although the results are less clear than in depression.[29] A systematic review that identified 40 studies of sedentary adults with chronic illness found exercise significantly reduced anxiety symptoms.[30] Other studies reveal that exercise can reduce tension/anxiety, depression, and other moods together with increasing perceived ability to cope with stress.[31] Small preliminary studies also suggest that exercise may be helpful for those suffering from post-traumatic stress disorder[32] and that adding exercise to group cognitive behavioral therapy can help relieve symptoms of generalized anxiety disorder, panic disorders, and phobias.[33] We need larger studies to better evaluate the role of exercise in these and other anxiety-related disorders.

SHAPING YOUR ATTITUDE
WITH TAI CHI

As you have read, the shapes you make with your body consciously or unconsciously affect how you breathe, your heart's efficiency, and the loads you place on your musculoskeletal system. Your body shape may also affect your attitude. You may use the word "attitude" to refer to a feeling, emotion, or mental state about an issue. For example, I regularly tell my teenage son, "Don't you give me any attitude." But the original use of attitude was in art as a technical term for the posture of a figure in a statue or a painting.

The relationship between shapes and emotional and energetic states is implicit in Tai Chi. For example, Master Yang Cheng Fu wrote, "If the crown of the head is not suspended lightly and alertly, the vital spirit cannot be raised." This relationship is also a fundamental tenet for many schools of manual therapy and body-centered psychotherapists that use body shape, in part, to diagnose emotional imbalances and guide treatment strategies.[34]

In 1872, Charles Darwin described how body language has evolved across many species to nonverbally communicate various emotions, such as aggressiveness and submissiveness. Contemporary researchers have shown that, for example, tilting the head slightly upward induces pride, and having a hunched posture elicits a more depressed feeling.[35]

Research by Amy Cuddy, a professor at the Harvard Business School, suggests that even short-term changes in how you carry yourself—your attitude—can markedly affect your emotions, including, for example, how you feel during a job interview or a key presentation.[36]

In a clever experimental design, researchers randomly assigned 42 participants to carry out poses that reflected a high-power or low-power person. Those in the high-power group held two poses for one minute each: the classic pose of sitting in a chair with feet up on the desk and hands behind the head, and then a standing pose with hands leaning on the desk. Those in the low-power group posed for the same period in two physically restrictive poses: sitting in a chair with arms held close to the side and hands folded on lap, and standing with arms and legs crossed tightly. The researchers took saliva samples before each pose and measured levels of testosterone and the stress hormone cortisol after the posing.

After controlling for the subjects' baseline hormone levels, the researchers found that high-power poses decreased cortisol by about 25 percent and increased testosterone by about 19 percent for both men and women. In contrast, low-power poses increased cortisol about 17 percent and decreased testosterone about 10 percent. Not surprisingly, high-power posers of both sexes also reported greater feelings of being powerful and in charge, and they were more likely to take risks as well.

Because of Tai Chi's emphasis on form and posture, and its explicit link to certain psychological states, it might be a great way to help you reshape your "attitude."

Stress Management

In the previous chapter, you learned that stress, especially chronic stress, can lead to heightened arousal that triggers stress hormones, such as cortisol, that are known to impact brain function. In addition, stress can alter other types of neurotransmitters in the brain, such as serotonin and dopamine, which, along with stress hormones, are linked to depression and other psychological disorders.[37]

Multiple active ingredients of Tai Chi are designed to reduce stress and, therefore, may help you manage stress and mood disorders. The slow, deep breathing associated with Tai Chi, for example, has been associated with reductions in anxiety and stress hormones (see Chapter 5). Another ingredient—imagery and visualization—leads to more positive thoughts; for example, imagining you are rooted like a tree creates a framework for releasing tensions down into the earth and offers more grounded sensations in the body. A third ingredient, discussed below, is through improved focus and attention, which helps to control the so-called monkey mind.

Meditative Focus and Taming the Monkey Mind

I was trying to daydream, but my mind kept wandering.

—Stephen Wright

One of the most profound ways Tai Chi affects psychological well-being is through mindfulness and focused attention. Meditation and cognitive behavioral research support that these meditative components of Tai Chi positively affect emotional well-being, as well as underlying brain circuitry.

RESTING IN THE MOMENT: GESTURE OF AWARENESS

During Tai Chi training, I regularly draw my students' attention to sensations in the present moment. I'll say, "Feel how your feet rest on the ground, feel the subtle movement your head makes (or does not make) as you shift from posture to posture, feel the movement of the breath in and out of your abdomen."

I regularly encourage them to "not think, but simply notice things as they are, without trying to fix or change them." In our everyday lives, we tend to always be doing or accomplishing something. The same may be true even during Tai Chi—you find yourself fixing the alignment of your feet or adjusting the posture of your spine. These adjustments can lead to greater efficiency and are part of training; but sometimes I find it valuable, if not essential, to encourage my students not to "fix" anything, but rather to just experience "being" during Tai Chi training.

One of my most influential teachers, Charles Genoud, developed and teaches "Gesture of Awareness," a practice that integrates principles of Eastern meditation and philosophy, sensory awareness, and movement.[38] His training emphasizes that the moment you actively attempt to fix or transform something—for example, your posture or breath, you leave that moment and embark on a journey toward an "imagined" future version of yourself—that is, one with better posture and more relaxed breathing. This practice is not necessarily bad, but for some people, it becomes a compulsive process and never stops. You can always attain a slightly better posture and deeper state of relaxation. With this behavior, even in Tai Chi, you may be attempting to reside in the present moment, but if, in your mind, you are always trying to catch up to an imaginary version of yourself, you cannot truly be present.

I used to live in Maine where the most famous line in answer to a question for directions is, "You can't get there from here." What I've learned from Gesture of Awareness and my Tai Chi training is that the exact opposite is true—you can only get "there" from "here." As you progress in your Tai Chi training, and relax and trust more of the yin, or non-doing, aspects of your practice, you will begin to cultivate a meditative curiosity or willingness to honestly meet and be yourself wherever you are. This mindful awareness, a resting and trusting of letting go into the sensations of the here and now, is a key active ingredient of Tai Chi that underlies many aspects of psychological and physical well-being.

Too much thinking, especially that endless chatter in your head as you wander from thought to thought analyzing relationships, worrying about the future, or simply daydreaming—what the Chinese call monkey mind—can affect your health.

According to a fascinating study by Harvard psychologists Matthew A. Killingsworth and Daniel T. Gilbert, it turns out that about half the time, you are thinking about something other than your immediate surroundings, and most of this daydreaming doesn't make you happy. In fact, the ability to think about what is not happening is a cognitive achievement, but one that comes at an emotional cost.[39]

To track mind-wandering behavior, they developed an app for the iPhone and asked more than 2,000 volunteers at random times how happy they were, what they were currently doing, and whether they were thinking about their current activity or about something else. During 47 percent of their waking hours, the volunteers were thinking about something other than what they were doing, and this mind-wandering typically made them unhappy. The more engaged they were in the activities in the here and now, the happier they were. Exercise was among a few of the activities that seemed to make people the happiest.

The bottom line: spend more time living in the moment, and you might be happier than if you are adrift in your thoughts and daydreams.

Improving mindfulness and focused attention indeed can improve your psychological well-being. One recent systematic review of mindfulness research concluded that a relationship exists between cultivating a more mindful way of being and a tendency to experience less emotional distress, more positive states of mind, and better overall quality of life.[40] In these studies, one of the main effects of mindfulness meditation appears to be reducing rumination—that is, taming the monkey mind.[41] These positive effects of meditation are further supported by research that shows mindfulness-based cognitive behavioral therapy prevents relapses in depressive symptoms.[42]

Together, these studies indicate that the active ingredients of mindfulness and focused attention in Tai Chi may help reshape the way you think and lead to enhanced emotional well-being.

Sleep and Health

Everyone needs an adequate amount of sleep. Sleep is no less important than air, water, and food. You most likely know what it's like to go without sleep and how lack of sleep affects your mood, stress level, and ability to function properly.

The National Sleep Foundation estimates that adults require seven to nine hours of sleep each night to stay healthy. Unfortunately, more than one-quarter of the US population reports not getting enough sleep on occasion, and from 10–15 percent of adults suffer from chronic insomnia. Insomnia is a particular problem among older adults—more than half of them suffer from insomnia. What's more, 85 percent of sleep problems remain untreated.[43]

The long-term effects of poor sleep have been implicated as a major contributor to chronic mental conditions, including depression, anxiety, and mental distress, as well as physical health issues, including diabetes, cardiovascular disease, and obesity. One recent study concluded that if you sleep less than six hours per night and have disturbed sleep, you stand a 48 percent greater chance of developing or dying from heart disease and a 15 percent greater chance of suffering or dying from a stroke.[44]

Treatment Options for Sleep Disorders

So-called "sleeping pills," usually sedative-hypnotic medications, remain the top choice to treat sleep disorders. These drugs may help some people for a short time, but their long-term use may have deleterious effects, particularly among older adults who may suffer from daytime confusion, falls and fractures, and adverse interactions with other medications. Some people also have what's known as rebound insomnia when they discontinue using these medications; that is, their sleep problems reoccur. Others develop tolerance to these powerful medications and need to use higher and higher doses, which can exacerbate the side effects.[45]

One alternative to drug therapy is cognitive behavior therapy. This type of psychotherapy shows results as robust as, if not more than, drug therapy.[46] However, physicians don't often prescribe cognitive behavioral therapy, which requires someone with advanced training and expertise. Tai Chi's active ingredients, which are similar to a number of components integrated in cognitive behavioral therapy, may help explain how Tai Chi favorably impacts sleep.

How Tai Chi Helps Sleep

> "Tai Chi to me is like a leaf that slowly floats down from a tree and then a cool breeze comes by. That is what Tai Chi is all about," says Ruth, a participant in our heart failure trial in her late eighties. "It is beginning to give to my body. I am able to sleep on my left side for the first time in four years. I feel fresher in the morning. It is loosening me up, and I am standing straighter."

Tai Chi can help you get a good night's sleep by reducing stress, improving your breathing, and relieving pain.

Stress

When you have had trouble sleeping, you may have tried a relaxation technique to reduce physical tension or intrusive thoughts. Not surprisingly, about one-quarter of insomniacs use relaxation techniques to help with their sleep problems, with deep breathing being the most commonly used relaxation technique. Other mind-body therapies, such as the relaxation response, progressive muscle relaxation, and hypnosis, have also shown promise in improving sleep.[47]

Middle-aged men, in particular, show an increased vulnerability of sleep to stress hormones, which may impair the quality of their sleep during times of stress. As men age, it appears they become more sensitive to the stimulating effects of corticotropin-releasing hormones. When Penn State researchers administered this arousal-producing stress hormone to both young and middle-aged men, the middle-aged men remained awake longer and slept less deeply. The researchers note that people who don't get enough of this "slow-wave" sleep may be more prone to depression. They suggest that stress may play a significant role in the marked increase of insomnia in middle-age men.[48] In another study, these Penn State re-

searchers compared patients with insomnia to those without sleep disturbances. They found that insomniacs with the highest degree of sleep
disturbance secreted the highest amount of cortisol, particularly in the
evening and nighttime hours. This data suggests that chronic insomnia
is partly related to the body's sustained state of hyperarousal in response
to stress.[49]

Breathing and Sleep Apnea

A serious concern for the brain is obstructive sleep apnea, a disorder of
interrupted breathing when muscles relax during sleep. It usually occurs in
association with fat buildup or loss of muscle tone with aging. The breathing pauses can last from a few seconds to minutes, often occurring 5 to 30
times or more an hour, according to the National Institutes of Health.
Typically, normal breathing then starts again, sometimes with a loud snort
or choking sound.

If you have sleep apnea, you often move from a deep sleep to a light
sleep when your breathing pauses or becomes shallow. As you might expect, the result is poor sleep quality that makes you tired during the day.
Sleep apnea is one of the leading causes of excessive daytime sleepiness.
Frequent awakenings due to sleep apnea may lead to personality changes
such as irritability or depression. Because it also deprives you of oxygen, it
can lead to a decline in mental functioning, as well as increase your risk of
a stroke or heart attack.[50]

Although no published studies have specifically evaluated Tai Chi for
sleep apnea, a few reasons suggest why it might help reduce the severity of
sleep apnea and improve sleep. First, Tai Chi training may lead to more
efficient posture, with greater muscle tone in the upper torso and neck. Tai
Chi, especially in sedentary people, may be a form of exercise that helps to
reduce or manage weight. Finally, Tai Chi includes rich breath training.[51]
Taken all together, these benefits may result in more open airways during
sleep, but research is needed to evaluate this hypothesis.

Pain and Sleep

Pain can lead to a serious intrusion into your sleep. If you have lower-back
pain, you likely experience intense microarousals (a change in the sleep

state to a lighter stage of sleep) each hour, which wake you up. Pain is frequently associated with insomnia and can be difficult to treat. Commonly prescribed medications, such as morphine and codeine, used to relieve pain can fragment sleep.

As discussed in Chapter 5, Tai Chi may reduce many forms of musculoskeletal pain and also improve the range of motion in your neck and back. Reduced pain and more relaxed sleeping postures may contribute to improved sleep seen in Tai Chi studies.

CLINICAL EVIDENCE FOR TAI CHI AND SLEEP

A few randomized trials have specifically studied the effects of Tai Chi on patients who had sleep problems; others have simply recorded sleep among healthy adults or noted the effects of sleep while evaluating Tai Chi for other conditions. University of California at Los Angeles researchers found 25 weeks of Tai Chi training helped 112 healthy older adults who had moderate sleep complaints to have better sleep quality as compared to controls enrolled in a health education program.[52] In another study of older adults who also complained of moderate sleep problems, researchers reported significant improvements in sleep for those who did an hour of Tai Chi three times a week for 24 weeks. The authors of these studies concluded that Tai Chi appears to be an effective, nonpharmacological approach to enhancing sleep, particularly for older adults.[53]

Other studies also show that Tai Chi seems to improve sleep quality. Our group observed more stable sleep among heart failure patients following three months of Tai Chi training.[54] Other studies have reported enhanced sleep following Tai Chi among those suffering with fibromyalgia and arthritis, as well as those recovering from cerebral vascular disorders, such as stroke.[55]

PART THREE

Integrating Tai Chi into Everyday Life

10

Tai Chi for Two

"I love Push Hands. After my first Push Hands class, I was laughing I was so happy," says Roger, age 47, a marketing manager. "It's easy to relax when you do solo Tai Chi, but when you match up with someone who is trying to push you, this challenges you to maintain what's going on both inside and outside of you. You have to be straightforward with your feelings, acknowledge where you are right away, and be honest with yourself."

"By nature, I'm not an extrovert, but my role at work is to do presentations and run meetings," continues Roger, who attends Tai Chi classes twice a week and does an hour of daily practice on his own. "I often found this was exhausting, but that doesn't happen anymore. I recently gave a presentation at a large conference, and I was completely unfazed. I attribute this to Tai Chi and Push Hands to helping me feel more comfortable in leading."

"I've also learned through Push Hands not to have an automatic defensive reflex when challenged, as happens to many people," says Roger. "One of the objectives of Push Hands is to yield, wait, and then return the force. This comes up all the time in my work. If I express an idea, and someone gets defensive, I don't get my hackles up any more.

I'm less apt to get into a cycle of defensiveness, and my meetings are more productive."

With diligent practice and a good teacher, and through the skillful application of active ingredients, Tai Chi can be a highly effective fighting art. To develop these skills, your Tai Chi training needs to include interactive partner exercises that complement your solo Tai Chi practice. "Tai Chi for two" exercises include techniques in simple pushing and yielding, rooting and strengthening, and both choreographed and free-form movements that stimulate dynamic balance, improve reflexes, and train your ability to neutralize and issue energetic attacks.

To become a good car driver, you need to learn more than the rules of the road. You need time behind the wheel, in traffic, and on the freeway to make progress. The same is true for developing martial arts skills in Tai Chi. You need substantial two-person training to apply Tai Chi principles effectively for self-defense. However, the benefits of partner work goes beyond martial training. Two-person Tai Chi exercises help you with your solo practice and your everyday life, even if you never thought about training in combat and self-defense.

For me, partner work is one of the most transformative and enjoyable aspects of practicing and teaching Tai Chi. Working with another person allows you to explore the application of Tai Chi movements and physical principles related to structure and movement. In addition, it provides a safe, structured, intimate framework to explore emotional and psychosocial issues. During physical interactions with others in Tai Chi, most people exhibit the same behaviors they adopt during encounters with people in general. Your emotional reactions to the physical, energetic pushing and pulling during two-person Tai Chi may mirror how you respond to suggestions from colleagues or advice from managers, or your preference to taking on a leadership or a subordinate role on work projects. You may learn how you typically handle uncertainty and how to learn from your mistakes. Partner work serves as a catalyst for progress in Tai Chi and, at the same time, can enhance your daily social encounters.

Most Tai Chi teachers integrate some form of two-person interaction in classes. Some teachers introduce these exercises early on in training as beginning students learn basic principles and solo forms. Others wait to teach these exercises to intermediate or advanced students who have already learned basic forms. In my Tai Chi school, I integrate interactive exercises into the most basic Tai Chi classes. Our Harvard team and other researchers have integrated simple two-person exercises into the protocols of clinical trials, including trials that target older or health-impaired adults.

This chapter delves into the advantages of partner work in Tai Chi. Partner work includes a great diversity of exercises and training goals. It is beyond the scope of this chapter to survey all of these exercises. Numerous excellent books are available that are entirely devoted to learning and mastering interactive Tai Chi exercises.[1] This chapter briefly introduces how working with a partner can be an excellent vehicle for exploring the active ingredients of Tai Chi, and how it can influence your health.

LEARNING THROUGH INTERACTIVE TAI CHI

Tai Chi has evolved over many generations through the transmission of kinesthetic knowledge passed down from teacher to student. A great deal of this transmission takes place nonverbally through mindful touch, heightened sensory awareness, and shared movement. In addition to developing your awareness and sensitivity, two-person exercises also enhance your strength and flexibility.

Mindful Touch

In working with some of my Tai Chi teachers and other high-level practitioners, I have had the sense that at the instant their hands touched my body, they knew a great deal about my physical and emotional state. Even before I could push them or evade their advance, they could sense my intention and "beat me to the punch." During these encounters, my teachers also seemed to convey nonverbal information intentionally; it was as if their touch and movements shared information with me about my movements and energy patterns. Becoming aware of their physical, energetic qualities provided me with a reference against which I could calibrate my own qualities and abilities.

Enhancing Form and Function

Touch is as important as vision and hearing for learning and retaining information. Tactile activities, such as playing with blocks, help children improve everything from their math abilities to thinking skills. Lack of touch can lead to emotional disturbances, as well as to lessened intellectual ability and physical growth, reduced sexual interest, and even immune system weaknesses.[2]

Educators increasingly appreciate what is called haptic or kinesthetic learning—that is, a learning style that occurs primarily through touch or movement. Hands-on physical engagement is the preferred learning style for approximately one out of every three people. The connection between touch and learning is instinctual, begins in infancy, and continues throughout life.[3]

Recent developments in robotic engineering have targeted haptic learning to teach people complex motor control skills. Subjects in studies have improved their piano playing by wearing a robotic glove that guides passive finger movement related to specific note sequences. Also, adults learning to write Japanese and Arabic characters have become more proficient when robotic devices applied provide gentle feedback to guide their hand movements during writing.[4]

Similarly, the tactile feedback you get from Tai Chi partner work can accelerate your understanding and practice of solo forms. Your body remembers the feelings of being rooted while pushing, of being relaxed and centered, and of being aligned while warding off an attack. Kinesthetically, your recall of these feelings adds intention and focus when you practice the solo form. Grand Master Cheng Man Ching regularly taught students to imagine an opponent in front of them while doing the solo form.

One of my teachers, Robert Morningstar, used a fun exercise to illustrate how essential tactile feedback is for learning Tai Chi. He would ask students to raise their right index finger in the air and, without thinking or planning, touch it to their navel. Then immediately after releasing the right hand, without thinking, they would repeat this with the left index finger. He called this his "Navel Academy Test." Some people said they could accurately touch their navel with both fingers, but I am not sure that all of them were being honest. Most people miss with one or both fingers.

Robert used this exercise to emphasize that even our own hands are not sure where our body's center is. Sometimes, one hand "thinks" it's in a different location than the other one does.

He argued that this is why you need a good Tai Chi teacher—to adjust your posture physically, to help calibrate your alignment, to point out where you are holding tensions, and to note any musculoskeletal imbalances. The nonverbal physical adjustments you get from your teachers, in addition to the kinesthetic feedback you get through partner practice, help you develop a level of self-awareness not accessible through solo practice alone.

Not surprisingly, research supports that Tai Chi training leads to heightened sensory awareness regarding the position and movement of the joints. This likely underlies Tai Chi's positive effects on balance and musculoskeletal health.[5] Other research conducted at Harvard Medical School by my colleague Dr. Cathy Kerr shows that experienced adult Tai Chi practitioners have greater tactile acuity—for example, heightened sensitivity in their fingertips to discriminate fine textures, compared to age-matched controls.[6]

Enhancing Strength and Flexibility

Continuously shifting your weight back and forth in concert with another person, including yielding to and issuing even the most gentle pushes, builds up your leg, arm, and core strength. Interactive Tai Chi exercises also expose you to a variety of movement patterns. As you practice with different partners in a class, your partner's size and movement patterns will vary. These variations in partners expand the diversity and range of motion of the joints you typically use during two-person Tai Chi, as compared with the solo form. With its emphasis on efficiency and minimizing muscular tension, interactive Tai Chi training enhances the Tai Chi principles of structural integration and connecting the body parts. The gains you make in strength and efficiency readily translate to everyday activities, such as lifting heavy objects without overtaxing or damaging individual body parts, in particular the back, shoulders, or knees.

To date, little research has specifically evaluated the potential benefits of interactive Tai Chi for musculoskeletal health. One small, randomized trial by researchers in China evaluated multiple forms of exercise for enhancing bone-mineral density in older post-menopausal women. Groups were assigned to rope skipping, Mulan Boxing (a Kung Fu–like dance form), Tai Chi solo form, Tai Chi Push Hands, and a control group that did no exercise. The Tai Chi Push Hands group made the greatest improvements in bone density.[7]

A second study helps interpret how Push Hands may improve bone density and highlights other unique features of interactive Tai Chi. In this study, researchers studied the biomechanics of a Tai Chi master who had 40 years' worth of experience as he defended himself against being pushed. His movements were compared to those inexperienced in Tai Chi. Movements were videotaped and digitized using a motion-analysis system, and the activity of muscle groups and the force of the feet on the ground were also measured.

Not surprisingly, the master maintained his balance by making multiple subtle adjustments in his posture, whereas those who had not done Tai Chi before fell over easily. The master shifted his body weight from the front to the rear foot and adjusted his center of gravity in response to the direction of incoming pushes. What's more, measurements showed the muscles in his arms and torso remained relaxed, while his leg muscles, in particular the hamstring muscles in the back of the leg, were very active. The combination of increased muscle and joint loading in the legs suggests that Push Hands may enhance the weight-bearing qualities of Tai Chi and therefore make it effective for maintaining bone health.[8]

Interactive Tai Chi as Applied Philosophy

"Push Hands gives you the opportunity to develop new capacities in yourself and to become more sensitive to others," says Florence, age 55, who started doing Push Hands one and a half years ago after practicing Tai Chi for 20 years. "I felt that I didn't get it at first, but it's a lesson in perseverance and building inner strength. You learn about yourself and other people when you're interacting."

"It's amazing how different everybody is. Push Hands shines a spotlight on different ways of feeling. It's an intimate experience," says Florence, who works in retailing. "Some people go hard and fast, others soft and slow, and this affects how you work with them. If I push with three people who are hard, I feel different when I push with someone who is a soft person. This puts a lens on their personalities, and my personality and habits, and how we all interact. I have to persevere through real difficulties at work, and Push Hands has given me more courage to try more, and to relax instead of being fearful."

Practicing interactive exercises can bring to life the philosophical wisdom inherent in Tai Chi. It's one thing to hear a phrase like "go with the flow" and think: okay, that makes sense. In two-person practice, you get to experience genuine physical and emotional yielding, to stay relaxed, yet alert, in the presence of an aggressive action. This type of Tai Chi training manifests what often sounds like lofty, esoteric principles. This embodied experience helps you progress with solo and interactive Tai Chi and can flow into other social interactions as well.

One of my teachers, Arthur Goodridge, often described interactive Tai Chi as a conversation or dialogue. He also emphasized the importance of "listening" with the entire body. Just as you must be a good listener to be fully engaged in a verbal conversation, you must develop what the Tai Chi classics call *tien jin* ("listening energy") to interact physically and energetically during two-person Tai Chi.

Tai Chi classics regard the ability to listen to your partner's movement and energy as one of the most fundamental skills. Of course, you do not do Tai Chi listening with the ears, but rather with the body. You listen with your skin, and with other poorly understood neurophysiological receptors, to detect what an opponent might do from the moment you make physical contact (commonly with forearm or palm, but it could be any body part). Listening provides information on the strength and direction of the upcoming attack. As you listen, you simultaneously tune in to your partner, and yourself. From this place of contact and with heightened sensitivity, you can apply many other Tai Chi techniques, such as yielding to neutralize and dissipate your opponent's force. Following an evasive action, you can take advantage of your partner's loss of mechanical advantage, which is often called "borrowing energy," and advance with your own mindful, strategically directed strength. The net result is that you lead by first following. Regardless of the techniques you use, listening is the key fundamental principle that underlies many practical and philosophical Tai Chi principles.

In introductory Tai Chi classes, I encourage students to explore a simple, informative exercise that involves leading and following. After pairing up in teams of two, one person, who is designated the leader, offers the top of the left wrist to the partner; the designated follower places his or her right palm on the leader's left wrist. The leader then is instructed to walk around the room freely and move the left limb up and down to provide a mild challenge for the partner to follow. The follower, without grasping, must stay attached to the leader's arm.

Many interesting things emerge from this simple exercise. First, beginning students often quickly forget Tai Chi principles when "attached" to another person. That happens even with my regular reminders to walk in a relaxed manner and maintain good posture, feel the feet on the ground, and keep breathing. The quality of their movements is far from meditative.

Afterward, some students say they had difficulty staying centered and grounded because of the physical challenges of unpredictable movements and concerns about balance. More frequently, they describe psychological challenges. Some students honestly admit it was very hard not to be in control, while others feel very uncomfortable taking the responsibility for leading. In both cases, the students recognize the challenge of staying mindful while being engaged with another. I suggest students learning Push Hands actively look for situations outside of class that challenge their ability to remain centered, or to play a leadership or subordinate role, at work or at home.

In practicing even the simplest of interactive Tai Chi exercises, like the one above, it becomes very obvious that learning is more than just physical. Touch and joined movement can catalyze emotional and psychosocial awareness. Angus Clark, a highly regarded Tai Chi teacher in England, nicely describes how partner work can raise awareness and help transform emotions and behaviors:

> Tai Chi is not a form of psychotherapy, but it reaches the art of dealing with emotions on a physical level. For example, partner practice encourages people to honestly look at themselves. The shape or position of the body and its effectiveness in dealing with a difficult situation, such as an incoming push, is a good indicator of a person's stance in life. In exchanges of pushing and yielding, receiving and giving, there are moments when partners of over- or under-assertiveness become clear. Tai Chi guides people toward achieving a balance.[9]

Social Support and Interaction

"My favorite thing to do with my two boys, Brian (age 9) and Jacob (age 6) is to wrestle with them," says Andy, a 43-year-old attorney, who has gone to Tai Chi class two or three times a week for the past two years. "Practicing Tai Chi has allowed me to play more actively with them. My older son now has a brown belt in karate, which is an outer martial art. I'm trying to give him a hint of the inner strength of Push Hands.

"It's fun to push around with someone. I remember that feeling from when I was a kid, now that I have my own kids. It's energizing and good exercise, too. The challenge of Push Hands is to draw on your energy and the other person's energy at the same time. When you go back to the Tai Chi form, it brings your form up to another level, and makes it more of a martial practice."

Safe, playful physical interactions in Tai Chi classes may help compensate for what may be a shortage of touching in contemporary Western society, particularly in America. One study observed sets of American, French, and Puerto Rican friends in coffee shops over the course of an hour to determine how frequently they made physical contact. Friends in the United States tend to touch each other an average of only twice an hour, whereas French friends touch 110 times, and Puerto Rican friends touch 180 times.[10] As discussed in earlier chapters, being a member of a community, like a Tai Chi school, provides important social support. The depth and intimacy of social interactions may become even greater when you regularly share physical contact with a Tai Chi partner.

However, know that even the simplest interactive exercises must be introduced in the context of safety and respect. Students may have undisclosed histories of abuse, trauma, or physical injuries, which make some aspects of interactive Tai Chi feel unsafe. For example, in my basic introductory Tai Chi classes, before starting an interactive exercise, I let everyone know what we are going to do and what the students can expect from the interactions. I emphasize that, like solo exercises that may cause discomfort, participation in interactive exercises is optional and sitting out is just fine.

The 70-percent rule of Tai Chi applies equally to emotional and social effort as it does to physical strain. For similar reasons, my more advanced Push Hands classes are limited to students who have been part of our community for an extended period, and we rarely allow "outsiders" to participate. We are not hiding training secrets, but respecting the intimacy of interactive Tai Chi work. Through long-standing relationships in class, students have the time to get to know each other. This time affords them a level of trust and familiarity, which is critical for our approach to partner work.

Partner work is a rich component of Tai Chi that goes well beyond martial training. It informs your understanding and depth of solo Tai Chi training, has health benefits, and can be applied to everyday activities. As you explore Tai Chi's interactive principles in everyday life, you may well see changes in activities as varied as how you open doors, walk down crowded, busy streets, and interact with colleagues and family members.

Cross-Train with Tai Chi

Martin, age 60, had played squash for most of his life until he was laid low by a serious shoulder injury that required rotator cuff surgery. "It was in the process of my pre-surgery that my Parkinson's disease was diagnosed. Between the shoulder surgery, the Parkinson's disease, not playing for more than a year, my advancing age, and my chronic arthritis, things didn't look good as far as returning to squash. So I cast around for some substitute activity when I found Tai Chi," he says. "At first, Tai Chi and squash seemed quite separate to me. Tai Chi was slow and graceful and followed a set form. Squash was fast and full of mad scrambles and improvising, delightfully chaotic with an edge related to the element of danger and risk of injury that is ever-present."

"Then, parallels began to emerge," he says. "Refining my ability to stay in the present with Tai Chi and to listen to my body's feedback was directly relevant to squash. So was the 70-percent rule. I consciously decided to let some points go and to prepare mentally for the next point. Using positive imagery to regulate mind-body boundaries was also relevant, as I relied less on combative self-talk and more on finding calmness and self-acceptance in the middle of the controlled chaos."

"Recently, I have been introduced to Push Hands, and the translation to squash is considerable," Martin continues. "I have learned to be receptive to the information my 'partner' is giving off, and learned to trust my intuitive integration of all that is happening and that needs to happen next. Being in the present instead of overthinking is most helpful. Now I await a serve without anticipation, balanced on my feet and confident that when the moment comes I will organize a coherent response that's suited to the moment—a plan but not a plan. And when I can do that, both my opponent and I are often surprised by what happens next, as I react more effectively than either of us thought possible."

Most people who succeed as an athlete cross-train—that is, participate in a variety of activities in addition to their chosen sport. Cross-training helps prevent you from suffering overuse injuries. Alternating activities also relieves the monotony of repeating the same training program over and over again. You can choose the best qualities of other sports to enhance your overall physical and mental skills.

Tai Chi offers many pluses to raise the level of your game. It provides flexibility, balance, and strength, as well as modest conditioning. Tai Chi can also help improve your focus and reflexes, enhance your range of motion, and open up new neuromuscular pathways. In addition, if you need to rehabilitate from a sports injury, such as muscle pulls, strains, or tears, Tai Chi allows you stay in shape and let your body heal while you recover.

For some athletes, Tai Chi becomes a lifetime sport. It's less physically taxing than most sports and can feed your body physically, emotionally, and spiritually as you age and move into the later stages of life. Tai Chi is a great sport to take into your retirement; you can keep doing it for as long as you live. In fact, many Chinese Tai Chi masters continue to practice Tai Chi into their eighties and nineties. Once you stop doing the jarring movements of other sports or more vigorous martial arts, you can use Tai Chi as a softer, yet still nourishing, exercise.

This chapter shows you how to incorporate the tools of Tai Chi to enhance your chosen sport. In sports and martial arts strength, stamina, coordination, speed, flexibility, balance, and resistance to injury are key. Tai Chi exercises can improve these elements as they essentially relate to all sports, whether it's the accuracy of your tennis serve, the length of your golf drive, or the carving of your ski turns.

Tai Chi's Synergy with Sports

> Extraordinary performances come out of a process of continuous, regular physical and mental practice. The mindset of an extraordinary athlete is relaxed but focused and open to ever higher achievements. Real success or victory is measured by the quality of that very process of attention and mindful involvement, practice, and commitment.
>
> —Chungliang Al Huang and Jerry Lynch,
> *Thinking Body, Dancing Mind*

Tai Chi training can help you develop the physical attributes and inner strength that you can apply to sports. It may help you expand your skill set to meet the challenges of athletic performance and learn how to react harmoniously to the stressful situations you may face during competitive sports. Tai Chi can create a synergy where the whole is greater than the parts.

Cross-training with Tai Chi helps you maintain balance and keeps you motivated, excited, and in good shape; it also serves as a hedge against burnout and fatigue. Within the martial arts, it's a tradition to cross-train. This rich tradition is now reflected in the increasingly popular mixed martial arts contests. Many mixed martial artists use Tai Chi to enhance their sensitivity and mental focusing skills. All of my Tai Chi teachers have cross-trained and studied other martial arts as well as Tai Chi. Currently, besides doing Tai Chi, I do Kung Fu, Bagua, Hsing Yi, and multiple forms of Qigong and meditation.

Many people learn more than one form of Tai Chi. Each style contributes to your general understanding of the Tai Chi principles and concepts. At first, a second style of Tai Chi may be difficult to learn. But after you become more familiar, you begin to see the similarities, and appreciate the differences, between styles. The new style may bring in new movements and ways of experiencing Tai Chi that can help you clarify what you have learned from the first style of Tai Chi.

Top athletes in competitive sports also have discovered the benefits of

Tai Chi. Former Boston Celtics star Robert Parish, who played in the National Basketball Association for 17 seasons, credited Tai Chi for his durability. Professional golfer Tiger Woods studied Qigong as a child, which his college golf coach at Stanford University believes may have contributed to his mental toughness and ability to hit a golf ball so far. Skier Ted Ligety was the most avid Tai Chi student among the members of the US Men's Alpine Ski team in 2005 and had a breakout season. In February 2006, he won a gold medal at the Winter Olympic Games in Turin, Italy.

How to Apply the Active Ingredients of Tai Chi

"I decided to take Tai Chi classes to build up my body for hip replacement surgery and also so I could get back onto the tennis court more quickly," says Susan, a 55-year-old businesswoman who started to play tennis seriously, five days a week, when she was 39. But ongoing, chronic pain in her right hip eventually led her to have a hip replacement. Six months after the surgery, "the richness of Tai Chi helped me regain physical balance and leg strength where my hip was replaced. Tai Chi made my body more ready for tennis," she says.

"There are many parallels between Tai Chi and tennis, which is one of the most demanding noncontact sports," adds Susan. "With tennis, the mental component is huge, and strength, particularly core strength, is extremely helpful. During competition, breathing is critical. The swinging movements of Tai Chi, the turning of the waist, and deep breathing, as well as doing Push Hands for faster reaction time, have all helped me up my game." Susan now plays three days a week post-surgery, including at a 4.0 level in her club championships.

Athletes can benefit from applying many of the ingredients of Tai Chi, including intention, deep breathing, integrated movement, and moderation.

Visualization and motor imagery are widely used to enhance sports performance. Tai Chi's use of visualization can train your mind as you would train a muscle. The deepened mind-body connection Tai Chi affords can help you see each movement of your chosen sport exactly as you would like it to be. This practice of visualization will help you carry out those movements during an actual performance. One of my Tai Chi teachers, Arthur Goodridge, encouraged us to play an imaginary video during all our Push Hands training and then review these tapes in our mind to learn about our physical and emotional patterns; then we could explore alternative strategies.

Tai Chi breathing can be used as a tool for relaxation; a relaxed athlete is a more efficient, better coordinated athlete. Relaxation can eliminate tension, stress, and anxiety that can impede your performance.

Musculoskeletal strength, flexibility, and neuromuscular coordination and reflexes are all integral parts of Tai Chi. Tai Chi training also helps you balance out both sides of the body. You are always ready to go left or right, and so never get stuck in an unbalanced position.

New computerized studies conducted by Professor William Tsang at Hong Kong University provide a hint of the advantages of Tai Chi in athletics. Tai Chi players viewed two random images on a computer screen. The researchers noted how quickly the subjects reacted to the images and how accurate they were in touching the right image on the screen. During the study, electrodes attached to the subjects' shoulders measured their muscle-reaction time. Feedback from the computer helped the subjects know whether they had made a good decision when they touched the screen. This study suggests that, with training, you can improve your reflexes. Improvement may allow, for example, a tennis player at the net to react more quickly to an approaching passing shot.[1]

Tai Chi's 70-percent rule prevents you from overtraining and allows you to recover from injuries. Practicing moderation teaches you what your limits are. If you know your limits, you honor the yin, the non-doing piece, of Tai Chi.

TAI CHI FOR TENNIS, GOLF, AND SKIING

Using Tai Chi techniques can help you "get in the zone" while playing any sport. Tai Chi has particular significance for tennis, golf, and skiing. For example, a tennis player could better focus on the tennis ball as it approaches. The golfer feels the golf club as a natural extension of the body. The skier feels the skis connected to the mountain.

Tennis

"Imagine that you're a person with preternaturally good reflexes and coordination and speed, and that you're playing high-level tennis. Your experience, in play, will not be that you possess phenomenal reflexes and speed; rather, it will seem to you that the tennis ball is quite large and slow-moving, and that you always have plenty of time to hit it."
—DAVID FOSTER WALLACE, "Federer as Religious Experience," *New York Times*, AUGUST 20, 2006

When I was growing up, I played on a youth tennis team in the Junior Tennis League in New York City, as well as on the tennis team at Stuyvesant High School. I started doing Tai Chi when I was 15, and it made me a better tennis player. My strokes were better, my reflexes faster, and I had more stamina. Now in my fifties, about once or twice a year, I play tennis with friends who play more regularly, and I can still give them a good game. I attribute that to my continuing Tai Chi training.

Tai Chi classics say that all movement is started in the feet, steered by the waist, and administered by the hand. Good ground strokes (forehand and backhand) in tennis use the same movements. You move your feet into position, turn your waist to begin the ground stroke, hit the ball with the racquet, and then follow through with the arm and hand. Tai Chi can also aid in conditioning and provide a strategy of how to use your body and recover after playing tennis.

Tai Chi helps you become more balanced physically and emotionally. Tennis requires a lot of balance as you shift from side to side chasing down your opponents' shots and getting yourself set to play the next stroke. You need to transfer your weight properly when you serve, hit ground strokes, or volley. The balanced stepping and weight transfer you learn in Tai Chi training transfers directly to the tennis court. When you are emotionally centered, you can focus more intently on your tennis game. A bad call or a poor shot played at a critical time is less likely to throw you off.

W. Timothy Gallwey's classic book, *The Inner Game of Tennis*, served up a unique way of looking at tennis when it was first published in 1974. This book concentrated on the "inner game," what goes on inside a player's mind, and how to apply that to the outer game, what happens on the tennis court. Much of Gallwey's thinking is similar to the Tai Chi concept of getting out of your own way to let your best game emerge. His theories are based on concentration, learning to trust oneself on the court, and awareness. He says the most beneficial first step is to see and feel what you are doing to increase your awareness of what actually is happening on the court.

Gallwey outlines his four-step approach to learn how to improve your game. The concepts he proposes follow some of the precepts of Tai Chi:

1. Observe, nonjudgmentally, existing behavior in an interested, some-what detached tone.
2. Ask yourself to change, programming with image and feel. If you wish the ball to go to the crosscourt corner, you simply imagine the necessary path of the ball to the target.
3. Let it happen. Having requested your body to perform a certain ac-tion, give it the freedom to do it.
4. Observe the results in a nonjudgmental, calm way. This leads to continuing observation of the process until behavior is automatic. Watch the results calmly and experience the process. Watch it change. Don't do the changing.[2]

TAI CHI TENNIS

As part of warm-up exercises in Tai Chi classes, I sometimes teach what I call Tai Chi Tennis. I also taught this approach at the Long-wood Tennis Club in Boston at a Tai Chi for Parkinson's disease fundraiser to give the participants a taste of Tai Chi.

Here's how to play Tai Chi Tennis:

Stand in a basic Tai Chi bow stance: left leg forward, feet shoul-der-width apart, the right, rear foot pointing at a 30- to 45-degree angle to the right, the left foot pointing forward. Begin with your weight on your back leg, navel pointing in the same direction as your right toes. Reach your right hand out to waist height. As you shift and pour your weight onto your left leg, imagine yourself hitting a tennis forehand without a racquet in your hand. The arm swing should be relaxed, continuous, and with a slight upward stroke (no higher than middle-of-chest height and with very relaxed shoulders).

Toward the end of the shift, there should be a slight turn into the left hip/kwah, and a release of the right heel as part of the follow through, so that the right knee hangs between the hip and the toe as in Tai Chi Swinging. Your feet then return to their starting position, and as the weight pours back to the rear leg, the right arm falls with a pendular motion back to its starting position.

As in Wave Hands Like Clouds, during your weight shifts forward, with the palm open, you can explore enhancing the flow of Qi into your hand, using attention and intention. After repeating this 6 to 9 times, do the mirror image of this move, with your right leg forward and play Tai Chi Tennis with your left hand.

As you do these exercises, bring in Tai Chi principles. Feel your feet rooted to the ground, and stand tall. Turn by using your waist. Stay focused. Integrate energy into the movement. You may feel that your hands are warmer after "playing" Tai Chi Tennis, which means you are feeling the Qi moving through your hands.

Golf

> First, I "see" the ball where I want it to finish, nice and white and sitting up high on bright green grass. Then the scene quickly changes, and I 'see' the ball going there: its path, trajectory, and shape, even its behavior on landing. Then there is a sort of fade-out, and the next scene shows me making the kind of swing that will turn the previous images into reality. —JACK NICKLAUS, *Golf My Way*

Tai Chi may be the perfect complement to your golf game. The key components of Tai Chi and a good golf swing are similar—a combination of relaxation, the mind and body working together, and balanced motion. The movements in Tai Chi and in golf both require a smooth acceleration to generate maximum power at the precise moment of contact—club on ball or fist on opponent.

All internal arts and the golf swing share basic principles. First, you relax into the initial stance. You shift your weight, coil your body around a vertical axis to build up power, and then uncoil your body to release the power. The power derives from the lower half of the body, flowing up from the feet, through the hips, and into the arms and hands.

Tai Chi can also increase your flexibility, build lower body strength, and improve your balance. Increased flexibility and improved leg strength will give you a more fluid swing, better tempo, and more distance on your shots. Better balance leads to a properly aligned stance and a solid swing.

The mental side of Tai Chi allows a golfer to maintain concentration. Tai Chi creates a quiet calm and confidence. With a positive attitude, your golf game will be less stressful, especially when you need to hit a good drive or make a crucial putt. Deep-breathing exercises help develop stamina so that you feel just as good on the last few holes as you did on the first ones.

Fluid Motion

Developing a fluid, powerful, consistent golf swing has as much to do with your mind-body connection as it does with your swing technique. Certain fundamentals learned from Tai Chi training translate directly into making a good golf shot. As you address the ball, relax to encourage a smooth swing. Feel your body in balance and your feet rooted into the ground. Quiet your mind with deep breathing to increase your positive attitude. Replicate these fundamentals as you set up to increase your chances of a fluid, effortless, repeatable swing.

Meditation

As you have learned in Tai Chi training, stillness is the master of motion. The simple practice of meditation produces calm, yet focused, awareness. This is the ideal performance state for golfers.

Relaxation helps minimize the "monkey mind," the internal dialogue and negative thoughts that often arise, particularly after you have played a poor shot. Return to a calmer state of mind so you can express your true skill level and passion for the game. Use mindfulness meditation to reduce performance anxiety, especially when the pressure is on to produce a good shot. The more you practice how to relax and quiet your mind in Tai Chi, the better your chances of using these techniques when you need them on the golf course. The regular practice of meditation is crucial when you want to perform fluidly.

Breathing

Deep breathing lowers your heart rate, relaxes your muscles, increases your mind-body connection, raises your confidence levels, and creates a calm, focused state from which to set up and swing a golf club. If you find yourself in a tough spot—for example, your ball is plugged in a bunker—focus on your breathing. Before your pre-shot routine, stop and take a few deep breaths. Do not let your stress response rule your brain and body. Take conscious control of your body through your breathing.

Bringing attention to your breath also helps to increase concentration. Your pre-shot routine is ideal for deep breathing to help you feel relaxed at address. Then breathe in as you move to the top of your backswing, and exhale all the way through striking the ball into your finish position. Focus entirely on your breath, and trust your swing.

Skiing

> Open your awareness, first, with attention to your breathing, noticing it, allowing its fullness. Follow it to your Center, then let it widen your receptivity to the sensations in the world around you and within you. Follow it to the extremities of your body, to your hands in your gloves, your toes in your boots, and the roots of your hair.
> —Denise McCluggage, *The Centered Skier*

Skiing is one of my favorite activities. For me, it brings together the mind, body, and spirit in an exhilarating sport that takes place in nature. Tai Chi training has made skiing a very rich, meditative experience for me, and it has allowed me to keep up with my teenage son, who has become an exceptional skier.

The carved turn is a perfect meditation, says Denise McCluggage in *The Centered Skier*. Your body is relaxed, alert, the arms (as you hold your ski poles) loosely embracing a ball of energy. Center your consciousness in the body's center. Breathe easily. Your shoulders should carry no tension.

Energy flows downward through the legs into the snow beneath the skis. Extend your awareness the length of the ski edges, sensing their cutting, carving capability. To initiate the turn, your thought directs the ski tips toward the fall line. The thought manifests in a sensation of pressure in the toes nudging the ski tips in the desired path. You expend no effort, and nothing shows, but the tips will fall away, yielding to gravity.

The constant shifting of weight from one leg to the other while carving turns is a direct expression of yin and yang. Led by the waist, as in Tai Chi, your weight shifts to the right or downhill ski as you turn to the left. Like a Taoist paradox, to go left, you must first shift to the right. Waist turning allows your downhill ski to advance through the turn, staying parallel and harmonious with the uphill ski. On a nice snowy day, if you get to make fresh tracks, you can look back uphill and see repeating S-shaped, yin-yang marks in the mountain.

Awareness

Tune in to your energy flow as you ski, just as you do when you practice Tai Chi. Sense the Qi as you breathe in the cool air. Feel the energy course through your body and tie you to the earth. Feel it through your legs and feet and into your skis. Feel the connection between the snow, the wind, and your own motion. Use all of your senses to relate to the elements and details as you ski gracefully.

Tai Chi can be an exceptional sports training tool. The basic message for all sports from Tai Chi is quite simple: cultivate awareness, pay attention to the rhythm of your body, and go with the energy flow.

12

On-the-Job Tai Chi

"When I'm at work, Tai Chi gives me the strength to function at my best," says Carol, age 52, an executive in a high-tech company. "I feel less diluted from things like office politics and the large workload. I know when I interact with someone at work I maintain a strong sense of self. Working in a demanding, competitive environment tests that constantly. Tai Chi is like an inner armor that helps me function."

Carol does Tai Chi warm-up exercises every day before heading to the office and attends Tai Chi classes twice a week at night. "I apply a lot of the aspects of flow I have learned in Tai Chi classes on the job, both consciously and unconsciously. I use Tai Chi exercises to calm my mind, particularly when it's racing. And I use Tai Chi for physical breaks at my desk just to take a moment and move my body. I wouldn't have that extra oomph if I didn't have Tai Chi in my life."

One of the motivations underlying the simplified approach to Tai Chi this book outlines is you can readily translate the key principles, and benefits, of Tai Chi into everyday daily activities. In one of our ongoing trials with chronic obstructive pulmonary disease patients, we have explicitly included time at the end of each Tai Chi training session to practice integrating Tai Chi principles into routine activities. We recently took a mini field trip immediately following a very deep, relaxing Tai Chi session. I led a group of five participants down the busy hallways of Beth Israel Deaconess Medical Center Hospital to the gift shop.

I felt like a first-grade schoolteacher leading a class trip; however, instead of repeatedly yelling at the patients to stay in line or stop chatting, I gently, repeatedly whispered to them, "Are you breathing?" "Can you feel your feet on the ground" "Are you standing tall?" None of the white-coated, stethoscope-wearing doctors and fast-moving nurses could figure out the purpose of our slow-moving, meditative parade. It didn't take long for us to shift out of the meditative state we had experienced during Tai Chi class, but we also saw how easy it was to integrate Tai Chi principles into routine activities using some simple reminders. The mini-field trip was a fun, profound revelation for all of us.

Work is an obvious, very relevant place to explore the integration of Tai Chi training. If you have a full-time job, you probably spend much of your day at work. Work is likely part of your identity. But work can be stressful. In fact, the Institute for Stress reports that job-related pressure is the top source of stress for Americans. Surveys of workers show that 80 percent feel stress on the job, nearly half say they need help learning how to manage it, and 42 percent say their coworkers need help in managing stress. Other ominous health statistics show that occupational pressures and hazards are responsible for 30 percent of workers' back pain, and that 60 percent of workers routinely complain of work-related neck pain, 44 percent say they have eyestrain, 38 percent feel hand pain, and 34 percent have difficulty sleeping.[1]

This chapter takes the principles of Tai Chi and suggests some ways to integrate them into your work. Corporate wellness programs have taken stress reduction directly into the workplace. Top corporations have learned to use wellness to their employees', and the company's, advantage. On a personal level, what you learn from Tai Chi training can help you manage both the physical and emotional stresses of work; for example, you might change how you sit and how you manage your time, including sneaking in Tai Chi breaks. This practice may make you more efficient and creative at work. The workplace may offer a new frontier for you to further develop and apply your Tai Chi skills.

Investing in Tai Chi

Nearly everyone struggles with having far too much work to do. Deadlines loom, fires need to be put out, and to-do lists stay too long while you try to maintain your regular, routine activities. So, the valid question comes up: Can I afford to make time for Tai Chi and other exercise, or am I better served working a bit earlier or staying later, sacrificing morning exercise or a lunch break, and crossing off a few more things from my to-do list?

From my own experience, and from what my students tell me, I find that making time for Tai Chi, exercise, and an occasional short relaxation break is a valuable investment of your time. Time spent practicing Tai Chi makes your time at work more focused and creative, helps you manage stress, makes your interactions with coworkers more efficient, and gives you the energy to work longer, more productive hours. Growing support for this "investment" perspective comes from those most concerned with the bottom line (money and productivity)—that is, the leaders of corporations and businesses who have invested in wellness programs.

The Corporate Wellness Movement

If you want to do better work, try Tai Chi, meditation, yoga, or other stress-reduction techniques. That's what Mayo Clinic researchers suggested after examining the relationship between stress levels and quality of life at a work-site wellness center. The researchers conducted a survey of more than 13,000 employees joining a wellness center, asking them about stress, health behaviors, and quality of life. More than 2,000 of these employees reported having high stress levels. Those under high stress had statistically significant lower quality of life, more fatigue, and poorer health compared with employees reporting low stress levels. They were also more likely to have high blood pressure, high blood sugar, high cholesterol, and to be overweight. The researchers concluded that tailored stress-reduction programs would be beneficial for these employees.[2]

Employers all across the nation are recognizing just how important a healthy workplace and a healthy workforce are to improving productivity, as well as to controlling health-care costs. The best employers establish workplace wellness programs, creating an environment that supports employees who are committed to long-term behavior changes, and launch programs or services to promote living a healthier lifestyle. Corporate wellness programs typically focus on physical fitness and weight loss initially, but some are also beginning to address other domains of wellness, including stress management, work-life balance, spirituality, and resilience. Not surprisingly, many now integrate mind-body therapies, such as Tai Chi, yoga, and relaxation training.

Currently, about two-thirds of large American companies offer some components of a wellness program, although only a little more than 10 percent have comprehensive wellness programs.[3] But the number of companies getting involved in workplace wellness is growing, driven by the rising costs they face in providing health-care coverage for their employees. Health-care reform also expands coverage for preventive services, which gives companies incentives to offer some kind of health-care screenings. The Patient Protection and Affordable Care Act mandated grants for small businesses to provide comprehensive workplace wellness programs. Some $200 million will be allocated from 2011 to 2015 for this purpose in businesses of 100 or fewer employees.

Businesses are about making money, and growing evidence suggests that investment in wellness pays back. A study mentioned in the December 2010 *Harvard Business Review*[4] found that the return on each dollar a large company invests in an employee wellness program might be as high as $6. Other studies show that wellness programs have achieved a rate of return on investment that ranges from $3 to $15 for each dollar invested, with savings realized within 12 to 18 months.[5]

Here are some reasons why investing in wellness programs pays off for both businesses and their employees.

- Reduced Medical Costs

    Comprehensive wellness programs typically aim at improving employees' cardiovascular and general health, according to a 2009 policy statement from the American Heart Association. These programs include regular physical activity, stress management/reduction, early detection/screening, nutrition education and promotion, weight management, tobacco cessation and prevention, disease management, cardiovascular disease education, and changes in the work environment to encourage healthy behaviors and promote occupational safety and health.[6] An estimated 25–30 percent of companies' medical costs each year are spent on employees who suffer with these major risk factors.[7] Some work-site wellness programs report some success in preventing major risk factors for cardiovascular disease and stroke, which include cigarette smoking, obesity, hypertension, dyslipidemia (abnormal cholesterol levels), physical inactivity, and diabetes.[8]

- Increased Productivity

    Estimates suggest that health-related productivity losses cost US employers $225.8 billion per year, or $1,685 per employee per year, of which 71 percent is due to reduced performance at work. Depression alone costs US employers approximately $35 billion in lost productivity. Studies evaluating productivity losses show links between these losses and absenteeism and associated health issues.[9]

    The good news is that your productivity improves along with your health. People who improve just one cardiovascular disease risk factor show a 2 percent increase in their productivity. This increase translates to an estimated health savings to companies of $950 per year per risk that was reduced.[10]

- Less Lost Time at Work

    Employees with the greatest health risks, poorest emotional health, and higher percentages of adverse behaviors have much higher rates of lost workdays and lower productivity. Exercise and other stress-management techniques can help ameliorate the effects of stress that manifest in back pain, migraines, and other symptoms of stress. A meta-analysis of corporate wellness programs has shown a 28 percent average reduction in sick leave absenteeism and a 30 percent decrease in workers' compensation and disability management claims costs.[11] One study among Japanese blue-collar workers shows how a stress-reduction program can reduce stress and the symptoms of depression, as well as sick leave. The electric company workers who scored high on a scale designed to diagnose depression and who participated in a year-long stress-reduction program showed a decrease in their depression compared to a similar group who did not go through the program. What's more, those who reduced their stress also had, on average, fewer sick days than the year before participation in the program.[12]

- Improved Morale

    Justice Ruth Ginsberg has her whole staff do yoga at the Supreme Court before work. She obviously understands the value of a healthy, happy staff. Wellness programs can also improve morale and camaraderie by getting workers to interact with one another. Other benefits to the companies that offer wellness programs are recruitment and retention of employees, as well as an improved company image.

    This investment in wellness on the part of corporations shares the same spirit of Tai Chi's 70-percent training principle. An executive who consistently pushes his staff to work extra hours may find that the more he pushes people, the less he gets out of them. In this case, more time chained to a desk may not necessarily translate to more productivity. Instead, an extra half hour for lunch that allows for some exercise or stress-reduction practices may help his staff refresh and balance themselves. Moderation at work—more of a yin-yang balance—may serve as a hedge against resistance, burnout, and fatigue.

INTEGRATING TAI CHI INTO THE WORKDAY

In addition to attending classes and maintaining a home practice, or participating in a wellness program at work, several approaches can help you integrate Tai Chi principles into your personal workday. What follows are some tips I've explored on my own and learned from my students.

Use Your Travel Time to and from Work to Practice Tai Chi Principles.

You probably spend a great deal of time traveling to and from work. I have learned to take advantage of my quiet time during my 30-minute drive. Sometimes on my way to work, I'll practice slow, deep-breathing exercises. While stopped at a red light, I do simple shoulder, neck, and hand stretches. Throughout the drive, I pay attention to my posture, including how I'm holding my arms on the steering wheel. I may also do some mental preparation and organize my thoughts. If I come across a stressful issue, such as a challenging presentation that I'm anxious about, I try to break down the issue into manageable pieces. I visualize doing the presentation with as little stress as possible. On the way home, or en route to an evening Tai Chi class, I use similar practices to decompress to leave the day's stress behind me.

Many of these practices are equally practical if you take public transportation, and perhaps even easier—you can close your eyes and go a little deeper into relaxation and meditation. Some of my Tai Chi students have purchased CDs or downloaded guided breathing or meditation tapes, or they simply relax with soothing music. If you have to stand a lot, for example, waiting for a bus or train, you can practice simple Tai Chi Pouring exercises, or do a simple standing meditation. A five- or 10-minute session each day on the way to and from work can make a huge difference. It sets the tone for your day or evening and can carry over into whatever comes next.

Set Up Your Work Space

Whether you work in a cubicle, a big private office, or behind a cash register at the mall, practicing Tai Chi principles can help you organize a healthier, energy-efficient environment.

For sedentary office workers, Tai Chi principles may mitigate what are now epidemic levels of occupational hazards—pain in the neck, back, shoulders, and hands—caused by sitting at a desk with inefficient posture. If you spend much of the day doing the same motions, you may be susceptible to repetitive stress injuries. One of the most common repetitive-stress injuries is carpal tunnel syndrome, which is often found among those who type or use the computer mouse for prolonged periods. This condition occurs from pressure on the median nerve, which is the nerve in the wrist that supplies feeling and movement to parts of the hand. The area in your wrist where the nerve enters the hand is called the carpal tunnel. This tunnel is normally narrow, so any swelling can pinch the nerve and cause pain, numbness, tingling, or weakness; the result is carpal tunnel syndrome. Other repetitive-stress injuries may arise from chopping vegetables, playing a musical instrument, or performing any other repetitive task.

The principles of efficient, supported postural alignment you learned in Tai Chi training translate directly into how you sit at your desk. An upright spine, relaxed shoulders, and feet grounded to the floor, among other postural principles, allow your neuromuscular and skeletal systems to work most efficiently. From the perspective of Chinese medicine, this good posture, combined with regular deep breathing, enhances the flow of blood and Qi and minimizes energy blockages that underlie physical injury, fatigue, and emotional imbalances.

These intuitive Tai Chi principles at your desk overlap with the rapidly growing field of ergonomics. Ergonomics is the science of designing user interaction with equipment and workplaces to fit the user.[13] Additional ergonomic principles that parallel the goals of Tai Chi include maintaining a proper height and distance of your computer screen relative to your eyes to minimize neck or eye strain and adapting the height and angle of your keyboard to minimize arm strain.

Heightened body awareness and sensitivity garnered through Tai Chi training may help you notice improper body alignment and strained postures at work. If you already have injuries due to repetitive strain on your joints, osteoarthritis, or back pain, Tai Chi may help you manage and minimize symptoms and allow you to work more easily. (Chapter 5 describes how Tai Chi helps reduce pain.) The ergonomic principles of Tai Chi apply not only to desk jobs but to physical tasks as well. One of my teachers, Robert Morningstar, has worked to integrate Tai Chi principles into vocations as diverse as those involving as aircraft pilots, assembly-line workers who lift heavy objects, and cashiers at supermarkets.

Occupational health research on Tai Chi is limited. One small study at York University in Toronto, Canada, examined the effects of Tai Chi in the workplace among female workers who used computers at the university. After taking two 50-minute Tai Chi classes a week for 12 weeks during their lunch hour, the 52 women who participated improved not only their fitness but also their psychological well-being.[14]

In another study, University of Vermont researchers investigated whether a Tai Chi workplace wellness program was a cost-effective way to improve physical and mental health, reduce work-related stress, and improve work productivity among older nurses (average age 54) who worked in a hospital. Six nurses attended Tai Chi classes once a week at the hospital and practiced on their own for 10 minutes each day at least four days per week for 15 weeks. Five other nurses (controls) did no Tai Chi. During the study, the Tai Chi group took no time off from work, whereas the controls were absent for 49 hours. Tai Chi also led to a 3 percent increase in work productivity and a significant improvement in the functional reach of the nurses compared with the control group.[15]

Move around When You Can

Although I essentially have a desk job, I have come to realize that I have many opportunities to move around at work. For example, during some teleconference calls, I turn on my speakerphone, stand, and do some simple stretching and Tai Chi movements that don't distract me from the call. Also, I know that I think better on my feet. If I am in the early stages of writing a journal article or a study grant, instead of sitting at my desk and jotting notes on small pieces of paper or a computer, I hang large sheets of blank paper on my office wall, or use a room with a white board, to organize my thoughts. I write down an outline of some ideas, step back and think about them, and move to different parts of room to see them from different perspectives. When I begin to get antsy or anxious, or when I want to be more creative, I often do a few Tai Chi–inspired movements and breathing exercises to keep the juices and Qi flowing.

I also like to develop and practice my academic talks while on a treadmill, walking at a modest pace with a draft of my PowerPoint slides in front of me. I silently imagine the words or ideas I wish to convey with each slide. In addition to squeezing in a little extra exercise into my day, I find that the flow of ideas is less inhibited while I am in motion, and I am better able to feel things I want to convey, in the spirit I want to convey them.

Mini Tai Chi Exercise Breaks

You can integrate a number of simple Tai Chi exercises you already have learned throughout your day to help avoid physical and emotional stress.

- Simple one- to three-minute stretches, every hour or two, while sitting at your desk. Some good stretches I particularly recommend include Spinal Cord Breathing, Hand Tai Chi, Neck and Shoulder Stretches, and Foot and Ankle Stretches.
- Mini-breathing meditations. Close your eyes at your desk, and practice renewing your body with your breath or using tan tien breathing for three to five minutes a few times a day.
- Walk mindfully to the water cooler or bathroom. Feel your feet on the ground. Notice the parts of your body that feel stressed, and

gently invite them to begin to relax. Move toward a feeling you might recall from a recent good Tai Chi practice.

- If you have enough room in your workspace, do a few minutes of Tai Chi Swinging and Drumming, followed by Washing Yourself with Qi from the Heavens. The Swinging and Drumming will get blood and Qi moving, and Washing with Qi will help balance and ground you.
- And, of course, if you can find an appropriate place and have 10 minutes, practice some formal Tai Chi moves.

If you look for them, many opportunities are available to practice Tai Chi principles and incorporate them into your workday. A short Tai Chi break may help you work harder and better, and even make you more creative, which is the topic of the next chapter.

13

Enhance Your Creativity
with Tai Chi

T'ai-chi ch'uan is an art in the deepest sense of the word. Aesthetically, it can be compared to a composition by Bach or a Shakespearian sonnet. However, t'ai-chi ch'uan is not art directed outward to an audience. It is an art-in-action for the doer; the observer, moved by its beauty, can only surmise its content. The experience of the form in process of change makes it an art for the self.

—DANCE AND TAI CHI MASTER SOPHIA DELZA,
T'ai-chi Ch'uan: Body and Mind in Harmony

It's not surprising that many people who practice Tai Chi are also involved in the creative arts. In addition, many creative arts programs draw from the East. Tai Chi is defined by yin and yang coming together, which, in effect, is creativity. The creativity that derives from Tai Chi leads to integration of complementary things—left brain (logic) and right brain (intuition), form and function, and body and mind.

Indeed, Tai Chi may be a key to unlocking creative consciousness. During Tai Chi practice, you are in a state of mind that allows creativity to flow naturally. Many Tai Chi students report improvements in mental clarity. If you can reduce tension and nervousness, you may be able to experience deeper thoughts and better tap into your creativity.

This chapter touches upon the principles of Tai Chi as they apply to painting (Qi flows through every brushstroke) and writing (posture, focusing skills); playing a musical instrument (breath and body shape); acting (honesty and patience); and dance (expression through movement).

How to Use the Eight Active Ingredients To Be Creative

Letting go and letting things happen naturally underlie any form of creativity. Many of the principles of Tai Chi can enhance your creativity, including development of focus; staying in the moment; concentration of energy; economy of movement; inner stillness; development of a flexible, balanced body; unification of mind and body; and appreciation and development of discipline.

Here are some ways the Eight Active Ingredients can lead to creativity:

You need to focus and pay attention to your art to be skillful, precise, and express yourself clearly. Be in touch with what you're feeling to engage in the artistic process. Also, listening skills, especially cultivated in interactive Tai Chi, come from mindfulness and attention. For example, good actors need to react honestly and spontaneously to interact with each other effectively, and jazz musicians need to listen and respond to one another to improvise.

Visualization helps shape your creativity. Most artists use their "inner" vision and imagination during the creative process.

Breath control is part of how instrumentalists and dancers maintain rhythm and balance. For singers and wind players, breath is what creates their sound and is essential to all aspects of their artistry.

Most sedentary artists, such as painters and writers, need to keep their bodies healthy to have the physical stamina to sustain long periods of creativity. Dancers can benefit directly from the strength and flexibility of Tai Chi training, and the protective and restorative effects it can have on recurrent injuries.

A relaxed posture is important for wielding sculpture tools or paintbrushes, as well as how you sit while playing a musical instrument or writing. Relaxed neuromuscular patterns can prevent repetitive-stress injuries that afflict piano or trumpet players in their hands, or violin players in their necks, or writers who spend a great deal of time sitting at computers and incur various types of injuries.

Tai Chi and the Arts

Painting and Writing

"Tai Chi is about getting flow to happen, from inside to outside, side to side, and top to bottom," says Michael, a 53-year-old painter. "This is the same as creativity—you are looking for a state of flow. When I'm creative and working, I'm in a flow state, a quiet place where energy flows freely."

"If I'm making a painting, a part of what I'm looking for in the painting is a dynamic movement from left to right, from the center to the periphery, from top to bottom," continues Michael, who often practices Tai Chi before painting. "I want the picture frame to pull the viewer into an energetic stream that enlivens him or her. I want the viewer to taste the state of consciousness that I have been living while I have been painting. This is a state of dynamic flow, which emerges out of stillness and expresses itself."

"The real joy in the creative act stems from just being," he says. "Part of resting into that creative state is letting go of all distractions, ideas, and agendas. When creativity emerges, it's an expression of that openness. That is the essence of both creativity and Tai Chi."

The life of Grand Master Cheng Man Ching is an excellent illustration of the interconnectedness of Tai Chi and the creative arts. Master Cheng was known as a scholar and the Master of Five Excellences—Tai Chi, calligraphy, medicine, philosophy, and poetry. However, as Cheng's biographer Mark Hennessy aptly wrote in the book *Master of Five Excellences*, "he was in essence a master of one thing—the unimpeded flow of ch'i."[1] This seamless integration of Tai Chi and artistic principles, combined with diligent study and practice, led Tam Gibbs, one of Master Cheng's senior students, to describe his calligraphy as "full, unified, even, and solid . . . his brush stroke seemed to penetrate through the paper . . . the ink seemed to maintain its freshness and even the water seemed to have body."[2] Perhaps, ironically, it was Professor Cheng's art—his painting and calligraphy—that brought him and Tai Chi to the West.

As in calligraphy, the painter strives for vigorous, rhythmic brushstrokes, flowing lines, and spirited projection of his or her thoughts onto the canvas. The positive energy and concentration accumulated in Tai Chi training may enable a painter to create with greater ease.

Similarly, mobilizing and maintaining energy plays a vital part in a writer's success. The process of writing takes tremendous concentration and perseverance. Tai Chi exercises can enhance energy while inducing a pleasant state of relaxation and help you develop your ability to let your thoughts flow naturally. Relaxation means slowing down the mind so that Qi can move smoothly. Just as the learning process for Tai Chi takes place on various levels—physical, emotional, and cognitive—so the writing process flows through physical, emotional, and cognitive phases. Tai Chi movements can help you slow down or quiet your mind, relax into the process, and dissolve psychological blockages, such as writer's block.

A writer often sits for long hours without moving. Simple Qigong or Tai Chi exercises can help move Qi after hours of sitting. Energy gained from Tai Chi's graceful movements not only helps focus the mind, but also can energize one's writing.

Music

"Learning Tai Chi was like stepping into very familiar territory," says Jackie, a 58-year-old music teacher who started playing violin at age 10 and has practiced Tai Chi for 17 years. "The experience felt so similar to playing music. Movement, rhythm, themes, and even vibrations, all come into play in both activities. When you play music, you have to play in tune, balance with your fellow players, and know where you are, but without thinking too much about it. Practicing Tai Chi teaches you to tune in to the mind-body, the sense of balance, of being in the moment, and nowhere else. Doing the Tai Chi form is a lot like playing chamber music!"

"As your Tai Chi practice deepens, you get more intimate with your mind and body," continues Jackie. "Complex movements become second nature, you learn to trust yourself, hold your own, stay open, and 'go with the flow.' In turn, this feeds back into your music-making. Rather than fixating on the difficulties in your part, for example, you can feel more confident and just let go. Accessing the Tai Chi way of being, you are more *in* the music. Any nervousness or performance anxiety tends to diminish and even just drop away!"

If you like music, you will probably like Tai Chi. You can learn to tune into your body and know what that means. When you learn to do Tai Chi well and correct your form, your whole body resonates. You can feel your body in tune, opening, and the Qi flowing. This dynamic expression of the moment is also what musicians strive to achieve.

It's no accident that many Tai Chi masters also study music. The right-brain, nonverbal, sensing patterns and the forms of expression are similar in both. Both involve fluidity within structure. The more fluid you become, the better you can sense the vibrational qualities. Musicians are tuned in to a kinesthetic style of learning, and they are familiar with the complex and dynamic process of learning new skills.

Many similarities exist between music and Tai Chi. Both need a body that is full of energy and yet soft. A musician must let go of tension to play well, just as Tai Chi will not flow with tension. Both music and Tai Chi require physical, mental, and emotional balance, as well as centeredness and focus. A musician strings together motifs and phrases, just as a Tai Chi player links movements in the form. Proper posture and body alignment are important for both.

If a musician's breath is open, the music flows freely. But, if any resistance to breathing occurs because the lungs are not working properly or because of holding in emotions, this resistance can subtly affect the quality of the musician's music. Poor breath control can also affect how a musician moves, stands, and interacts with other performers.

Tai Chi breathing, learned in training, can help you to relax. Doing breathing and other Tai Chi exercises is a super way to warm up for a performance. Already, before you begin to play, you are in the flow. The experience of having just done Tai Chi makes you more centered, more open to the music you are performing, and less distracted by performance jitters. Practicing Tai Chi may well increase your ability to play and appreciate music.

Long practice hours, awkward body positions, heavy instruments, repetitive movements, and the stress of performance and competition can take a toll on a musician's health. Musicians are at high risk of developing musculoskeletal disorders, but preventive measures, including Tai Chi, might reduce the chance and intensity of an injury. Researchers at the University of California Medical Center and the University of California San Francisco School of Nursing recommend that musicians take up body posture work, such as the Alexander Technique, yoga, Tai Chi, or Feldenkrais, as well as mindfulness stress management. These techniques can help musicians identify their strength and flexibility, improve their posture, and learn to be more mindful/aware of how working with their particular instrument plays out in their whole body. The researchers also encourage musicians to take rest breaks; use ergonomic aids to lift, carry, and support instruments; and incorporate targeted warm-up exercises, stretches, and movement practices that improve postural awareness and movement efficiency.[3]

Some rock musicians have taken to Tai Chi. Lou Reed, the singer and guitarist from The Velvet Underground, says he has tamed the "rock and roll animal" by practicing Tai Chi for three hours a day. He cowrote and performed backup music for a Chen-style Tai Chi instructional DVD. Robert Diggs, better known as RZA, is the leader of the Wu Tan Clan rap group. This Grammy-winning music producer, rapper, and actor trained in Kung Fu and Tai Chi for several years.

Acting

"In Tai Chi, you learn to stay balanced, find your center, and be in the moment," says John, a 47-year-old actor. "As an actor, you have to feel your body, your own weight, find where you are feeling tension, and let it go. Then you look up at the other actors, and something starts to happen. Being present in your own body and being aware of someone else stems from stripping off the exterior to allow you to be in the moment. That's the most important thing in acting—to be human, in the moment."

"Tai Chi is not just a physical practice," continues John, who has practiced Tai Chi on and off for more than 25 years. "You become aware of your body and send energy to parts of the body. This leads to a heightened state of insights and a deep spiritual sense. Tai Chi is about getting rid of external hardness and developing inner softness, to approach life with an open, genuine heart, and therefore experience the world in a more open way. If you can do that, then art expression comes from a genuine place inside."

Actors need to be present, open, and in the moment to perform at their best. Even when acting from a script, they seek to go from moment to unanticipated moment. As they express their character's emotions in the moment, they also have to move and fit in nonverbal communication as well.

Tai Chi is an excellent form of movement and mental training for actors. Regular Tai Chi practice helps to improve body centering, coordination, accuracy, and fluency of movements; arouses bodily awareness; and develops physical and mental endurance. In addition, Tai Chi teaches how to interact with people. So much of what Tai Chi is about, particularly in Push Hands, is becoming sensitized to other people's energy. Students learn to recognize and manage their own feelings and become more sensitive to other people's feelings as well. This sensitivity is essential for an actor to be able to "feel" and respond to the other actors at hand.

Famous actors have also taken up Tai Chi as a relaxing, yet highly structured, Chinese martial art. Jet Li, the Chinese martial artist–turned–movie star, is starting a Tai Chi school that he hopes will break the stereotypes of Tai Chi as an art practiced only by old people in parks. The late David Carradine popularized Taoist thinking when he was the star of the television series *Kung Fu,* and later made several Tai Chi instruction videos. Movie star Mel Gibson reportedly is well versed in both Brazilian Jiu-Jitsu and Tai Chi. Another Tai Chi practitioner is Adrian Paul, an actor best known for his role on the television series *Highlander: The Series.*

Dance

The practice of Tai Chi has much to teach any student of dance. There are obvious things—balance, centeredness, and continuity of motion.

The slowness of the motion of Tai Chi, moving as if under water, heightens the body's consciousness of space. The air around the body takes on a viscous quality. Space, the dancer's medium, becomes real and substantial.

—TEM HOROWITZ AND SUSAN KIMMELMAN, *Tai Chi Ch'uan*

To become really effective at Tai Chi or any martial art requires hard work, discipline, intelligence, and perseverance. Even practicing a Tai Chi short form promotes regular rhythms in a dancer's body and mind. This makes it easier to keep up other rhythms related to dance.

—BRUCE FRANTZIS IN *Tai Chi for Health*

The connection between dance and Tai Chi in America goes back to before Professor Cheng's arrival when Sophia Delza taught and wrote about Tai Chi. Delza had lived in Shanghai in the late 1940s and early 1950s when her husband worked for the United Nations. She was fascinated by the Tai Chi she saw practiced in the parks, but was unable to find anyone willing to teach a Westerner. A back injury during a Chinese dance class led to referral to a Chinese master who agreed to allow her to become his student. When she returned to New York City, she continued to seek out teachers in Chinatown. She wrote magazine articles and books and made television appearances promoting Tai Chi. Delza, who became the head of the dance program at Hunter College in New York, taught Tai Chi, sword and knife forms, and Qigong, informing her teaching with her own training as a dancer.

Modern dance and ballet are based on similar principles of body alignment as Tai Chi. The joints are relaxed and the body "hangs" from the crown of the head as if suspended from above. The arms rarely move in isolation from the rest of the body. All movement begins in the center as the waist swings with no strain. As in Tai Chi, a dancer integrates the torso with legs. Both dancers and Tai Chi practitioners cultivate the skill of balancing on one leg. The "empty" leg is freed to extend and rotate at the hip.

The Tai Chi 70-percent principle is also very helpful for dancers, who tend to suffer injuries through overexertion and overstretching. In working to stretch their muscles even further, they may go beyond their body's natural ability to compensate. Tai Chi can help soften muscles and connective tissues so they can stretch further without using as much force. Tai Chi also offers some rest and protection against injury for the hard-working dancer. Therefore, the healing, stress-relieving, and meditative qualities of Tai Chi may be especially appealing to dancers.

Tai Chi may help improve a dancer's performance. Tai Chi relaxes and opens the joints and ligaments, allowing movements that are more fluid. It strongly develops whole-body coordination through the integration of the upper and lower body. Tai Chi increases leg strength, reflexes, and lightness, all valuable for dancers.

Whether you express artistically or not, cultivating a regular Tai Chi practice, which you learn how to do in the following chapter, is beneficial.

14

Lifelong Learning with Tai Chi

"I was in a musical group 20 years ago, and the leader introduced us to some Tai Chi exercises," says Pam, a 55-year-old real estate agent. "I thought I'd like to study Tai Chi, so I found a teacher through a friend and studied for a few years with the teacher until he moved to another studio and I lost track of him."

Over the next 10 years, Pam sporadically studied with Tai Chi teachers at adult education courses; then she was invited to participate in a Harvard Tai Chi study about bone health. "Being in the study, Tai Chi became a habit. After the study ended, I tried out several classes in a few local Tai Chi schools," says Pam, who takes classes three or four days a week and practices at home whenever she can. "I read about each school on the Internet, the school's approach, and what style it teaches, and found one that felt comfortable and very welcoming to a new person."

The two factors needed to learn Tai Chi, according to Professor Cheng Man Ching, are perseverance and right teaching. To progress in your Tai Chi training, you need to practice. Even with the right teachers, you are responsible for what you get out of Tai Chi. I often jokingly say to my students, "When you sign up for a Tai Class, it's good for my health (meaning financial health). But, for it to be good for your health, you have to practice and mine the benefits." As a teacher, I respect every person who comes to class. Those who are more committed and appreciative of the art are the easiest to teach. With the right teachers, you can go far with Tai Chi.

Now that you have familiarized yourself with the active ingredients and basic principles of Tai Chi, this chapter will help you develop a formal Tai Chi practice that is sustainable and matches your goals. For those of you who want to add to the practices introduced in this book, you will also learn how to find a good Tai Chi program to maintain and further your practice.

DEVELOP A TAI CHI PRACTICE

"When I first started taking Tai Chi classes, I didn't remember right away what I had learned. But within a few weeks, I had a nice rhythm going," says Linda, a 53-year-old saleswoman. "I could do little segments on my own—the opening of the form, ward off right and left, and Grasp Sparrow's Tail."

"I found the best time for me to practice at home was first thing in the morning before breakfast," says Linda, who also takes Tai Chi classes several days a week. "I shoot for 30 minutes at a time. It's fun to put on some soft music, or try it outside with my shoes off, either on the beach or in the yard. When I practice in nature, things drop away, the air flows through my lungs, and I feel the air on my skin. Without the familiar references from my classes, I may have to work a little harder, but to do Tai Chi and see a beautiful view can be quite inspiring."

"Tai Chi has become part of my life," Linda says. "I read about, think about, bring in the elements of Tai Chi into my day. I use Tai Chi breathing to relax at work, and do exercises to align my body while I'm at my desk. I do simple Tai Chi Pouring all the time. I never have to just stand in line again!"

Some basic rules apply in developing a Tai Chi practice. You need to find your own optimal frequency and duration to practice, the best times of day, and the most convenient places to do Tai Chi, whether in a class, at home, or in a local park.

Here's what I share with my Tai Chi students:

- *Some practice is better than no practice.* Like any learning process, the more you put into it, the more you get out of it. The regimen you choose depends on what your goals are. One of my teachers, Arthur Goodridge, said that learning Tai Chi is like learning to play the piano. To learn enough to play a few songs for your friends requires different training than to become a concert pianist. If you are drawn to Tai Chi as a way to maintain wellness and manage the minor stresses of life, then practicing for 30 minutes a day for a few days a week, in addition to other exercise regimens, will likely lead to substantial benefits. If you are working through a serious illness, or are highly deconditioned and want to make major health changes, and/or if you wish to mine the deeper martial and spiritual dimensions of Tai Chi, then you will need a more rigorous practice regimen.

- *Pace yourself.* Like most exercises, it's better to do a little Tai Chi frequently than to do a lot all at once and nothing in between. Part of the 70-percent rule is that your body needs time to absorb and adapt to the changes set in motion by your Tai Chi practice. A young tree requires a certain amount of water to thrive, but the timing of the water is just as important. Intermittent rain that seeps through the soil allows the young tree to grow better than one rain shower burst.

- *Be patient with your progress.* Change happens slowly with Tai Chi. At certain stages, your learning curve may become relatively flat, and you many even feel as if you are going backward. Then one day, you notice a change and you can perform a certain movement more efficiently or smoothly. Or, maybe it's a simple real-life change, such as being able to pull your pants up while standing on one leg instead of sitting down. Look for ways to mark your progress. Many of my students get frustrated, despite my words encouraging patience. They ask, "Is there something else I can use? A book, a DVD, a pill?" With Tai Chi, you must learn to learn slowly, organically, and develop patience.

- *Don't compare yourself to others.* People learn in different ways and at different rates. You may extract different elements from Tai Chi than someone else does. Some people are good at learning the choreography of a Tai Chi form, but their minds race a mile a minute. Others can physically embody some of the mind-body principles, but find it a challenge to coordinate the movements.

• *Don't be too overly self-critical.* I often have to remind my students (and myself) to be gentle regarding their progress or the quality of practice in any given class. Sometimes I suggest they turn off their "internal scoreboards." You want to be aware of the inefficiencies and inaccuracies in your techniques and do your best to rectify them. But, most of the time, you also want to simply enjoy what is going well, the basic feeling of even a little flow or getting a movement sort of right. You even feel good for simply showing up. Negative self-chatter scatters your Qi and worsens your practice. Being kind and gentle with yourself is better for your Qi and for relaxation, and makes it more likely you will improve.

• *Make Tai Chi part of your regular routine.* A structured routine will help you prioritize your practice. It's like putting "Go to the gym" on your calendar. Pick a regular place and time to practice Tai Chi so that it becomes a kind of ritual. For some people, the act of taking off their shoes or putting on Tai Chi slippers gets them into the right frame of mind to practice. Find something that anchors you and helps you recall previous good experiences as you prepare to practice. Choosing a common place and time, working out with a friend, wearing comfortable clothes, and turning off your cell phone can all add a sense of ritual and purpose to your practice.

• *Keep a notebook or sketchbook.* As you learn new movements, take notes. Translate the movements into your own words, or draw sketches. The process of filtering an intangible experience through your own words or pictures helps to incorporate it into your body. This tool is a particularly good one early on in your practice, instead of just relying on your memory. Later in your training, this is good for reflecting on richer, more subtle principles. Many of the books written by today's Tai Chi masters draw on journals they kept and impart "aha" moments and pearls of wisdom they heard in their weekly classes.

• *Find ways to integrate Tai Chi throughout the day.* The simple protocol in this book allows you to focus on the key active ingredients of

Tai Chi, not on the choreography of a long Tai Chi form. Find places to apply these active ingredients in your daily life. As you wait on line at the supermarket or bank, pour your weight back and forth, feel your feet on the ground, and be aware of how you are breathing. Without looking weird, you are practicing Tai Chi and doing some moving meditation. While watching TV, do mindful stretches for your feet, ankles, and shoulders. At work, take a two-minute break every hour to do some deep breathing. If you need to, set a timer or download a software program to your computer or smart phone to remind you to take a breathing break. Just as a computer has a screen saver to protect against certain pixels becoming overused, you can establish an internal "screen saver" so you don't fry too many brain cells.

- *Join a Tai Chi program.* Find a place to practice Tai Chi with others. Doing so will add social support to your structured practice. It's very important to find the right teacher to help you to continue to grow into your practice.

How to Find a Tai Chi Program

"I learned a few Tai Chi movements from a woman who was taking care of my grandmother when I was a teenager. Twenty-five years later, when my son Brandon was starting first grade, I asked one of the class fathers who was into martial arts about Tai Chi, and he suggested a school right in the neighborhood," says Sunny, a 50-year-old artist. "I learned the Yang style short form over the next several years at that school. When I joined my local Y, I found there were free Tai Chi classes, so I started going there, too. And that's where I ran into the same dad, who told me he was now teaching Tai Chi. I started going to his classes as well, and learned how to do Push Hands and a sword form," says Sunny, who now does Tai Chi for about one hour almost every day.

Just as it is when you shop for a doctor, a home, or a car, it's worth doing some research to find a Tai Chi teacher. Several factors come into play. Check out several Tai Chi classes, and talk to the teachers and students to get a feel for the class and to gather more information. Look at your resources in terms of time and money, and consider practical constraints, such as travel distance to a class. If the Tai Chi studio is on the other side of town, the class is held during rush hour, and it's hard to park there, this choice may not be the ideal place to learn Tai Chi.

The first place to look for a Tai Chi teacher or program is on the Internet. The Tai Chi school's website will give you some clues about the type of training, how long the teacher has trained, and with whom. Be aware that on the Internet, teachers can portray themselves in whatever way they want. The best way to check out the teacher is to attend a class, where you can see the teacher's style and demeanor, and interact with and receive feedback from other students. Feel the vibe of the class. Finding a teacher is done more by feel than as an exact science.

Here's what to look for when you search for a Tai Chi teacher or Tai Chi program:

- *An experienced teacher.* All things being equal, someone with more experience is likely to teach you more effectively. An experienced Tai Chi teacher should be intimately familiar with and embody the Tai Chi exercises he or she teaches and be able to guide you into the deeper experience of Tai Chi. The teacher may also have training in related internal arts, like Qigong, and have training in traditional Chinese medicine, or even biomedical training (for example, physical therapy). This range of knowledge is important, especially if you have health issues. Also, consider the opportunity for long-term growth of your Tai Chi practice. If the teacher or program offers multiple Tai Chi forms (including weapons forms like a sword form) and interactive training like Push Hands, this both reflects a rich diversity in the teacher's Tai Chi training and opportunities for you to learn a diversity of techniques. Lineage is emphasized by many teachers, and many had the opportunity to study directly with renowned masters. But, keep in mind that there are no formal criteria to earn the title of master, and anyone can say he or she is a Tai Chi master, so this can be tricky. You have to feel out the teacher. Most schools will allow you to take a trial class. This will give you the best opportunity to experience the program firsthand. Afterward, talk to students in the class about their experience with the teacher.

- *Good teachers tend to have long-term students.* If students have made a commitment to stay with a teacher, this commitment reflects well upon the teacher. Visit a class, and ask other students how long they have been studying with that teacher. If the students are open and friendly, ask them about the teacher's strengths and weaknesses to get a sense of how the teacher runs the class. The students should be happy and appear in good spirits. A good program will have an obvious sense of community, with lots of social interaction before and after classes.

- *A teacher with good teaching skills and good people skills.* Some of the best Tai Chi practitioners do not make the best teachers. A teacher needs to have good communication skills, not only to teach you the outer movements but, more importantly, to guide you so that you can experience the meditative and energetic internal qualities of Tai Chi. For some teachers, good communication might include clear verbal articulation and a meditative voice. Other teachers communicate very effectively by illustrating movements, embodying principles, and making physical and energetic adjustments to your postures. Just as importantly, the teacher needs to be able to convey this information in a style that makes it easy for you to understand. Since you will probably have a long, intimate relationship with your teacher, find one who matches your learning style, whether it's someone who is verbal or nonverbal, articulate or quiet. If you have unique medical issues or limitations, you need to feel safe when you take a Tai Chi class. Make sure the teacher knows your needs, has experience with your condition, and is willing to accommodate.

- *A comfortable environment in a practical location.* You should feel comfortable in the class's environment. If a clean, lighted space is important to you, then don't pick a class in a grungy, dark space. If you find a class that is inconvenient to your schedule, it can derail your practice. You don't want the class to turn you off from doing Tai Chi. If you have a health issue and the class requires you to climb four flights of stairs, this probably is not the best location to take a class.

- *Look for the right size class.* Some people like small classes, while others prefer large classes. Large classes may reflect the teacher's popularity, but you may not get a lot of one-on-one attention. Some large classes break out into smaller groups to afford more personal, hands-on instruction with each student. In a small class, you will likely get special attention, but if you are self-conscious, you may stand out like a sore thumb. Visit a number of Tai Chi schools to get a sense of what size class you prefer.

- *Trust your instincts.* If you find a teacher, but it doesn't feel right, respect your instincts. The richer aspects of Tai Chi require lengthy training to achieve, so you may have to stick with a teacher for a while to reach these levels. If you trust the teacher, expect to be challenged and maybe even pushed to your best level of achievement.
- *Consider the costs.* If cost is an issue, find an affordable class. Most Tai Chi classes are not too expensive, and many health clubs, gyms, and YMCAs offer free group classes.
- *Understand your goals.* Are you practicing Tai Chi to improve your health, add to your martial arts skills, or explore your spirituality? Assess the teacher's skills according to your intentions. If you are taking the class to rehabilitate a significant health issue, you want a teacher who not only is proficient in Tai Chi but also understands some aspects of biomedicine, as well as body mechanics and skeletal alignment and structure. Many Tai Chi teachers have direct training in rehabilitation medicine, sports medicine, or acupuncture and can adapt their teaching to someone with special needs. If you are attracted to Tai Chi for the martial arts aspect, find a teacher with martial arts skills as part of his or her pedigree. If the spiritual tradition of Tai Chi is important to you, make sure the teacher has sound character, embodies listening skills, and has a sense of warmth and empathy.
- *Pick a style.* Tai Chi comes in many different styles. While systematic differences occur among these styles in the stances and training, the principles of Tai Chi are the same throughout all styles. No hard-and-fast rule dictates which style you should try first. After you have learned one style well, you can expand and learn another one. If you spend enough time learning one style, you may appreciate the differences of another style.

Your progress in Tai Chi will depend on your ongoing commitment and perseverance. Like any exercise or self-improvement activity, sustaining your practice and keeping it fresh and engaging can be a challenge. The exercises and ideas developed in this book and the tips outlined above will help you develop your Tai Chi practice. Joining an ongoing class or Tai Chi program led by an experienced teacher will provide you with in-person instruction, the ability to learn new material, and the social support of a Tai Chi community. Now that you have learned and practiced the general Tai Chi exercises and principles in this book, you will be prepared to move further along in your learning about Tai Chi and become a more discerning shopper as you seek out a Tai Chi program that matches your interest and learning style.

Afterword

Tai Chi and Twenty-First-Century Medicine

The doctor of the future will give no medicine but will interest his patients in the care of the human frame, in diet and in the cause and prevention of disease. —THOMAS EDISON

The US health-care system is in serious trouble. Americans spend significantly more per capita on health care than do the citizens of any other nation in the world, and medical costs continue to spiral out of control. A 2009 study by Harvard Medical School faculty found that more than 60 percent of personal bankruptcies are due to medical costs, and in the majority of these cases, those claiming bankruptcy were medically insured.[1]

What's even more disturbing is that these massive expenditures for health do not translate into making US citizens the healthiest people in the world. Using virtually every measure of health-care outcome, including longevity, infant mortality, fitness, and chronic disease rates, the United States appears at or near the bottom compared to other developed countries. The World Health Organization recently rated America thirty-seventh in health outcomes, on a par with Serbia. In addition, for the first time in history, Americans are witnessing a decline in life expectancy. We are paying more and more for health care and have less and less to show for it. Something needs to change in twenty-first-century medicine to avert this continuing crisis.

The Chinese word for crisis (*wēijī*; 危机) is sometimes interpreted as being composed of two characters, one representing "danger" and the other "opportunity." More generally, according to the yin-yang principle, when a system becomes imbalanced and unstable, it affords an opportunity for transformation or change. Our current health-care system is at such a juncture, and one of the solutions is a greater emphasis on self-care and prevention.

HEALTH CARE VS. "SICK" CARE

In a provocative article by Susan Blumenthal, MD, former Assistant Surgeon General of the United States, who is a widely respected health-care leader, she stated, "Today's health-care reform efforts must reestablish public health and prevention as priorities—transforming our country from a 'sick'-care system to a health-care system."[2] Dr. Blumenthal highlights the major causes of death and disability in America today, including chronic diseases such as heart disease, cancer, stroke, diabetes, and lung disease. These diseases affect the lives of 40 percent of Americans and contribute to our high and still rising health-care costs.

Sadly, the prevalence, onset, and severity of all of these and many other conditions can be improved upon by lifestyle changes, including physical activity, weight control, smoking cessation, and healthy diets. Most striking is that chronic conditions contribute to 75 percent of health-care costs in the United States, yet only 2–3 percent of the US government's health-care budget is invested in prevention—a percentage that has not changed since 1934. Importantly, Dr. Blumenthal went on to write that a re-energized focus on prevention cannot be the purview of physicians alone. I couldn't agree more. Each of us has a personal responsibility for lifestyle choices, and all sectors of society, including families, schools, businesses, health-care providers, foundations, media, and the government, will have to play a role.

Greater Emphasis on Self-Care and Prevention

A great deal of health-care reform discussion has been focused on how to make our current system more efficient, but we haven't devoted enough time and effort to the fundamentals of self-care and prevention.

Medical professionals commonly classify levels of care according to primary, secondary, and tertiary care. At the bottom of this pyramid of care is primary care. Primary care typically represents your first level of contact with the health-care system. For example, you may seek treatment for new symptoms, such as the flu or a strained muscle, or go for your annual physical. Your primary care provider may be a doctor, nurse practitioner, or physician assistant. The next step up the pyramid is secondary care, which refers to referrals by your primary care provider to receive treatment from a medical specialist. For example, your primary care provider might refer you to a cardiologist for a heart condition or an endocrinologist for a hormone-related disease like diabetes. The top tier of the pyramid is tertiary care. This level refers to highly specialized care, often based in academic medical centers. For example, you may need a complicated procedure such as knee replacement surgery that requires a team of highly specialized medical personnel.

Two additional tiers should be included in the health-care pyramid—self-care and prevention—suggests my colleague Donald Levy, MD, Director of Osher Clinical Center for Complementary and Integrative Medical Therapies at Brigham and Women's Hospital. In both his academic lectures and clinical consultations, Dr. Levy emphasizes the fundamental importance of physical exercise, stress reduction, psychosocial support, healthy eating habits, weight management, and a good night's sleep. He gives this advice to patients who already have chronic illnesses, such as cardiovascular disease or back pain, as well those seeking his advice on how to prevent chronic conditions so they can live long, healthy, medically uncomplicated lives. Dr. Levy, along with a growing number of practitioners of integrative medicine, believes that by involving patients in their own self-care, they are more likely not only to improve their health, but also to learn more about how their bodies work to maintain health. The result is that they feel more empowered, become better patients, and advocate for themselves as they navigate through the health-care system.

One of the more versatile self-care tools in Dr. Levy's toolbox for lifestyle change is Tai Chi. Typically, patients looking to manage their blood pressure without medications, ease and rehabilitate chronic back pain, or manage chronic depression or anxiety leave with a "prescription" to learn Tai Chi as part of an integrated health-care strategy. Because Dr. Levy practices in an evidence-based manner, patients who are "prescribed" Tai Chi often leave with a research article that supports the application of Tai Chi for their specific medical condition. I, too, often share research articles about Tai Chi to those referred to me with specific medical issues. Providing this evidence engenders patient buy-in, and better follow-though and long-term compliance.

Integrating Tai Chi and Related Mind-Body Practices across the Entire Human Life Span

Up until now, the majority of Tai Chi research has targeted the potential health benefits for relatively older adults, as well as for those managing or rehabilitating a variety of illnesses. However, in order for Tai Chi and related practices to influence our current health-care crisis significantly, we need to include people of all ages. This broader view will help us greatly expand the potential for impact on a much wider population and therefore reduce health-care costs. To prevent chronic diseases and enhance healthy lifestyles effectively, I believe that Tai Chi and related mind-body practices should begin in childhood. My research is moving in this direction—that is, to study how the integration of mind-body practices can meaningfully affect all age groups, including children. Tai Chi can help kids lay down lifelong skills early on when led by their schoolteachers and parents.

As I look to the future, I see seeds of this approach already sprouting up across the United States and the world.

Integration of Tai Chi and Mind-Body Exercise for Grade-School Kids

Physical education increasingly is being short-changed in schools for budgetary and curriculum-based reasons. The short-sightedness of cutting out gym class is an example of the limited appreciation of the mind-body connection. Lack of exercise during school likely contributes to the current childhood obesity epidemic and likely hurts the academic performance of kids.[3] Multiple studies show that exercise is essential for an adolescent's mind-body health and sets a trajectory for lifelong healthy behaviors.

It turns out that children are remarkably receptive and responsive to mind-body exercises like Tai Chi. About 15 years ago, I had the opportunity to teach Tai Chi to fourth graders in the Cambridge, Massachusetts, public school system. I was initially brought in to teach Tai Chi to help kids manage their anxieties and focus better on new standardized tests. I developed a playful curriculum that focused on simple Tai Chi–inspired animal movements, body awareness, and breathing exercises. And, contrary to my initial expectations, the kids were very open not only to the movements of Tai Chi, but also to the meditation, imagery, and the experience of energy.

Since then, while raising my son, I have felt a greater appreciation for teaching the active ingredients of Tai Chi to children. In addition to encouraging my son to learn martial arts and be athletically active, my wife and I have combined bedtime stories with breathing exercises, visualizations, body awareness, and relaxation techniques. Watching my son grow up with these resources has reinvigorated my interest in making Tai Chi and related mind-body practices an integral part of grade-school education. Learning how to stand and move with ease and confidence, breathe deeply, and be able to sense and manage emotions should be just as an important part of school as the classic Three Rs. All of my adult students agree that they wish they had been taught some of the active ingredients of Tai Chi when they were children.

My vision is that Tai Chi and related mind-body exercises will become deeply integrated into the grade-school curriculum, and not only in physical education classes or during recess. Mind-body practices can become part of modules related to learning about human biology—how we breathe, how muscles and bones relate to each other, and how flexibility and balance, as well as focus, impact sports performance. They can be woven into science curricula that test hypotheses about the impact of health-promoting activities on human physiology. As kids learn about Asian culture in social studies classes, they can learn about different ways of viewing the body for a healthy, balanced lifestyle.

Several Tai Chi programs for kids currently are available, and many have been successfully implemented in public schools. Little research evidence is available, but anecdotal observations suggest regular Tai Chi practice leads kids to better focus and behavior.[4] Some studies suggest Tai Chi helps children with special needs, including those with ADHD, deal with anxiety and moods.[5] In addition, a growing body of research on Qigong, yoga and other mind-body practices, including a review our group conducted, adds further support for Tai Chi-like exercise in the classroom.[6]

Tai Chi Is a Nice Alternative to High School Gym Class

A handful of high schools in the Greater Boston area already give students the option of taking a Tai Chi or yoga class instead of participating in standard gym classes. I think it would be great if this option became more widely available.

A small study conducted by my colleague Robert Wall combined Tai Chi with mindfulness-based stress reduction. He found that these high school students felt calmer, more relaxed, had improved sleep, were less reactive, and took better care of themselves.[7]

Similarly, a randomized control trial of yoga versus physical education by fellow researchers at Harvard Medical School showed that high school students who practiced yoga had a better mood overall and felt less anxiety, while the typical gym class group showed a worsening of these symptoms over the course of the 10-week study.[8]

Tai Chi Goes to College and Medical School

College is often a stressful time. It may be the first time a student has been on his or her own. The study workload may be heavy. Then there's the lack of sleep and temptations to drink and do drugs. Tai Chi may be a helpful stress-reduction antidote.

In fact, Tai Chi is becoming increasingly popular in colleges across the country. Many college physical education departments now include Tai Chi, yoga, or meditation alternatives. In China, Tai Chi has found its way into the curriculum of nearly all universities. Researchers have begun to show the benefits of Tai Chi for college students. A growing number of studies have reported that college students who do Tai Chi for a few months have improved sleep quality and mood, and feel less stress.[9]

In the United States, Tai Chi is also beginning to make its way into medical schools and nursing schools as part of the trend toward more mind-body training. Andrew Weil, MD, Clinical Professor of Medicine and Director and Founder, Arizona Center for Integrative Medicine in Tucson, Arizona, introduces all of his internal medicine fellows to Tai Chi and related practices. Some 80 percent of Georgetown University School of Medicine students undergo 11 weeks of mind-body training during their first academic semester, showing marked changes in their reported levels of stress.[10] I expose all the fellows in the Harvard Medical School Research Training Program in Complementary and Integrative Medicine to Tai Chi and Qigong, and teach these practices to more than 200 health professionals each year who participate in Dr. Herbert Benson's continuing medical education program in mind-body medicine at Harvard Medical School.

Integration of Tai Chi into medical professional training is especially valuable. A high level of burnout occurs among medical and nursing students because of their rigorous course load and lack of sleep.[11] The stress-reduction skills they learn through Tai Chi and other mind-body exercises will carry over into their practices to make them better health professionals. A new generation of doctors and nurses will have the knowledge of how and when to prescribe mind-body therapies to improve the health of their patients. Those who practice these skills also become better advisors to their patients. Good evidence suggests that patients are more likely to follow those who lead by example. That is, a slim, trim doctor gets better buy-in when asking an overweight patient to lose weight than an overweight doctor does. A healthy-looking doctor who presents in a grounded, centered manner is likely to have better success "prescribing" Tai Chi, yoga, or meditation to patients.[12]

Tai Chi—The Eastern Ambassador to Self-Care and Prevention

Tai Chi is helping to transform Western health care toward integrative medicine. Claims of Tai Chi's health benefits are increasingly evidence-based, with more than 700 peer-reviewed, scientific publications in print and more than 180 randomized trials conducted, to date. You might say Tai Chi plays an ambassadorial role, helping to integrate Eastern and Western approaches to optimize health.

Tai Chi not only serves as a catalyst and example of integrative medicine but also holds a unique niche. Tai Chi has something to offer you whether you are young or old, hoping to prevent disease or rehabilitating from one, trying to manage everyday stress more gracefully, or interested in self-discovery, enhancing creativity, or improving sports performance. Because of this versatility, Tai Chi has the potential to impact Western health care and help keep you and the rest of society physically and psychologically healthy.

While we all know that lifestyle changes, such as exercise and stress reduction, can help lengthen your life, it's hard to change your behavior. An important part of the future work of Tai Chi researchers and the developers of Tai Chi programs for people of all ages will be to analyze what motivates people to change their lives for the better. Tai Chi may offer a different enough approach to exercise and self-care to inspire people to sustain healthy lifestyle changes.

One reason for this is that Tai Chi cultivates self-responsibility and self-empowerment. When you do Tai Chi, you feel healthier, partly because you are participating in your own health care. You are also more likely to become physically active and engage in other forms of exercise. Self-discovery is an appealing, lifelong learning skill. Tai Chi can be a lot more fun and meaningful than walking on a treadmill day after day, so you are more likely to stick with it.

But our Western culture may need to find new ways of teaching and marketing Tai Chi for even greater buy-in and longer-term adherence. The emphasis on scientific evidence and more knowledge about how the body works, paired with Eastern wisdom, may make Tai Chi even more attractive to new or potential Tai Chi students, as well as to referring health-care professionals. We also need more teachers who can build the bridge between East and West.

My hope is that this book contributes to this bridging concept and inspires you to take up Tai Chi and learn more about it, and perhaps become a teacher yourself. One of my greatest experiences as a Tai Chi teacher and researcher was learning that participants of our clinical trials—who originally volunteered to be in our study for health reasons—have continued their training and became Tai Chi teachers themselves. Perhaps you will be among the next generation of Tai Chi teachers who work with school kids, in a corporate wellness center, with doctors, or in a senior center, and contribute to the integration of Tai Chi into twenty-first-century health care.

Notes

Introduction

1. Ted Kaptchuk, *The Web That Has No Weaver: Understanding Chinese Medicine* (New York: McGraw-Hill, 2000).
2. A. C. Ahn et al., "The Limits of Reductionism in Medicine: Could Systems Biology Offer an Alternative?" *Public Library of Science Medicine* 3, no. 6 (2006). e208.
3. Ibid.

Chapter 1

1. There are two systems for translating Chinese characters into phonetic words. One is the Wade-Giles system developed by academic thinkers in the Western tradition. A second, more widely used system today is Pinyin. Throughout this book, we will largely follow the Pinyin system, for example, writing Qigong (vs. Chi Kung) and Beijing (vs. Peking). However, because the term is already so widely accepted in the West, we will continue to use the Wade-Giles term "Tai Chi" vs. the Pinyin "taiji."
2. Douglas Wile, *T'ai Chi's Ancestors: The Making of an Internal Art* (Brooklyn: Sweet Chi Press, 1999).
3. Readers interested in more scholarly discussions of Tai Chi's history should see Douglas Wile, *Lost T'ai-chi Classics from the Late Ch'ing Dynasty* (Albany:

SUNY Press, 1996); Douglas Wile, *Tai Chi Touchstones: Yang Family Secret Transmissions*, Sweet Chi Press: Brooklyn, 2010; Douglas Wile, *T'ai Chi's Ancestors: The Making of an Internal Art* (Brooklyn: Sweet Chi Press: Brooklyn, 1999); Barbara Davis, *The Taijiquan Classics, An Annotated Translation* (Berkeley: North Atlantic Books, 2004); and Benjamin Lo, Martin Inn, Susan Foe, and Robert Amacker, *The Essence of T'ai Chi Ch'uan: The Literary Tradition* (Berkeley: North Atlantic Books, 1993).

4. For more on the history of Shaolin, and more generally, the history of Chinese martial arts, see Meir Shahar, *The Shaolin Monastery: History, Religion, and the Chinese Martial Arts* (Honolulu: University of Hawaii Press, 2008); David Chow and Richard Spangler, *Kung Fu: History, Philosophy, and Techniques* (Dallas: Unique Publications, 1989); Donn Draeger and Robert Smith, *Comprehensive Asian Fighting Arts (Bushido—The Way of the Warrior)*, (New York: Kodansha USA, 1981); and Robert Smith, *Chinese Boxing Masters and Methods* (Berkeley: North Atlantic Books, 1993).

5. For a more scholarly historic account on Chang San-feng, see Anna Seidel, "A Taoist Immortal of the Ming Dynasty: Chang San-feng," in William DeBary, *Self and Society in Ming Thought* (New York: Columbia University Press, 1970), 483–531.

6. In reality, the classification of martial arts as internal vs. external represents a gradient. An excellent discussion of this topic can be found in: Barbara Davis, *The Taijiquan Classics: An Annotated Translation* (Berkeley: North Atlantic Books, 2004). Also see Stanley Henning, "Chinese Boxing: The Internal vs. External Schools in Light of History and Theory," *Journal of Asian Martial Arts* 6, no. 3 (1997): 10–19.

7. Other accounts suggest that Yang Lu-chan was an indentured servant to Master Chen Chang Shing; see Barbara Davis, *The Taijiquan Classics, An Annotated Translation* (Berkeley: North Atlantic Books, 2004).

8. For a nice introduction to the animal frolics, see Kenneth S. Cohen, *The Way of Qigong: The Art and Science of Chinese Energy Healing*, (New York: Ballantine Books, 1997). Also see: Yang Jwing-Ming, *The Root of Chinese Chi Kung*, (Boston: YMAA Publications, 1989).

9. It would be misleading not to acknowledge the long history of Tai Chi masters known to love their booze, food, and tobacco, along with other unhealthy lifestyle choices. The association of Tai Chi with healthy living may be more greatly emphasized in today's Western society.

10. The poem is anonymous and likely written in late nineteenth or early twentieth century. From Barbara Davis, *The Taijiquan Classics: An Annotated Translation* (Berkeley: North Atlantic Books, 2004).

11. For a good summary of history and development of standardized short forms, see Alexandra Ryan, "Globalization and the 'Internal Alchemy' in

Chinese Martial Arts: The Transmission of Taijiquan to Britain," *East Asia Science, Technology, and Society* 2, no. 4, (2008): 525–43.

12. Like Tai Chi itself, Taoism is quite pluralistic, with some branches being more secular and others more spiritual and esoteric. Some excellent references on Taoism include Livia Kohn, *Introducing Daoism* (London: Routledge, 2008) and Eva Wong, *Taoism: An Essential Guide* (Boston: Shambhala, 2011).

13. Stephen Mitchell, *The Tao Te Ching* (New York: Harper Perennial, 1992).

14. Ibid.

15. Douglas Wile, *Lost T'ai-chi Classics from the Late Ch'ing Dynasty* (Albany: SUNY Press, 1996).

16. Hall of Happiness is a good example of how philosophies other than Taoism, in this case, Confucianism, affected the evolution of Tai Chi. Many of Master Cheng's writings further develop this link. See Cheng Man Ching Enterprise, "Hall of Happiness," www.chengmanching.com/hallofhappiness.html.

17. Another noteworthy teacher in the United States, prior to Cheng Man Ching, is the dancer Sophia Delza, who opened the first Tai Chi school in New York in 1954 and wrote the first English language book on the art in 1961: Sophia Delza, *Tai Chi Chuan: Body and Mind in Harmony* (N. Canton, Ohio: Good News Publishing, 1961). For a more general discussion of history of traditional Chinese medicine in the United States, see Linda Barnes *Needles, Herbs, Gods, and Ghosts: China, Healing, and the West to 1842* (Cambridge, Mass.: Harvard University Press, 2005).

18. For more on the life of Cheng Man Ching, see Barbara Davis, "In Search of a Unified Dao: Zheng Manqing's Life and Contributions to Taijiquan," *Journal of Asian Martial Arts* 5, no. 2 (1996): 36–59; and Cheng Man-ching and Mark Hennessey, *Master of Five Excellences* (Berkeley: North Atlantic Books, 1995).

19. Douglas Wile, *Lost T'ai-chi Classics from the Late Ch'ing Dynasty* (Albany: SUNY Press, 1996).

20. See http://worldtaichiday.org.

21. An excellent discussion on the impact of the West on Chinese practices like Tai Chi can be found in Alexandra Ryan, "Globalization and the 'Internal Alchemy' in Chinese Martial Arts: The Transmission of Taijiquan to Britain," *East Asia Science, Technology, and Society* 2, no. 4 (2008): 525–43. Also see Nancy Chen, *Breathing Spaces* (New York: Columbia University Press, 2003); Elizabeth Hsu, *The Transmission of Chinese Medicine (Cambridge Studies in Medical Anthropology),* (Cambridge, U.K.: Cambridge University Press, 1999); and Heiner Freuhauf, "Chinese Medicine in Crisis: Science, Politics, and the Making of TCM," *Journal of Chinese Medicine,* (October 1999).

22. For example, see Joseph Needham, *Science and Civilization in China,* vol. 6,

Biology and Biological Technology, part 1, *Botany* (Taipei: Caves Books, 1986); Robert K. G. Temple, *The Genuis of China: 3,000 Years of Science, Discovery, and Invention* (New York: Simon and Schuster, 1986).

23. J. Van Deusen and D. Harlowe, "The Efficacy of the ROM Dance Program for Adults with Rheumatoid Arthritis," *American Journal of Occupational Therapy* 41, no. 2 (1987): 90–95.

24. G. S. Birdee, P. M. Wayne, R. B. Davis, R. S. Phillips, and G. Y. Yeh, "T'ai Chi and Qigong for Health: Patterns of Use in the United States," *Journal of Alternative and Complementary Medicine* 15, no. 9 (2009): 969–73.

25. S. L. Wolf et al., "Reducing Frailty and Falls in Older Persons: An Investigation of Tai Chi and Computerized Balance Training. Atlanta FICSIT Group. Frailty and Injuries: Cooperative Studies of Intervention Techniques," *Journal of the American Geriatrics Society* 44, no. 5 (1996): 489–97.

26. Examples of research on Qigong and Qi include G. Yount et al., "In Vitro Test of External Qigong," *BMC Complementary and Alternative Medicine* 4, no. 5 (2004): 1–8; K. W. Chen et al., "A Preliminary Study of the Effect of External Qigong on Lymphoma Growth in Mice," *Journal of Alternative and Complementary Medicine* 8, no. 5 (2002): 615–21; A. P. Colbert, "Electrodermal Activity at Acupoints: Literature Review and Recommendations for Reporting Clinical Trials," *Journal of Acupuncture and Meridian Studies* 4, no. 1 (2011), 5–13; A. C. Ahn et al., "Electrical Impedance of Acupuncture Meridians: the Relevance of Subcutaneous Collagenous Bands," *PLoS One* 5, no. 7 (2010): e11907; A. C. Ahn et al., "Electrical Properties of Acupuncture Points and Meridians: A Systematic Review," *Bioelectromagnetics* 29, no. 4 (2008), 245–56; N. T. Jou and S. X. Ma, "Responses of Nitric Oxide-cGMP Release in Acupuncture Point to Electroacupuncture in Human Skin in Vivo Using Dermal Microdialysis," *Microcirculation* 16, no. 5 (2009): 434–43; P. L. Faber et al., "EEG Source Imaging during Two Qigong Meditations," *Cognitive Processing* 13, no. 3 (2012): 255–65. For good reviews, see Wayne B. Jonas and Cindy C. Crawford, *Healing, Intention, and Energy Medicine: Science, Research Methods, and Clinical Implications* (Philadelphia: Churchill Livingstone, 2003); and K. W. Chen, "An Analytic Review of Studies on Measuring Effects of External QI in China," *Alternative Therapies in Health and Medicine* 10, no. 4 (2004): 38–50; D. L. Fazzino et al., "Energy Healing and Pain: A Review of the Literature," *Holistic Nursing Practice* 24, no. 2 (2010): 79–88; S. Jain and P. J. Mills. "Biofield Therapies: Helpful or Full of Hype? A Best Evidence Synthesis, *Internal Journal of Behavioral Medicine,* 17, no. 1 (2010): 1–16; J. Levin, "Energy Healers: Who They Are and What They Do," *Explore* 7, no. 13 (2011): 13–26; B. Rubik "The Biofield Hypothesis: Its Biophysical Basis and Role in Medicine, *Journal of Alternative and Complimentary Medicine,* 8, no. 6 (2002): 703–17.

Chapter 2

1. Our approach paralleled one developed by S. L. Wolf and colleagues in their landmark Tai Chi for balance study at Emory University: S. L. Wolf et al., "Reducing Frailty and Falls in Older Persons: An Investigation of Tai Chi and Computerized Balance Training. Atlanta FICSIT Group. Frailty and Injuries: Cooperative Studies of Intervention Techniques," *Journal of the American Geriatrics Society* 44, no. 5 (1996): 489–97. Also see S. L. Wolf et al., "Exploring the Basis for Tai Chi Chuan," *Archives of Physical Medicine Rehabilitation* 78, no. 8 (1997): 886–92.

2. Wolfe Lowenthal, *There Are No Secrets: Professor Cheng Man Ch'ing and His T'ai Chi Chuan* (Berkely: North Atlantic Books, 1993), chap. 23.

3. The language related to awareness I have adopted in my teaching is greatly influenced by my study of Gesture of Awareness, developed by my teacher Charles Genoud. See Charles Genoud, *Gesture of Awareness: A Radical Approach to Time, Space, and Movement* (Somerville, Mass.: Wisdom Publications, 2006).

4. Systematic reviews of studies evaluating aspects of meditative mindfulness and awareness include P. Grossman, et al., "Mindfulness-Based Stress Reduction and Health Benefits: A Meta analysis," *Journal of Psychosomatic Research* 57, no. 1 (2004): 35–43; and A. Chiesa and A. Serretti, "A Systematic Review of Neurobiological and Clinical Features of Mindfulness Meditations," *Psychological Medicine* 40, no. 8 (2010): 1239–52. Also see M. E. Teixeira, "Meditation as an Intervention for Chronic Pain: An Integrative Review," *Holistic Nursing Practice* 22, no. 4 (2008): 225–34.

5. L. Li and B. Manor, "Long Term Tai Chi Exercise Improves Physical Performance among People with Peripheral Neuropathy," *American Journal of Chinese Medicine* 38, no. 3 (2010): 449–59.

6. Examples of studies proprioception and kinesthetic sense include W. W. Tsang and C. W. Hui-Chan, "Effects of Tai Chi on Joint Proprioception and Stability Limits in Elderly Subjects, *Medicine, Science, Sports, and Exercise* 35, no. 12 (2003): 1962–71; B. H. Jacobson et al., "The Effect of T'ai Chi Chuan Training on Balance, Kinesthetic Sense, and Strength," *Perception and Motor Skills* 84, no. 1 (1997): 27–33; D. Xu et al., "Effect of Tai Chi Exercise on Proprioception of Ankle and Knee Joints in Old People," *British Journal of Sports Medicine* 38, no. 1 (2004): 50–54; and S. M. Fong and G. Y. Ng, "The Effects on Sensorimotor Performance and Balance with Tai Chi Training," *Archives of Physical Medicine Rehabilitation* 87, no. 1 (2006): 82–87.

7. M. A. Killingsworth and D. T. Gilbert, "A Wandering Mind Is an Unhappy Mind," *Science* 330, no. 6006 (2010): 932. Further discussed in Chapter 8 "Sharpen Your Mind."

8. Some recent examples of meditation research include F. Zeidan et al., "The Effects of Brief Mindfulness Meditation Training on Experimentally Induced Pain," *Journal of Pain* 11, no. 3 (2010): 199–209; R. J. Davidson et al., "Alterations in Brain and Immune Function Produced by Mindfulness Meditation," *Psychosomatic Medicine* 65, no. 4 (2010): 564–70; L. E. Carlson et al., "One Year Pre–Post Intervention Follow-up of Psychological, Immune, Endocrine, and Blood Pressure Outcomes of Mindfulness-Based Stress Reduction (MBSR) in Breast and Prostate Cancer Outpatients," *Brain, Behavior, and Immunology* 21, no. 8 (2007): 1038–49; J. Carmody and R. Baer, "Relationships between Mindfulness Practice and Levels of Mindfulness, Medical and Psychological Symptoms, and Well-Being in a Mindfulness-Based Stress Reduction Program," *Journal of Behavioral Medicine* 31, no. 1 (2007): 23–33.

9. For a longer discussion of the inability to use placebo controls in trials evaluating Tai Chi, see P. M. Wayne and T. J. Kaptchuk, "Challenges Inherent to Tai Chi Research: Part 2—Defining the Intervention and Optimal Study Design," *Journal of Alternative and Complementary Medicine* 14, no. 2 (2008): 191–97.

10. Jeanne Achterberg, *Imagery and Healing* (Boston: Shambhala, 2002). For excellent discussions of imagery as it relates to Tai Chi, also see Martin Mellish, *A Tai Chi Imagery Workbook: Spirit, Intent, and Motion* (London: Jessica Kingsley, 2010); Bruce McFarlane, "Notes on Anatomy and Physiology: Using Imagery to Relax the Weight," *From the Tiger's Mouth: Official Blog of the International Taoist Tai Chi Society*, April 25, 2010, http://ittcs. wordpress.com/?s=imagery.

11. Good examples include E. Lang et al., "Adjunctive Self-Hypnotic Relaxation for Outpatient Medical Procedures: A Prospective Randomized Trial with Women Undergoing Large Core Breast Biopsy," *Pain* 126, nos. 1–3 (2006): 155–64; O. Eremin, "Immuno-Modulatory Effects of Relaxation Training and Guided Imagery in Women with Locally Advanced Breast Cancer Undergoing Multimodality Therapy: A Randomized Controlled Trial, *Breast* 18, no. 1 (2009): 17–25.

12. Evidence for this idea comes from the field of motor imagery. Some representative studies include T. Mulder et al., "Observation, Imagination, and Execution of an Effortful Movement: More Evidence for a Central Explanation of Motor Imagery," *Experimental Brain Research* 163, no. 3 (2005): 344–51; C. Schuster et al., "Best Practice for Motor Imagery: A Systematic Literature Review on Motor Imagery Training Elements in Five Different Disciplines," *BMC Medicine* 17, no. 9 (2011): 75; M. Jeannerod, "Neural Simulation of Action: A Unifying Mechanism for Motor Cognition," *Neuroimage* 14, no. 1 pt. 2, (2001): S103–9; and S. J. Page et al., "Mental Practice in Chronic Stroke: Results of a Randomized, Placebo-Controlled Trial," *Stroke* 38, no.

4 (2007): 1293–97. More discussion of motor imagery research is included in Chapter 8, "Sharpen Your Mind."

13. A good review of this topic is H. A. Shlagter et al., "Mental Training as a Tool in the Neuroscientific Study of Brain and Cognitive Plasticity," *Frontiers in Human Neuroscience* 10, no. 5 (2011): 17.

14. Summaries of placebo research can be found in Anne Harrington, *The Placebo Effect: An Interdisciplinary Exploration* (Cambridge, Mass.: Harvard University Press, 1999); Fabrizio Benedetti, *Placebo Effects: Understanding the Mechanisms in Health and Disease* (Oxford: Oxford University Press, 2008).

15. T. T. Liang, *Imagination Becomes Reality* (Little Canada: Dragon Door Publications, 1992).

16. T. J. Kaptchuk, J. M. Kelley, A. Deykin, P. M. Wayne, L. C. Lasagna, I. O. Epstein, I. Kirsch, M. E. Wechsler. "Do 'Placebo Responders' Exist?" *Contemporary Clinical Trials* 29 (2008): 587–95.

17. For a deeper discussion of imagery and Tai Chi, see: Martin Mellish, *A Tai Chi Imagery Workbook: Spirit, Intent, and Motion* (London: Jessica Kingsley, 2010).

18. For example, see A. C. Ahn et al., "Electrical Properties of Acupuncture Points and Meridians: A Systematic Review," *Bioelectromagnetics* 29, no. 4 (2008): 245–56; A. C. Ahn et al., "Electrical Impedance of Acupuncture Meridians: The Relevance of Subcutaneous Collagenous Bands," *PLoS One* 5, no. 7 (2012): e11907; H. M. Langevin and J. A. Yandow, "Relationship of Acupuncture Points and Meridians to Connective Tissue Planes," *The Anatomical Record* 269, no. 6 (2002): 257–65.

19. James Oschman, *Energy Medicine: The Scientific Basis* (Philadelphia: Churchill Livingstone, 2000).

20. The central role of connective tissue in this matrix, and its potential to bridge both Western mechanical and Eastern energy-based concepts of integration, is beautifully captured in the following quote from Dr. James Oschman:

> The connective tissue forms a continuously interconnected system throughout the living body. All movements, of the body as a whole and of its smallest parts, are created by tensions carried through the connective tissue fabric. It is a liquid crystalline material and its components are semiconductors, properties that give rise to many remarkable properties. One of the semiconductor properties of connective tissue is piezoelectricity, from the Greek, meaning "pressure electricity." Because of piezoelectricity, every movement of the body, every pressure and every tension anywhere, generates a variety of oscillating bioelectric signals or microcurrent and other kinds of signals . . . Because of the continuity and conductivity of the connective tissue, these signals spread through the tissues . . . and are also conducted into the cells. If parts of the organism are cooperative in their

functioning and every cell knows what every other cell is doing, it is due to the continuity and signaling properties of connective tissue.

James Oschman, *Energy Medicine: The Scientific Basis* (Philadelphia: Churchill Livingstone, 2000). Also see: Emily Conrad, *Life on Land: The Story of Continuum* (Berkeley: North Atlantic Books, 2007) and Bonnie Gintis, *Engaging the Movement of Life* (Berkeley: North Atlantic Books, 2007).

21. Chen Wei-Mind, Benajmin Pang Jeng Lo, and Robert W. Smith, *T'ai Chi Ch'uan Ta Wen: Questions and Answers on T'ai Chi Ch'uan* (Berkeley: North Atlantic Books, 1993).

22. Cheng Man Ching, trans. Mark Hennessy, *Master Cheng's New Method of Taichi Ch'uan Self-Cultivation* (Berkeley: Blue Snake Books, 1999).

23. Charles Darwin, *The Expression of Emotions in Man and Animals* (London: Penguin Classics, 2009); Paul Eckman, *What the Face Reveals: Basic and Applied Studies of Spontaneous Expression Using the Facial Action Coding System (FACS)* (Series in Affective Science) (New York: Oxford University Press, 2005).

24. D. R. Carney et al., "Power Posing: Brief Nonverbal Displays Affect Neuroendocrine Levels and Risk Tolerance," *Psychological Sciences* 21, no. 10 (2010): 1363–68.

25. For a systematic review of Tai Chi for pain conditions that highlights Tai Chi's safety, see C. Wang, "Tai Chi and Rheumatic Diseases," *Rheumatological Disease Clinics of North America* 37, no. 1 (2010): 19–32.

26. Surprisingly, the scientific understanding of the physiology of stretching, and hence, what types of stretching are safest and most effective is not conclusive and debated. For summaries of this research, see L. C. Decoster et al., "The Effects of Hamstring Stretching on Range of Motion: A Systematic Literature Review," *Journal of Orthopaedic & Sports Physical Therapy* 35, no. 6 (June 2005): 377–87; L. E. Hart, "Effect of Stretching on Sport Injury Risk: A Review," *Medicine and Science in Sports and Exercise* 15, no. 2 (2005): 113; R. Shehab et al., "Pre-Exercise Stretching and Sports Related Injuries: Knowledge, Attitudes and Practices," *Clinical Journal of Sport Medicine* 16, no. 3 (May 2006): 228–31.

27. L. Sheppard et al., "The National Blueprint Consensus Conference Summary Report: Strategic Priorities for Increasing Physical Activity among Adults Aged ≥50," *American Journal of Preventive Medicine* 25, no. 3, suppl. 2 (2001): 209–13.

28. For a good summary of the aerobic intensity of Tai Chi, see C. Lan et al., "The Exercise Intensity of Tai Chi Chuan," *Medicine and Sport Science* 52, (2008): 12–19.

29. G. Y. Yeh, E. P. McCarthy, P. M. Wayne, L. W. Stevenson, M. J. Wood, D. Forman, R. B. Davis, and R. S. Phillips, "Tai Chi Exercise in Patients with

Chronic Heart Failure: A Randomized Clinical Trial," *Archives of Internal Medicine* 171, no. 8 (2011): 750–57; J. A. Fontana et al., "Tai Chi as an Intervention for Heart Failure," *Nursing Clinics of North America* 35 (2000): 1031–46.

30. Systematic reviews of Tai Chi for patients with cardiovascular disease or risk factors support that Tai Chi is safe for this population. See: G. Y. Yeh, C. Wang, P. M. Wayne, and R. Phillips, "Tai Chi Exercise for Patients with Cardiovascular Conditions and Risk Factors: A Systematic Review," *Journal of Cardiopulmonary Rehabilitation Prevention* 29, no. 3 (2009): 152–60; R. E. Taylor-Pillae and E. S. Froelicher, "The Effectiveness of Tai Chi Exercise in Improving Aerobic Capacity: A Meta Analysis," *Journal of Cardiovascular Nursing* 19, no. 1 (2004): 48–57.

31. For examples, see G. Wu and D. Mellon, "Joint Kinetics During Tai Chi Gait and Normal Walking Gait in Young and Elderly Tai Chi Chuan Practitioners," *Clinical Biomechanics* 23, no. 6 (2008): 787–95; G. Wu and J. Hitt, "Ground Contact Characteristics of Tai Chi Gait," *Gait Posture* 22, no. 1 (2005): 32–39; P. M. Wayne, D. P. Kiel, J. E. Buring, E. M. Connors, P. Bonato, G. Y. Yeh, C. J. Cohen, C. Mancinelli, and R. B. Davis, "Impact of Tai Chi Exercise on Multiple Fracture-Related Risk Factors in Post-Menopausal Osteopenic Women: A Pilot Pragmatic, Randomized Trial. *BMC Complementary and Alternative Medicine* 12, no. 7 (2012); P. M. Wayne, D. E. Krebs, S. L. Wolf, K. M. Gill-Body, D. M. Scarborough, C. A. McGibbon, T. J. Kaptchuk, and S. W. Parker, "Can Tai Chi Improve Vestibulopathic Postural Control?" *Archives of Physical Medicine Rehabilitation* 85, no. 1 (2004): 142–52; P. M. Wayne, D. P. Kiel, D. E. Krebs, R. B. Davis, J. Savetsky-German, M. Connolly, and J. E. Buring, "The Effects of Tai Chi on Bone Mineral Density in Postmenopausal Women: A Systematic Review," *Archives of Physical Medicine Rehabilitation* 88, no. 5 (2007): 673–80.

32. S. L. Wolf et al., "Reducing Frailty and Falls in Older Persons: An Investigation of Tai Chi and Computerized Balance Training," *Journal of the American Geriatrics Society* 44, no. 5 (1996): 489–97.

33. See C. Wang, "Tai Chi and Rheumatic Diseases," *Rheumatological Disease Clinics of North America* 37, no. 1 (2010): 19–32, as well as chapter 4.

34. For an excellent history of breathing in Western traditions, see Don Hanlon Johnson, *Bone, Breath, and Gesture: Practices of Embodiment Volume 1* (Berkeley: North Atlantic Books, 1995).

35. See A. W. Chan et al., "Tai Chi Qigong Improves Lung Functions and Activity Tolerance in COPD Clients: A Single Blind, Randomized Controlled Trial," *Complementary Therapies in Medicine* 19, no. 1 (2011): 3–11; R. W. Leung et al., "A Study Design to Investigate the Effect of Short-Form Sun-Style Tai Chi in Improving Functional Exercise Capacity, Physical Performance, Balance, and Health-Related Quality of Life in People with Chronic

Obstructive Pulmonary Disease (COPD)," *Contemporary Clinical Trials* 32, no. 2 (2011): 267–72; S. Kiatboonsri et al., "Effects of Tai Chi Qigong Training on Exercise Performance and Airway Inflammation in Moderate to Severe Persistent Asthma," *CHEST* 134 (2008): s54003.

36. Support for this statement comes from large-scale epidemiological studies, including G. D. Friedman et al., "Lung Function and Risk of Myocardial Infarction and Sudden Cardiac Death," *New England Journal of Medicine* 294, no. 20 (1976): 1071–75; P. C. Hall, "Impaired Lung Function and Mortality Risk in Men and Women: Findings from the Renfrew and Paisley Prospective Population Study," *British Medical Journal* 313, no. 7059 (1996): 21; 711–15; and J. Weuve et al., "Forced Expiratory Volume in 1 Second and Cognitive Aging in Men," *Journal of the American Geriatrics Society* 59, no. 7 (2011): 1283–92.

37. For example, see E. H. Hulzebos et al., "Preoperative Intensive Inspiratory Muscle Training to Prevent Postoperative Pulmonary Complications in High-Risk Patients Undergoing CABG Surgery: A Randomized Clinical Trial," *Journal of the American Medical Association* 296, no. 15 (2006): 1851–57.

38. T. Raupach et al., "Slow Breathing Reduces Sympathoexcitation in COPD," *European Respiratory Journal* 32, no. 2 (2008): 387–92.

39. For examples, see E. Agostoni and H. Rand, "Abdominal and Thoracic Pressures at Different Lung Volumes," *Journal of Applied Physiology* 15 (1960): 1087–92; G. E. Tzelepis et al., "Transmission of Pressure within the Abdomen," *Journal of Applied Physiology* 81, no. 3 (1996): 1111–14; and J. Mead et al., "Abdominal Breathing Transmission in Humans during Slow Breathing Maneuvers," *Journal of Applied Physiology* 68, no. 5 (1990): 1850–53.

40. T. Osada et al., "Determination of Comprehensive Arterial Blood Inflow in Abdominal-Pelvic Organs: Impact of Respiration and Posture on Organ Perfusion," *Medical Science Monitor* 17, no. 2 (2011): CR57–66.

41. W. E. Mehling et al., "Randomized Controlled Trial of Breath Therapy in Patients with Chronic Low Back Pain," *Alternatives Therapies for Health and Medicine* 11, no. 4 (2005): 44–52. Also see W. E. Mehling, "The Experience of Breath as a Therapeutic Intervention—Psychosomatic Forms of Breath Therapy. A descriptive study about the actual situation of breath therapy in Germany, its relation to medicine, and its application in patients with back pain." *Forsch Komplementarmed Klass Naturheilkd* 8, no. 6 (2001): 359–67.

42. B. N. Uchino, "Understanding the Links between Social Support and Physical Health," *Perspectives on Psychological Science* 4 (2009): 236–55; F. Mookadam and H. M. Arthur, "Social Support and Its Relationship to Morbidity and Mortality after Acute Myocardial Infarction: Systematic Overview," *Archives of Internal Medicine* 164 (2004): 1514–18.

43. T. J. Kaptchuk et al., "Components of Placebo Effect: Randomised Controlled Trial in Patients with Irritable Bowel Syndrome," *British Medical Journal* 336, no. 7651 (2008): 999–1003; L. A. Conboy et al., "Which Patients Improve: Characteristics Increasing Sensitivity to a Supportive Patient-Practitioner Relationship," *Social Sciences and Medicine* 70, no. 3 (2010): 479–84.

44. M. H. Huffman, "Health Coaching: A Fresh, New Approach to Improve Quality Outcomes and Compliance for Patients with Chronic Conditions," *Home Healthcare Nurse* 27, no. 8 (2009): 490–96; T. G. Wetzel, "Health Coaching," *Hospital Health Networks* 85, no. 5 (2011): 20–24.

45. Harold George Koenig and Harvey Jay Cohen, *The Link between Religion and Health: Psychoneuroimmunology and the Faith Factor* (New York: Oxford University Press, 2002).

46. Like Tai Chi, Taoist philosophy is quite diverse. For good introductions to Taoism, see Livia Kohn, *Introducing Daoism* (London: Routledge, 2008); Eva Wong, *Taoism: An Essential Guide* (Boston: Shambhala, 2011).

47. J. A. Astin, "Why Patients Use Alternative Medicine: Results of a National Study," *Journal of the American Medical Association* 279, no. 19 (1998): 1548–53. Also see T. J. Kaptchuk and D. Eisenberg, "The Persuasive Appeal of Alternative Medicine," *Annals of Internal Medicine* 129, no. 12 (1998): 1061–65.

48. Jeffrey S. Levin and Wayne B. Jonas, *Essentials of Complementary and Alternative Medicine*, (Philadelphia: Lippincott Williams & Wilkins, 1999). The introductory chapter to this book provides a nice overview of the holistic approach to health and health care.

49. A. L. Goldberger, "Giles F. Filley Lecture: Complex Systems," *Proceedings of the American Thoracic Society* 3, no. 6 (2006): 467–71; A. L. Goldberger, "Fractal Dynamics in Physiology: Alterations with Disease and Aging," *Procedures of the National Academy of Science USA* 99, suppl. 1 (2002): 2466–72; B. Manor et al., "Physiological Complexity and System Adaptability: Evidence from Postural Control Dynamics of Older Adults," *Journal of Applied Physiology* 109, no. 6 (2010): 1786–89; P. H. Chaves et al., "Physiological Complexity Underlying Heart Rate Dynamics and Frailty Status in Community-Dwelling Older Women," *Journal of the American Geriatrics Society* 56, no. 9 (2008): 1698–703; P. M. Wayne et al. "A Systems Biology Approach to Studying Tai Chi, Physiological Complexity and Healthy Aging: Design and Rationale of a Pragmatic Randomized Controlled Trial," *Contemporary Clinical Trials* (e-pub October 9, 2012).

50. M. Sasagawa, "Positive Correlation between the Use of Complementary and Alternative Medicine and Internal Health Locus of Control," *Explore* 4, no. 1 (2008): 38–41.

51. R. E. Taylor-Piliae and E. S. Froelicher, "Measurement Properties of Tai Chi

Exercise Self-Efficacy among Ethnic Chinese with Coronary Heart Disease Risk Factors: A Pilot Study," *European Journal of Cardiovascular Nursing* 3, no. 4 (2004): 287–94; F. Li et al., "Tai Chi, Self-Efficacy, and Physical Function in the Elderly," *Prevention Science* 2, no. 4 (2001): 229–39.

52. C. Wang, "Tai Chi and Rheumatic Diseases," *Rheumatological Disease Clinics of North America* 37, no. 1 (2010): 19–32; G. Y. Yeh, C. Wang, P. M. Wayne, and R. Phillips, "Tai Chi Exercise for Patients with Cardiovascular Conditions and Risk Factors: A Systematic Review," *Journal of Cardiopulmonary Rehabilitation Prevention* 29, no. 3 (2009): 152–60; R. W. Motl and E. McAuley, "Physical Activity, Disability, and Quality of Life in Older Adults," *Physical Medicine and Rehabilitation Clinics of North America* 21, no. 2 (2010): 299–308.

53. S. Kliewer, "Allowing Spirituality into the Healing Practice," *Journal of Family Practice* 53, no. 8 (2004): 616–24.

54. George Gallup and D. Michael Lindsay, *Surveying the Religious Landscape: Trends in US Beliefs* (New York: Morehouse Group, 1999); S. Kliewer, "Allowing Spirituality into the Healing Practice," *Journal of Family Practice* 53, no. 8 (2004): 616–24.

55. A. H. Fortin VI and K. G. Barnett "Medical School Curricula in Spirituality and Medicine," *Journal of the American Medical Association* 291, no. 23 (2004): 2883.

56. Harold George Koenig, *Handbook of Religion and Health* (New York: Oxford University Press, 2001). Harold George Koenig and Harvey Jay Cohen, *The Link between Religion and Health: Psychoneuroimmunology and the Faith Factor* (New York: Oxford University Press, 2002).

57. For example, see Robert Ader, *Psychoneuroimmunology*, 4th ed. (Salt Lake City: Academic Press, 2006).

58. William James, *The Varieties of Religious Experience* (New York: Cosimo, 2007).

Chapter 4

1. "Bone Health and Osteoporosis: A Report of the Surgeon General," Rockville, Md.: U.S. Department of Health and Human Services, 2004.

2. The framework for discussing postural control in this chapter largely follows the model of Anne Shumway-Cook and Marjorie Woollacott, *Motor Control: Translating Research into Clinical Practice,* 4th ed. (Philadelphia, Lippincott Williams & Wilkins 2011).

3. Stephen R. Lord et al., *Falls in Older People: Risk Factors and Strategies for Prevention*, 2nd ed., (Cambridge, Mass.: Cambridge University Press 2007); W. R. Frontera et al., "Aging of Skeletal Muscle: A 12-Year Longitudinal Study," *Journal of Applied Physiology* 88, no. 4 (2000): 1321–26; Lewis C. Bottomley, "Musculoskeletal Changes with Age," in C. Lewis, ed., *Aging:*

Health Care's Challenge, 2nd ed. (Philadelphia: F. A. Davis, 1990); A. A. Vandervoort et al., "Age and Sex Effects on Mobility of the Human Ankle," *Journal of Gerontology* 47, no. 1 (1992): M17–21.

4. W. M. Paulus et al., "Visual Stabilization of Posture. Physiological Stimulus Characteristics and Clinical Aspects," *Brain* 107, pt. 4 (1984): 1143–63.

5. M. Magnusson et al., "Significance of Pressor Input from the Human Feet in Lateral Postural Control: The Effect of Hypothermia on Galvanically Induced Body-Sway," *Acta Oto-Laryngologica* 110, nos. 5–6 (1990): 321–27.

6. Anne Shumway-Cook and Marjorie Woollacott, *Motor Control: Translating Research into Clinical Practice,* 4th ed. (Philadelphia, Lippincott Williams & Wilkins, 2011).

7. D. G. Pitts, "Visual Acuity as a Function of Age," *Journal of American Optometric Association* 53, no. 2 (1982): 117–24; N. S. Gittings and J. L. Fozard, "Age-Related Changes in Visual Acuity," *Experimental Gerontology* 21, no. 4–5 (1986): 423–33; S. L. Lord, "Vision, Balance, and Falls in the Elderly," *Geriatric Times* 4, no. 6 (2003): 9–10.

8. P. F. Meyer et al., "Reduced Plantar Sensitivity Alters Postural Responses to Lateral Perturbations of Balance," *Experimental Brain Research* 157, no. 4 (2004): 526–36; P. F. Meyer et al., "The Role of Plantar Cutaneous Sensation in Unperturbed Stance," *Experimental Brain Research* 154, no. 4 (2004): 505–12; L. Li and B. Manor, "Long Term Tai Chi Exercise Improves Physical Performance among People with Peripheral Neuropathy," *American Journal of Chinese Medicine* 38, no. 3 (2010): 449–59; G. C. Gauchard et al., "Beneficial Effect of Proprioceptive Physical Activities on Balance Control in Elderly Human Subjects," *Neuroscience Letters* 273 (1999): 81–84.

9. B. M. Tourtillott et al., "Age-Related Changes in Vestibular Evoked Myogenic Potentials Using a Modified Blood Pressure Manometer Feedback Method," *American Journal of Audiology* 19, no. 2 (2010): 100–108; T. Brandt et al., "Long-Term Course and Relapses of Vestibular and Balance Disorders," *Restorative Nerology and Neuroscience* 28, no. 1 (2010): 69–82.

10. Anne Shumway-Cook and Marjorie Woollacott, *Motor Control: Translating Research into Clinical Practice,* 4th ed. (Philadelphia: Lippincott Williams & Wilkins, 2011).

11. A. C. Scheffer et al., "Fear of Falling: Measurement Strategy, Prevalence, Risk Factors and Consequences among Older Persons," *Age and Ageing* 37, no. 1 (2008): 19–24; J. Visschedijk et al., "Fear of Falling after Hip Fracture: A Systematic Review of Measurement Instruments, Prevalence, Interventions, and Related Factors," *Journal of the American Geriatrics Society* 58, no. 9 (2010): 1739–48.

12. T. Herman et al., "Executive Control Deficits as a Prodrome to Falls in Healthy Older Adults: A Prospective Study Linking Thinking, Walking, and Falling," *Journals of Gerontology: Series A: Biological Sciences and Medical*

Sciences 65, no. 10 (2010): 1086–92; G. Yogev-Seligmann et al., "The Role of Executive Function and Attention in Gait," *Movement Disorders* 23, no. 3 (2008): 329–42.

13. A. J. Campbell et al., "Falls in Old Age: A Study of Frequency and Related Clinical Factors," *Age and Ageing* 10, no. 4 (1981): 264–70; M. E. Tinetti et al., "Risk Factors for Falls among Elderly Persons in the Community," *New England Journal of Medicine* 319, no. 26 (1988): 1701–7; L. A. Lipsitz et al., "Causes and Correlates of Recurrent Falls in Ambulatory Frail Elderly," *Journal of Gerontology* 46, no. 4 (1991): M114–22.

14. L. Z. Rubenstein, "Falls in Older People: Epidemiology, Risk Factors and Strategies for Prevention," *Age and Ageing* 35, suppl. 2 (2006): ii37–ii41.

15. L. D. Gillespie et al., "Interventions for Preventing Falls in Older People Living in the Community," *Cochrane Database of Systematic Reviews* 15, no. 2 (2010): CD007146; M. M. Gardner et al., "Exercise in Preventing Falls and Fall Related Injuries in Older People: A Review of Randomized Controlled Trials," *British Journal of Sports Medicine* 34 (2000): 7–17; D. J. Rose, "Preventing Falls among Older Adults: 'No One Size Suits All' Intervention Strategy," *Journal of Rehabilitation Research and Development*, 45, no. 8 (2008): 1153–66; E. Costello and J. E. Edelstein, "Update on Falls Prevention for Community-Dwelling Older Adults: Review of Single and Multifactorial Intervention Programs," *Journal of Rehabilitation Research and Development* 45, no. 8 (2008): 1135–52; C. Sherrington et al., "Exercise to Prevent Falls in Older Adults: An Updated Meta-Analysis and Best Practice Recommendations," *New South Wales Public Health Bulletin* 22, nos. 3–4 (2011): 78–83.

16. I. H. Logghe et al., "The Effects of Tai Chi on Fall Prevention, Fear of Falling and Balance in Older People: A Meta-Analysis," *Preventive Medicine* 51, nos. 3–4 (2010): 222–27; L. D. Gillespie et al., "Interventions for Preventing Falls in Older People Living in the Community," *Cochrane Database of Systematic Reviews* 15, no. 2 (2010): CD007146; F. Li and P. A. Harmer, "Tai Chi and Falls Prevention in Older People," *Medicine Sports and Science* 52 (2008): 124–134; H. Lui and A. Frank, "Tai Chi as a Balance Improvement Exercise for Older Adults: A Systematic Review," *Journal of Geriatric Physical Therapy* 33, no. 3 (2010): 103–9; M. M. Schleicher et al., "Review of Tai Chi as an Effective Exercise on Falls Prevention in Elderly," *Research in Sports Medicine* (2011); D. P. K. Leung, "Tai Chi as an Intervention to Improve Balance and Reduce Falls in Older Adults: A Systematic and Meta-analytical Review," *Alternative Therapies in Health and Medicine* 17, no. 1 (2011): 40–48; S. Low et al., "A Systematic Review of the Effectiveness of Tai Chi on Fall Reduction among the Elderly," *Archives of Gerontology and Geriatrics* 48, no. 3 (2009): 325–31; M. M. Schleicher, L. Wedam, G. Wu, "Review of Tai Chi as an Effective Exercise on Falls Prevention in Elderly," *Research in Sports Medicine* 20, no. 1 (2012): 37–58.

17. F. Li et al., "Tai Chi and Fall Reductions in Older Adults: A Randomized Controlled Trial," *Journal of Gerontology* 60A, no. 2 (2005): 187–194; F. Li et al., "Tai Chi: Improving Functional Balance and Predicting Subsequent Falls in Older Persons," *Medical Science Sports Exercise* 36 (2004): 2046–52; F. Li et al., "Translation of an Effective Tai Chi Intervention into a Community-Based Falls-Prevention Program," *American Journal of Public Health* 98, no. 7 (2008): 1195–98.

18. S. L. Wolf et al., "Reducing Frailty and Falls in Older Persons: An Investigation of Tai Chi and Computerized Balance Training. Atlanta FICSIT Group. Frailty and Injuries: Cooperative Studies of Intervention Techniques," *Journal of the American Geriatrics Society* 44, no. 5 (1996): 489–97. S. L. Wolf et al., "The Effect of Tai Chi Quan and Computerized Balance Training on Postural Stability in Older Subjects. Atlanta FICSIT Group. Frailty and Injuries: Cooperative Studies on Intervention Techniques," *Physical Therapy* 77, no. 4 (1997): 371–84.

19. Some recent large-scale randomized clinical trials have not observed Tai Chi to be superior in randomized trials. These include I. H. Logghe et al., "Lack of Effect of Tai Chi Chuan in Preventing Falls in Elderly People Living at Home: A Randomized Clinical Trial," *Journal of the American Geriatrics Society* 57, no. 1 (January 2009): 70–75; D. Taylor et al., "Effectiveness of Tai Chi as a Community-Based Falls Prevention Intervention: A Randomized Controlled Trial," *Journal of the American Geriatrics Society* 60, no. 5 (May 2012): 841–48. For a discussion of these negative results, see: I. H. Logghe et al., "Explaining the Ineffectiveness of a Tai Chi Fall Prevention Training for Community-Living Older People: A Process Evaluation alongside a Randomized Clinical Trial (RCT)," *Archives of Gerontology and Geriatrics* 52, no. 3 (2011): 357–62.

20. C. J. Wilson and S. K. Datta, "Tai Chi for the Prevention of Fractures in a Nursing Home Population: An Economic Analysis," *Journal of Clinical Outcomes Management* 8 (2001):19–27; J. Church et al., "An Economic Evaluation of Community Residential Aged Care Falls Prevention Strategies in NSW," *New South Wales Public Health Bulletin* 22, nos. 3–4 (2011): 60–68; K. D. Frick et al., "Evaluating the Cost-Effectiveness of Fall Prevention Programs that Reduce Fall-Related Hip Fractures in Older Adults," *Journal of the American Geriatrics Society* 58, no. 1 (2010): 136–41; L. Day et al., "Modelling the Population-level Impact of Tai-Chi on Falls and Fall-related Injury among Community-Dwelling Older People," *Injury Prevention* 16 (2010): 321–26.

21. Professor Ge Wu at the University of Vermont has documented increased single-stance time and associated load and torque while doing Tai Chi compared to walking: G. Wu, "Muscle Action Pattern and Knee Extensor Strength of Older Tai Chi Exercisers," *Medicine and Sport Science* 52

(2008): 20–29; G. Wu and D. Millon, "Joint Kinetics during Tai Chi Gait and Normal Walking Gait in Young and Elderly Tai Chi Chuan Practitioners," *Clinical Biomechanics* (Bristol, Avon) 23, no. 6 (2008): 787–95. Representative studies demonstrating increased strength are D. Q. Xu et al., "Tai Chi Exercise and Muscle Strength and Endurance in Older People," *Journal of Biomechanics* 29, no. 8, pt. 42 (2009): 967–71; J. X. Li et al., "Changes in Muscle Strength, Endurance, and Reaction of the Lower Extremities with Tai Chi Intervention," *Journal of Biomechanics* 42, no. 8 (2009): 967–71; W. W. Tsang and C. W. Hui-Chan, "Comparison of Muscle Torque, Balance, and Confidence in Older Tai Chi and Healthy Adults," *Medicine and Science in Sports and Exercise* 37, no. 2 (2005): 280–89. Studies showing increased flexibility include C. Lan et al., "12-month Tai Chi Training in the Elderly: Its Effect on Health Fitness," *Medicine and Science in Sports and Exercise* 30, no. 3 (1998): 345–51; E. N. Lee et al., "Tai Chi for Disease Activity and Flexibility in Patients with Ankylosing Spondylitis—a Controlled Clinical Trial," *Evidence-Based Complementary and Alternative Medicine* 5, no. 4 (2008): 457–62.

22. A. L. Gyllensten et al., "Stability Limits, Single-Leg Jump, and Body Awareness in Older Tai Chi Practitioners," *Archives of Physical Medicine and Rehabilitation* 91, no. 2 (2010): 215–20.

23. D. Xu et al., "Effect of Tai Chi Exercise on Proprioception of Ankle and Knee Joints in Old People," *British Journal of Sports Medicine* 38 (2004): 50–54. Also see J. X. Li et al., "Effects of 16-Week Tai Chi Intervention on Postural Stability and Proprioception of Knee and Ankle in Older People," *Age and Ageing* 37, no. 5 (2008): 575–78; S. M. Fong and G. Y. Ng, "The Effects on Sensorimotor Performance and Balance with Tai Chi Training," *Archives of Physical Medicine Rehabilitation* 87, no. 1 (2006): 82–87; W. W. Tsang and C. W. Hui-Chan, "Effects of Tai Chi on Joint Proprioception and Stability Limits in Elderly Subjects," *Medicine and Science in Sports and Exercise* 35 (2003): 1962–71; W. W. Tsang and C. W. Hui-Chan, "Effect on Exercise on Joint Sense and Balance in Elderly Men: Tai Chi versus Golf," *Medicine and Science in Sports and Exercise* 36 (2004): 658–67.

24. B. Manor and L. Li, "Characteristics of Functional Gait among Older Adults with and without Peripheral Neuropathy," *Gait and Posture* 30, no. 2 (2009): 253–56.

25. L. Li and B. Manor, "Long Term Tai Chi Exercise Improves Physical Performance among People with Peripheral Neuropathy," *American Journal of Chinese Medicine* 38, no. 3 (2010): 449–59.

26. J. W. Hung et al., "Effect of 12-Week Tai Chi Chuan Exercise on Peripheral Nerve Modulation in Patients with Type 2 Diabetes Mellitus," *Journal of Rehabilitation Medicine* 41, no. 11 (2009): 924–29.

27. C. E. Kerr et al., "Tactile Acuity in Experienced Tai Chi Practitioners: Evi-

dence for Use Dependent Plasticity as an Effect of Sensory-Attentional Training," *Experimental Brain Research* 188, no. 2 (2008): 17–22. And another prospective study showed Tai Chi can improve kinesthetic sense of shoulder joints: Jacobson et al., "The Effect of T'ai Chi Chuan Training on Balance, Kinesthetic Sense, and Strength," *Perception and Motor Skills* 84, no. 1 (1997): 27–33.

28. C. A. McGibbon et al., "Effects of Tai Chi and Vestibular Rehabilitation on Gaze and Whole-Body Stability during a Repeated Stepping Task in Patients with Vestibulopathy, *Journal of Vestibular Research* 14 (2004): 467–78; P. M. Wayne et al., "Tai Chi for Vestibulopathic Balance Dysfunction: A Case Study," *Alternative Therapies in Health and Medicine* 11, no. 2 (2005): 60–66.

29. W. W. Tsang et al., "Tai Chi Improves Standing Balance Control under Reduced or Conflicting Sensory Conditions," *Archives of Physical Medicine Rehabilitation* 85 (2004): 129–37; W. W. Tsang and C. W Hui-Chan, "Standing Balance after Vestibular Stimulation in Tai Chi–Practicing and Nonpracticing Healthy Older Adults," *Archives of Physical Medicine Rehabilitation* 87 (2006): 546–53.

30. S. K. Gatts and M. H. Woollacott, "How Tai Chi Improves Balance: Biomechanics of Recovery to a Walking Slip in Impaired Seniors," *Gait and Posture* 25, no. 2 (2007): 205–1; Also see D. Q. Xu et al., "Effect of Regular Tai Chi and Jogging Exercise on Neuromuscular Reaction in Older People," *Age and Ageing* 34, no. 5 (2005): 439–34; A. K. Ramachandran et al., "Effect of Tai Chi on Gait and Obstacle Crossing Behaviors in Middle-Aged Adults," *Gait and Posture* 26, no. 2 (2007): 248–55; G. Wu, "Biomechanical Characteristics of Stepping in Older Tai Chi Practitioners," *Gait and Posture* no.3 (2012).

31. C. J. Hass et al., "The Influence of Tai Chi Training on the Center of Pressure Trajectory during Gait Initiation in Older Adults," *Archives of Physical Medicine and Rehabilitation* 85, no. 10 (2004): 1593–98.

32. C. A. McGibbon et al., "Tai Chi and Vestibular Rehabilitation Improve Vestibulopathic Gait via Different Neuromuscular Mechanisms: Preliminary Report," *BMC Neurology* 18, no. 5 (2005): 3.

33. R. W. Sattin et al., "Reduction in Fear of Falling through Intense Tai Chi Exercise Training in Older, Transitionally Frail Adults," *Journal of the American Geriatrics Society* 53, no. 7 (2005): 1168–78; S. L. Wolf et al., "Reducing Frailty and Falls in Older Persons: An Investigation of Tai Chi and Computerized Balance Training. Atlanta FICSIT Group. Frailty and Injuries: Cooperative Studies of Intervention Techniques," *Journal of the American Geriatrics Society*, 44, no. 5 (1996): 489–97; S. L. Wolf et al., "The Effect of Tai Chi Quan and Computerized Balance Training on Postural Stability in Older Subjects. Atlanta FICSIT Group. Frailty and Injuries: Cooperative Studies on Intervention Techniques," *Physical Therapy* 77, no. 4 (1997): 371–84.

34. T. T. Huang et al., "Reducing the Fear of Falling among Community-Dwelling Elderly Adults through Cognitive-Behavioural Strategies and Intense Tai Chi Exercise: A Randomized Controlled Trial," *Journal of Advanced Nursing* 67, no. 5 (2011): 961–71.

35. W. W. Tsang et al., "Effects of Tai Chi on Pre-landing Muscle Response Latency during Stepping Down While Performing a Concurrent Mental Task in Older Adults," *European Journal of Applied Physiology* (November 2011).

36. F. Li, et al., "Tai Chi and Postural Stability in Patients with Parkinson's Disease," *New England Journal of Medicine* 366, no. 6 (2012) : 511–19.

37. P. J. Klein and L. Rivers, "Taiji for Individuals with Parkinson Disease and their Support Partners: A Program Evaluation," *Journal of Neurologic Physical Therapy* 30, no. 1 (March 2006): 22–27; M. E. Hackney and G. M. Earhart, "Tai Chi Improves Balance and Mobility in People with Parkinson Disease," *Gait and Posture* 28 (2008): 456–60; T. Schmitz-Hubsch et al., "Qigong Exercise for the Symptoms of Parkinson's Disease: A Randomized, Controlled Pilot Study." *Movement Disorders,* 21, no. 4 (2006): 543–48; M. Venglar, "Case Report: Tai Chi and Parkinsonism,"*Physiotherapy Research International*10 (2005):116–21.

38. M. M. Matthews and H. G. Williams, "Can Tai Chi Enhance Cognitive Vitality? A Preliminary Study of Cognitive Executive Control in Older Adults after a Tai Chi Intervention," *Journal of the South Carolina Medical Association* 104 (2008): 255–57.

39. C. D. Hall et al., "Effects of Tai Chi Intervention on Dual-Task Ability in Older Adults: A Pilot Study," *Archives of Physical Medicine and Rehabilitation* 90, no. 3 (2009): 525–29.

40. "Bone Health and Osteoporosis: A Report of the Surgeon General," October 14, 2004.

41. Ibid.

42. Ibid.

43. P. M. Wayne et al., "The Effects of Tai Chi on Bone Mineral Density in Postmenopausal Women: A Systematic Review," *Archives of Physical Medicine and Rehabilitation* 88, no. 5 (May 2007): 673–80; Also see: M. S. Lee, "Tai Chi for Osteoporosis: A Systematic Review," *Osteoporosis International* 19, no. 2 (2008): 139–46.

44. L. Qin et al., "Beneficial Effects of Regular Tai Chi Exercise on Musculoskeletal System," *Journal of Bone and Mineral Metabolism* 23 (2005): 186–190.

45. Y. Zhou, "The Effect of Traditional Sports on the Bone Density of Menopausal Women," *Journal of Beijing Sport University* 27 (2004): 354–360.

46. J. Woo et al., "A Randomised Controlled Trial of Tai Chi and Resistance Exercise on Bone Health, Muscle Strength and Balance in Community-Living Elderly People," *Age and Ageing* 36, no. 3 (2007): 262–268.

47. P. M. Wayne et al., "Tai Chi for Osteopenic Women: Design and Rationale

of a Pragmatic Randomized Controlled Trial," *BMC Musculoskeletal Disorders* 11 (2010): 40; P. M. Wayne et al., "Impact of Tai Chi Exercise on Multiple Fracture-Related Risk Factors in Postmenopausal Osteopenic Women: A Pilot Pragmatic, Randomized Trial" *BMC Complementary and Alternative Medicine* 12 (January 30, 2012): 7.

48. C. L. Shen et al., "Effect of Green Tea and Tai Chi on Bone Health in Postmenopausal Osteopenic Women: A 6-Month Randomized Placebo-Controlled Trial," *Osteoporosis International* 23 (2011): 1541–52; C. L. Shen et al., "Green Tea Polyphenols Supplementation and Tai Chi Exercise for Postmenopausal Osteopenic Women: Safety and Quality of Life Report," *BMC Complementary and Alternative Medicine* 9 (2010): 76; M. C. Chyu et al., "Effects of Tai Chi Exercise on Posturography, Gait, Physical Function and Quality of Life in Postmenopausal Women with Osteopaenia: A Randomized Clinical Study," *Clinical Rehabilitation* 24, no. 12 (2010): 1080–90.

49. Although this is quite different from Tai Chi shaking, there is some evidence to suggest mechanical vibration of bones may enhance bone health. For example, see: J. O. Totosy de Zepetnek, "Whole-Body Vibration as Potential Intervention for People with Low Bone Mineral Density and Osteoporosis: A Review," *Journal of Rehabilitation Research and Development* 46, no. 4 (2009): 529–42.

Chapter 5

1. A. Malmivaara et al, "The Treatment of Acute Low Back Pain—Bed Rest, Exercises, or Ordinary Activity," *New England Journal of Medicine*, 332, no. 6 (1995): 351–55.

2. M. Lethbridge-Cejku and J. Vickerie, "Summary Health Statistics for U.S. Adults: National Health Interview Survey, 2003. National Center for Health Statistics," *Vital Health Statistics* 10 (2005): 225); S. M. Schappert, "Ambulatory Care Visits to Physicians' Offices, Hospital Outpatient Departments, and Emergency Departments: United States, 1996," *Vital and Health Statistics* 13, no. 134 (1998): 1–80; C. Harstall, "How Prevalent Is Chronic Pain?" *Pain: Clinical Updates* 9, no. 2 (2003): 1–4.

3. P. M. Wolsko et al, "Use of Mind-Body Medical Therapies," *Journal of General Internal Medicine* 19, no. 1 (2004): 43–50; D. M. Eisenberg, "Trends in Alternative Medicine Use in the United States, 1990–1997: Results of a Follow-Up National Survey," *Journal of the American Medical Association* 208 (1998): 1569–75; S. M. Bertisch et al., "Alternative Mind-Body Therapies Used by Adults with Medical Conditions," *Journal of Psychosomatic Research* 66, no. 6 (2009): 511–19.

4. A. K. Kanodia et al., "Perceived Benefit of Complementary and Alternative Medicine (CAM) for Back Pain: A National Survey," *Journal of the American Board of Internal Medicine* 23, no. 3 (2010): 354–62; H. A. Tindle et al.,

"Factors Associated with the Use of Mind-Body Therapies among United States Adults with Musculoskeletal Pain," *Complementary Therapies in Medicine* 13, no. 3 (2005): 155–64.

5. R. L. Nahin et al., "Costs of Complementary and Alternative Medicine (CAM) and Frequency of Visits to CAM Practitioners: United States, 2007," *National Health Statistics Reports,* no. 18 (Hyattsville, Md.: National Center for Health Statistics, 2009).

6. "Exploring the Science of Complementary and Alternative Medicine: Third Strategic Plan 2011–2015," http://nccam.nih.gov/about/plans/2011.

7. R. Chou et al., "Diagnostic Imaging for Low Back Pain: Advice for High-Value Health Care from the American College of Physicians," *Annals of Internal Medicine* 154 (2011): 181–89.

8. W. E. Mehling and N. Krause, "Alexithymia and 7.5-Year Incidence of Compensated Low Back Pain in 1207 Urban Public Transit Operators," *Journal of Psychosomatic Research* 62, no. 6 (2007): 667–74; T. Pincus et al., "Cognitive-Behavioral Therapy and Psychosocial Factors in Low Back Pain: Directions for the Future," *Spine* 27, no. 5 (2002): E133–38; S. J. Linton, "A Review of Psychological Risk Factors in Back and Neck Pain," *Spine* 25, no. 9 (2000): 1148–56; S. J. Keefe et al., "Psychological Aspects of Persistent Pain: Current State of the Science," *Journal of Pain*, 5, no. 4 (2004): 195–211.

9. For motor imagery and pain, see G. L. Mosely, "Imagined Movements Cause Pain and Swelling in a Patient with Complex Regional Pain Syndrome," *Neurology* 62, no. 9 (2004): 1644.

10. B. M. Wand and N. E. O'Connell, "Chronic Non-specific Low Back Pain—Sub-groups or a Single Mechanism," *BMC Musculoskeletal Disorders* 25, no. 9 (2008): 11; J. M. Fritz et al., "Subgrouping Patients with Low Back Pain: Evolution of a Classification Approach to Physical Therapy," *Journal of Orthopedic Sports and Physical Therapy* 37, no. 6 (2007): 290–302; S. Z. George and A. Delitto, "Clinical Examination Variables Discriminate among Treatment-based Classification Groups: A Study of Construct Validity in Patients with Acute Low Back Pain," *Physical Therapy* 85, no. 4 (2005): 306–14.

11. H. M. Langevin and K. J. Sherman, "Pathophysiological Model for Chronic Low Back Pain Integrating Connective Tissue and Nervous System Mechanisms," *Medical Hypotheses* 68, no. 1 (2007): 74–80.

12. H. M. Langevin et al., "Reduced Thoracolumbar Fascia Shear Strain in Human Chronic Low Back Pain," *BMC Musculoskeletal Disorders* 19, no. 12 (2011): 203.

13. S. M. Corey et al., "Stretching of the Back Improves Gait, Mechanical Sensitivity and Connective Tissue Inflammation in a Rodent Model," *PLoS One* 7, no. 1 (2012): e29831.

14. For additional reading on fascia, see Tom Myers *Anatomy Trains: Myofascial Meridians for Manual and Movement Therapists* (Philadelphia: Churchill

Livingstone, 2008); R. L Schultz and R. Fcitus, *The Endless Web: Fascial Anatomy and Physical Reality* (Berkeley: North Atlantic Books, 1996); H. M. Langevin, "Connective Tissue: A Body-wide Signaling Network?" *Medical Hypotheses* 66 (2006): 1074–77; R. Schleip, "Fascial Plasticity–a New Neurobiological Explanation: Part 1," *Journal of Bodywork and Movement Therapies* 7 (2003): 11–19.

15. Developing a strong vertical structure is a key element in many movement and healing arts therapies such as Structural Integration, Alexander Technique, and Awareness through Movement.

16. For a good review of the possible role of musculoskeletal patterns and back pain, see S. F. Nadler et al., "Relationship between Hip Muscle Imbalance and Occurrence of Low Back Pain in Collegiate Athletes: A Prospective Study," *American Journal of Physical Medicine and Rehabilitation* 80, no. 8 (2001): 572–77; J. H. Abbott et al., "Lumbar Segmental Mobility Disorders: Comparison of Two Methods of Defining Abnormal Displacement Kinematics in a Cohort of Patients with Non-specific Mechanical Low Back Pain," *BMC Musculoskeletal Disorders* 19 (2006): 45; P. H. Ferreira et al., "Changes in Recruitment of Transversus Abdominis Correlate with Disability in People with Chronic Low Back Pain," 44, no. 16 (2010): 1166–72. For a good discussion on the kwa and its central importance in Tai Chi, see Bruce Frantzis, *Opening the Energy Gates of Your Body: Chi Gung for Lifelong Health*, (Berkeley: Blue Snake Books, 1993); also see William Chen, "The Vastus Medialis and Inner Thigh," *T'AI CHI Magazine* 35, no. 1 (2011).

17. Improve ankle range of motion has been reported by Wu et al., "Spatial, Temporal and Muscle Action Patterns of Tai Chi Gait," *Journal of Electromyography and Kinesiology* 14, no. 3 (2004): 343–54; D. W. Mao et al., "Plantar Pressure Distribution during Tai Chi Exercise," *Archives of Physical Medicine and Rehabilitation* 87, no. 6 (2006) 814–20. More general studies of foot biomechanics and Tai Chi include D. W. Mao et al., "The Duration and Plantar Pressure Distribution during One-leg Stance in Tai Chi Exercise," *Clinical Biomechanics* 21 (2006): 640–45.

18. Bruce Frantzis, *Tai Chi: Health for Life* (Berkeley: Blue Snake Books, 2006).

19. For good review of kinesiophobia, see M. Leeuw et al., "The Fear-Avoidance Model of Musculoskeletal Pain: Current State of Scientific Evidence," *Journal of Behavioral Medicine* 30, no. 1 (2007): 77–94.

20. Some examples include J. Kingston et al., "A Pilot Randomized Control Trial Investigating the Effect of Mindfulness Practice on Pain Tolerance, Psychological Well-being, and Physiological Activity," *Journal of Psychosomatic Research* 62, no. 3 (2007): 297–300; K. H. Kaplan et al., "The Impact of a Meditation-based Stress Reduction Program on Fibromyalgia," *General Hospital Psychiatry* 15, no. 5 (1993): 284–89; P. Creamer et al., "Sustained Improvement Produced by Nonpharmacologic Intervention in Fibromyalgia:

Results of a Pilot Study," *Arthritis Care and Research* 13, no. 4 (2000): 198–204; S. E. Sephton et al., "Mindfulness Meditation Alleviates Depressive Symptoms in Women with Fibromyalgia: Results of a Randomized Clinical Trial," *Arthritis and Rheumatism* 57, no. 1 (2007): 77–85; E. Lush et al., "Mindfulness Meditation for Symptom Reduction in Fibromyalgia: Psychophysiological Correlates," *Journal of Clinical Psychology in Medical Settings* 16, no. 2 (2009): 200–207; F. Zeidan et al., "The Effects of Brief Mindfulness Meditation Training on Experimentally Induced Pain," *Journal of Pain* 11, no. 3 (2010): 199–209.

21. L. E. Carlson et al., "One Year Pre-post Intervention Follow-up of Psychological, Immune, Endocrine and Blood Pressure Outcomes of Mindfulness-based Stress Reduction (MBSR) in Breast and Prostate Cancer Outpatients," *Brain Behavior and Immunity* 21, no. 8 (2007): 1038–49; L. Witek-Janusek et al., "Effect of Mindfulness Based Stress Reduction on Immune Function, Quality of Life and Coping in Women Newly Diagnosed with Early Stage Breast Cancer," *Brain Behavior and Immunity* 22, no. 6 (2008): 969–81.

22. M. R. Irwin and R. Olmstead, "Mitigating Cellular Inflammation in Older Adults: A Randomized Controlled Trial of Tai Chih," *American Journal of Geriatric Psychiatry* 20, no. 9 (2012): 764–72. M. C. Janelsins et al., "Effects of Tai Chi Chuan on Insulin and Cytokine Levels in a Randomized Controlled Pilot Study on Breast Cancer Survivors," *Clinical Breast Cancer* 11 (2011): 161–70; B. Oh et al., "Effect of Medical Qigong on Cognitive Function, Quality of Life, and a Biomarker of Inflammation in Cancer Patients: A Randomized Controlled Trial," *Supportive Care in Cancer* 20 (2012): 1235–42; H. H. Chen et al., "The Effects of Baduanjin Qigong in the Prevention of Bone Loss for Middle-Aged Women," *American Journal of Chinese Medicine* 34 (2006): 741–47.

23. J. A. Grant and P. Rainville, "Pain Sensitivity and Analgesic Effects of Mindful States in Zen Meditators: A Cross-sectional Study," *Psychosomatic Medicine* 71, no. 1 (2008): 106–14.

24. F. Zeidan et al., "Brain Mechanisms Supporting the Modulation of Pain by Mindfulness Meditation," *Journal of Neuroscience* 31, no. 14 (2011): 5540–48; J. A. Grant et al., "A Non-elaborative Mental Stance and Decoupling of Executive and Pain-related Cortices Predicts Low Pain Sensitivity in Zen Meditators," *Pain* 152, no. 1 (2011): 150–56.

25. For good reviews, see D. G. Finniss et al., "Biological, Clinical, and Ethical Advances of Placebo Effects," Lancet 375, no. 9715 (February 20, 2010): 686–95; Fabrizio Benedetti, Placebo Effects: Understanding the Mechanisms in Health and Disease (Oxford: Oxford University Press, 2008); Anne Harrington, The Placebo Effect (Cambridge, Mass.: Harvard University Press, 1999).

26. F. Benedetti et al., "Somatotopic Activation of Opioid Systems by Target-

directed Expectations of Analgesia," *Journal of Neuroscience* 19, no. 9 (1999): 3639–48. Of note, and unintentionally, researcher used key energy centers focused on in Tai Chi practice. The palm centers in Chinese medicine are referred to as "Laogong" and help regulate fire energy of the heart. Foot sole points used correspond with "Yongquan" or bubbling wells, and help ground the body and regulate kidney energy. Both receive significant attention during Tai Chi training, so it is not surprising that intention focused on these sites results in a significant physiological effect.

27. W. E. Mehling et al., "Randomized, Controlled Trial of Breath Therapy for Patients with Chronic Low-back Pain," *Alternative Therapies in Health and Medicine* 11, no. 4 (2005): 44–52.

28. A. J. Zautra et al., "The Effects of Slow Breathing on Affective Responses to Pain Stimuli: An Experimental Study," *Pain* 149, no. 1 (2010): 12–18.

29. N. I. Eisenberger and M. D. Lieberman, "Why It Hurts To Be Left Out: The Neurocognitive Overlap between Physical and Social Pain" in K. D. Williams, J. P. Forgas, and W. van Hippel (eds.), *The Social Outcast: Ostracism, Social Exclusion, Rejection, and Bullying* (New York: Cambridge University Press, 2005), 109–27.

30. A. M. Hall et al., "Tai Chi Exercise for Treatment of Pain and Disability in People with Persistent Low Back Pain: A Randomized Controlled Trial," *Arthritis Care and Research* 3, no. 11 (2011): 1576–83.

31. E. N. Lee et al., "Tai Chi for Disease Activity and Flexibility in Patients with Ankylosing Spondylitis—a Controlled Clinical Trial," *Evidence-Based Complementary and Alternative Medicine* 5, no. 4 (2008): 457–62.

32. H. W. Tian et al., "Taijiquan as Adjuvant Treatment of Senility and Middle-age Lumbar Vertebrae Disease," *Journal of Hubei Institute for Nationalities, Medical Edition* 21 (2004): 24–26; C. Y. Chin, "Prevention of Falls in the Elderly with Taijiquan," *Chinese Aging* 28 (2008): 2055–56.

33. Y. Liu and C. G. Wang, "Clinicial Observation on Rectifying Spinal Curvature by Practicing Chenshe Hexagram Boxing (Taijiquan) and Athletic Rehabilitation," *Guiding Journal of TCM* 21 (2007): 24–26; S. L. Hou and Y. Ding, "Benefits of Long-term Taijiquan Practice for Lumbosacral Health," *J Qigong* 19 (1988): 483–85; L. W. Zhang et al., "Clinical Observation of Combined Tuina and Taijiquan for Lumbosacral Conditions," *China Medical Herald* 5 (2008): 82–83; C. F. Yue et al., "Clinical Observation on Combined Acupuncture and Taijiquan for Lumbosacral Conditions," *China Medical Herald* 5 (2008): 86–87.

34. K. J. Sherman et al., "A Randomized Trial Comparing Yoga, Stretching, and a Self-care Book for Chronic Low Back Pain," *Archives of Internal Medicine* 171 (2011): 2019–26; K. J. Sherman et al., "Comparing Yoga, Exercise, and a Self-care Book for Chronic Low Back Pain: A Randomized, Controlled Trial," *Annals of Internal Medicine* 143, no. 12 (2005): 849–56. Also see R. Saper et al., "Yoga for Chronic Low Back Pain in a Predominantly Minority

Population: A Pilot Randomized Controlled Trial," *Alternative Therapies in Health and Medicine* 15 (2009): 18–27.

35. M. A. Minor et al., "Exercise Tolerance and Disease Related Measures in Patients with Rheumatoid Arthritis and Osteoarthritis," *Journal of Rheumatology* 15, no. 6 (1988): 905–11.

36. G. Jamtvedt et al., "Physical Therapy Interventions for Patients with Osteoarthritis of the Knee: An Overview of Systematic Reviews," *Physical Therapy* 88, no. 1 (2008): 123–36; A. K. Lange, "Strength Training for Treatment of Osteoarthritis of the Knee: A Systematic Review," *Arthritis and Rheumatism* 59, no. 10 (2008): 1488–94.

37. C. Wang, "Tai Chi and Rheumatic Diseases," *Rheumatic Diseases Clinics of North America* 37, no. 1 (2011): 19–32; M. S. Lee et al., "Tai Chi for Osteoarthritis: A Systematic Review," *Clinical Rheumatology* 27, no. 2 (2008): 211–18.

38. C. Wang et al., "Tai Chi is Effective in Treating Knee Osteoarthritis: A Randomized Controlled Trial," *Arthritis and Rheumatism* 61, no. 11 (2009): 1545–53.

39. M. Fransen et al., "Physical Activity for Osteoarthritis Management: A Randomized Controlled Clinical Trial Evaluating Hydrotherapy or Tai Chi Classes," *Arthritis and Rheumatism* 57, no. 3 (2007): 407–14.

40. R. Song et al., "Effects of Tai Chi Exercise on Pain, Balance, Muscle Strength, and Perceived Difficulties in Physical Functioning in Older Women with Osteoarthritis: A Randomized Clinical Trial," *Journal of Rheumatology* 30, no. 9 (2003): 2039–44; R. Song et al., "A Randomized Study of the Effects of T'ai Chi on Muscle Strength, Bone Mineral Density, and Fear of Falling in Women with Osteoarthritis," *Journal of Alternative and Complementary Medicine* 16, no. 3 (2010): 227–33.

41. J. M. Brismee et al., "Group and Home-based Tai Chi in Elderly Subjects with Knee Osteoarthritis: A Randomized Controlled Trial," *Clinical Rehabilitation* 21, no. 2 (2007): 99–111; C. L. Shen et al., "Effects of Tai Chi on Gait Kinematics, Physical Function, and Pain in Elderly with Knee Osteoarthritis—a Pilot Study," *American Journal of Chinese Medicine* 36, no. 2 (2008): 219–32.

42. Other Tai Chi and Qigong studies of note related to arthritis include C. A. Hartman et al., "Effects of T'ai Chi Training on Function and Quality of Life Indicators in Older Adults with Osteoarthritis," *Journal of American Geriatrics Society* 48, no. 12 (2000): 1553–59; H. J. Lee et al., "Tai Chi Qigong for the Quality of Life of Patients with Knee Osteoarthritis: A Pilot, Randomized, Waiting List Controlled Trial," *Clinical Rehabilitation* 23, no. 6 (2009): 504–11; P. F. Tsai et al., "The Effect of Tai Chi on Knee Osteoarthritis Pain in Cognitively Impaired Elders: Pilot Study," *Geriatric Nursing* 30, no. 2 (2009): 132–39.

43. For systematic reviews on Tai Chi for rheumatoid arthritis, see C. Wang, "Tai Chi and Rheumatic Diseases," *Rheumatic Disease Clinics of North*

America 37, no. 1 (2011): 19–32; M. S. Lee et al., "Tai Chi for Rheumatoid Arthritis: Systematic Review," *Rheumatology* 46, no. 11 (2007): 1648–50.

44. C. Wang et al., "Effect of Tai Chi in Adults with Rheumatoid Arthritis," *Rheumatology* 44, no. 5 (2005): 685–87.

45. In another randomized, controlled trial evaluating Tai Chi for rheumatoid arthritis in Korea, 42 patients received either 12 weeks of Tai Chi training or usual care. Those in the Tai Chi group experienced significantly improved mood, but no changes in pain or fatigue. (E. N. Lee et al., "Effects of a Tai-Chi Program on Pain, Sleep Disturbance, Mood and Fatigue in Rheumatoid Arthritis Patients," *Journal of Muscle and Joint Health* 12 (2005): 57–68. Another larger randomized, controlled trial in the United States evaluated a Tai Chi–"inspired" dance program. This study found that the Tai Chi dance group exhibited significant improvement in range of motion in the upper body and the ankle: J. Van Deusen and D. Harlow, "The Efficacy of the ROM Dance Program for Adults with Rheumatoid Arthritis," *American Journal of Occupational Therapy* 41, no. 2 (1987): 90–95. Also see A. E. Kirstein et al., "Evaluating the Safety and Potential Use of a Weight-bearing Exercise, Tai-Chi Chuan, for Rheumatoid Arthritis Patients," *American Journal of Physical Medicine and Rehabilitation* 70, no. 3 (1991): 136–41; T. Uhlig et al., "No Improvement in a Pilot Study of Tai Chi Exercise in Rheumatoid Arthritis," *Annals of the Rheumatic Diseases* 64, no. 3 (2005): 507–9; T. Uhlig et al., "Exploring Tai Chi in Rheumatoid Arthritis: A Quantitative and Qualitative Study," *BMC Musculoskeletal Disorders* 5 (2010): 43.

46. C. Wang et al., "A Randomized Trial of Tai Chi for Fibromyalgia," *New England Journal of Medicine* 363, no. 8 (2010): 743–54.

47. H. M. Taggart et al., "Effects of T'ai Chi Exercise on Fibromyalgia Symptoms and Health-Related Quality of Life," *Orthopaedic Nursing* 22, no. 5 (2003): 353–60; A. Carbonell-Baeza et al., "T'ai-Chi Intervention in Men with Fibromyalgia: A Multiple-Patient Case Report," *Journal of Alternative and Complementary Medicine* 17, no. 3 (2011): 187–89.

48. J. A. Astin et al., "The Efficacy of Mindfulness Meditation plus Qigong Movement Therapy in the Treatment of Fibromyalgia: A Randomized Controlled Trial," *Journal of Rheumatology* 30, no. 10 (2003): 2257–62.

49. K. H. Kaplan et al., "The Impact of a Meditation-based Stress Reduction Program on Fibromyalgia," *General Hospital Psychiatry* 15, no. 5 (1993): 284–89; P. Creamer et al., "Sustained Improvement Produced by Nonpharmacologic Intervention in Fibromyalgia: Results of a Pilot Study," *Arthritis Care and Research* 13, no. 4 (2000): 198–204; S. E. Sephton et al., "Mindfulness Meditation Alleviates Depressive Symptoms in Women with Fibromyalgia: Results of a Randomized Clinical Trial," *Arthritis and Rheumatism* 57, no. 1 (2007): 77–85; E. Lush et al., "Mindfulness Meditation for

Symptom Reduction in Fibromyalgia: Psychophysiological Correlates," *Journal of Clinical Psychology in Medical Settings* 16, no. 2 (2009): 200–207.

50. If the hand joints are highly inflamed and feel too hot, adding more warmth may not be optimal, according to traditional Chinese medicine theory. In this case, one might explore using imagery with a cooler quality, such as bathing the tissues with soothing "blue sky" energy.

Chapter 6

1. P. Taggart et al., "Anger, Emotion, and Arrhythmias: from Brain to Heart," *Frontiers in Physiology* 2 (2011): 67; A. Golabchi and N. Sarrafzadegan, "Takotsubo Cardiomyopathy or Broken Heart Syndrome: A Review Article," *Journal of Research in Medical Sciences* 16, no. 3 (2011): 340–45; J. Macleod, "Commentary: Broken Hearts and Minds—Depression and Incident Heart Disease and Stroke," *International Journal of Epidemiology* 39, no. 4 (2010): 1025–26.

2. Ted Kaptchuk, *The Web That Has No Weaver* (New York: McGraw-Hill, 2000); Thomas Ots, "The Angry Liver, the Anxious Heart, and the Melancholy Spleen: The Phenomenology of Perception in Chinese Culture," *Culture, Medicine, and Psychiatry* 14, no. 1 (1990): 21–58.

3. W. Rosamond et al., "Heart Disease and Stroke Statistics—2007 Update: A Report from the American Heart Association Statistics Committee and Stroke Statistics Subcommittee," *Circulation* 115, no. 5 (2007): e69–171.

4. Ibid.

5. For example, see "Your Guide to Lowering Your Cholesterol with TLC," U.S. Department of Health and Human Services, National Institutes of Health National Heart, Lung, and Blood Institute (NIH Publication No. 06–5235, December 2005); D. J. Becker et al., "Simvastatin vs. Therapeutic Lifestyle Changes and Supplements: Randomized Primary Prevention Trial," *Mayo Clinic Proceedings* 83, no. 7 (2008): 758–64; N. F. Gordon et al., "Effectiveness of Therapeutic Lifestyle Changes in Patients with Hypertension, Hyperlipidemia, and/or Hyperglycemia," *American Journal of Cardiology* 94, no. 12 (2004): 1558–61.

6. G. Y. Yeh et al., "Use of Complementary Therapies in Patients with Cardiovascular Disease," *American Journal of Cardiology* 98, no. 5 (2006): 673–80; Y. W. Leung et al., "The Prevalence and Correlates of Mind-Body Therapy Practices in Patients with Acute Coronary Syndrome," *Complementary Therapies in Medicine* 16, no. 5 (2008): 254–61.

7. US Department of Health and Human Services, *Physical Activity and Health: A Report of the Surgeon General* (Atlanta, Ga. Public Health Service, CDC, National Center for Chronic Disease Prevention and Health Promotion, 1996).

8. G. Wannamethee et al., "Changes in Physical Activity, Mortality, and Inci-

dence of Coronary Heart Disease in Older Men," *Lancet* 351, no. 9116 (1998): 1603–8.

9. See reviews by C. Lan et al., "The Exercise Intensity of Tai Chi Chuan," *Medicine and Sport Science* 52 (2008): 12–19.

10. W. J. Kop, "Chronic and Acute Psychological Risk Factors for Clinical Manifestations of Coronary Artery Disease," *Psychosomatic Medicine* 61, no. 4 (1999): 476–87; A. Rozanski et al., "Impact of Psychological Factors on the Pathogenesis of Cardiovascular Disease and Implications for Therapy," *Circulation* 99, no. 16 (1999): 2192–217; D. S. Krantz, "Mental Stress as a Trigger of Myocardial Ischemia and Infarction," *Cardiology Clinics* 14, no. 2 (1996): 271–87; J. Suls and J. Bunde, "Anger, Anxiety, and Depression as Risk Factors for Cardiovascular Disease: The Problems and Implications of Overlapping Affective Dispositions," *Psychological Bulletin* 131, no. 2 (2005): 260–300; Willem J. Kop and Jennifer L. Francis, "Psychological Risk Factors and Pathophysiological Pathways Involved in Coronary Artery Disease: Relevance to Complementary Medicine Interventions," in Vogel and Krucoff, eds., *Integrative Cardiology: Complementary and Alternative Medicine for the Heart* (New York: McGraw-Hill Medical); B. W. Penninx et al., "Effects of Social Support and Personal Coping Resources on Mortality in Older Age: The Longitudinal Aging Study Amsterdam," *American Journal of Epidemiology* 146, no. 6 (1997): 510–19.

11. D. E. Ford et al., "Depression is a Risk Factor for Coronary Artery Disease in Men: the Precursors Study," *Archives of Internal Medicine* 158 (1998): 1422–26; A. H. Glassman, "Depression and Cardiovascular Comorbidity," *Dialogues in Clinical Neuroscience* 9, no. 1 (2007): 9–17.

12. M. A. Mittleman et al., "Triggering of Acute Myocardial Infarction Onset by Episodes of Anger: Determinants of Myocardial Infarction Onset Study Investigators," *Circulation* 92, no. 7 (1995): 1720–25.

13. D. R. Witte et al., "A Meta-Analysis of Excess Cardiac Mortality on Monday," *European Journal of Epidemiology* 20, no. 5 (2005): 401–6.

14. T. Raupach et al., "Slow Breathing Reduces Sympathoexcitation in COPD," *European Respiratory Journal* 32, no. 2 (2008): 387–92; L. Bernardi et al., "Effect of Rosary Prayer and Yoga Mantras on Autonomic Cardiovascular Rhythms, Comparative Study," *BMJ* 323, no. 7327 (2001): 1446–49; K. Narkiewicz et al., "Sympathetic Neural Outflow and Chemoreflex Sensitivity Are Related to Spontaneous Breathing Rate in Normal Men," *Hypertension* 47, no. 1 (2006): 51–55; B. Oneda et al., "Sympathetic Nerve Activity Is Decreased during Device-guided Slow Breathing," *Hypertension Research* (2010): 1–5; R. Jerath et al., "Physiology of Long Pranayamic Breathing: Neural Respiratory Elements May Provide a Mechanism that Explains How Slow Deep Breathing Shifts the Autonomic Nervous System," *Medical Hypotheses* 67, no. 3 (2006): 566–71.

15. For example, see F. Li et al., "Tai Chi, Self-efficacy, and Physical Function in the Elderly," *Prevention Science* 2, no. 4 (2001): 229–39; R. E. Taylor-Piliae and E. S. Froelicher, "Measurement Properties of Tai Chi Exercise Self-efficacy among Ethnic Chinese with Coronary Heart Disease Risk Factors: A Pilot Study," *European Journal of Cardiovascular Nursing* 3, no. 4 (2004): 287–94; F. Li et al., "Falls Self-efficacy as a Mediator of Fear of Falling in an Exercise Intervention for Older Adults," *Journals of Gerontology Series B: Psychological Sciences and Social Sciences* 60, no. 1 (2005): 34–40.

16. B. N. Uchino. "Understanding the Links between Social Support and Physical Health," *Perspectives on Psychological Science* 4 (2009): 236–255; F. Mookadam and H. M. Arthur, "Social Support and Its Relationship to Morbidity and Mortality after Acute Myocardial Infarction: Systematic Overview," *Archives of Internal Medicine* 164 (2004): 1514–18.

17. G. Y. Yeh, C. C. Wang, P. M. Wayne, R. Phillips, "Tai Chi Exercise for Patients with Cardiovascular Conditions and Risk Factors: A Systematic Review," *Journal of Cardiopulmonary Rehabilitation and Prevention* 29, no. 3 (2009): 152–60; R. E. Taylor Pillie and E. S. Froelicher, "Effectiveness of Tai Chi Exercise in Improving Aerobic Capacity: A Meta-Analysis," *The Journal of Cardiovascular Nursing* 19, no. 1 (2004): 48–57; G. Y. Yeh, C. C. Wang, P. M. Wayne, R. Phillips, "The Effect of Tai Chi Exercise on Blood Pressure: A Systematic Review," *Preventive Cardiology* 11, no. 2 (2008): 82–89; M. S. Lee et al., "Tai Chi for Cardiovascular Disease and Its Risk Factors: A Systematic Review," *Journal of Hypertension* 25 (2007): 1974–77; M. S. Lee et al., "Tai Chi for Lowering Resting Blood Pressure in the Elderly: A Systematic Review," *Journal of Evaluation in Clinical Practice* 16, no. 4 (2010): 818–24; R. E. Taylor Pilliae, "Tai Chi as an Adjunct to Cardiac Rehabilitation Exercise Training," *Journal of Cardiopulmonary Rehabilitation* 23, no. 2 (2003): 90–96.

18. G. Y. Yeh, C. C. Wang, P. M. Wayne, R. Phillips, "The Effect of Tai Chi Exercise on Blood Pressure: A Systematic Review," *Preventive Cardiology* 11, no. 2 (2008): 82–89; M. S. Lee et al., "Tai Chi for Cardiovascular Disease and Its Risk Factors: A Systematic Review," *Journal of Hypertension* 25 (2007): 1974–77; M. S. Lee et al., "Tai Chi for Lowering Resting Blood Pressure in the Elderly: A Systematic Review," *Journal of Evaluation in Clinical Practice* 16, no. 4 (2010): 818–24.

19. D. R. Young et al., "The Effects of Aerobic Exercise and T'ai Chi on Blood Pressure in Older People: Results of a Randomized Trial," *Journal of the American Geriatrics Society* 47, no. 3 (1999): 277–84.

20. J. C. Tsai et al., "The Beneficial Effects of Tai Chi Chuan on Blood Pressure and Lipid Profile and Anxiety Status in a Randomized Controlled Trial," *Journal of Alternative and Complementary Medicine* 9 (2003): 747–54; G. N. Thomas et al., "Effects of Tai Chi and Resistance Training on Cardiovascular Risk Factors in Elderly Chinese Subjects: A 12-Month Longitudinal,

Randomized, Controlled, Intervention Study," *Clinical Endocrinology* 63 (2005): 663–69; Z. S. Sheng and X. H. Su, "The Effect of Tai Chi Qigong Form 18 on Hypertension," *Modern Rehabilitation* 4 (2000): 33–34; S. L. Wolf et al., "The Influence of Intense Tai Chi Training on Physical Performance and Hemodynamic Outcomes in Transitionally Frail, Older Adults," *Journals of Gerontology Series A: Biological Sciences and Medical Sciences* 61, no. 2 (2006): 184–89.

21. In one RCT, researchers in Taiwan recruited 76 older sedentary adults, average age 51, with borderline or stage I hypertension who were not taking medications. They were assigned to either 12 weeks of Tai Chi three times a week or no intervention (controls). The authors reported a number of improvements in lipid profiles in the Tai Chi group, including a reduction in total cholesterol (–15.2 md/dL), LDL cholesterol (–20 md/dL), triglycerides (–23.8 mg/dL), and increases in HDL cholesterol (+4.7 mg/dL): J. C. Tsai et al., "The Beneficial Effects of Tai Chi Chuan on Blood Pressure and Lipid Profile and Anxiety Status in a Randomized Controlled Trial," *Journal of Alternative and Complementary Medicine* 9 (2003): 747–54).

22. T. M. Liu and S. X. Li, "Effect of Shadow Boxing on the Cardiovascular Excitability, Adaptability and Endurance in Middle-aged and Elderly Patients with Hypertension," *Chinese Journal of Clinical Rehabilitation* 8 (2004): 7508–09; S. C. Chen et al., "Effect of Tai Chi on Biochemical Profiles and Oxidative Stress Indicators in Obese Patients with Type 2 Diabetes," *Journal of Alternative and Complementary Medicine* 16 (2010): 1153–59; C. Lan et al., "Effect of T'ai Chi Chuan Training on Cardiovascular Risk Factors in Dyslipidemic Patients," *Journal of Alternative and Complementary Medicine* 14 (2008): 813–19; G. T. Ko et al., "A 10-Week Tai-Chi Program Improved the Blood Pressure, Lipid Profile and SF-36 Scores in Hong Kong Chinese Women," *Medical Science Monitor* 12, no. 5 (2006): CR196–99.

23. G. N. Thomas et al., "Effects of Tai Chi and Resistance Training on Cardiovascular Risk Factors in Elderly Chinese Subjects: A 12-Month Longitudinal, Randomized, Controlled, Intervention Study," *Clinical Endocrinology* 63 (2005): 663–69; Y. Zhang and F. H. Fu, "Effects of 14-Week Tai Ji Quan Exercise on Metabolic Control in Women with Type 2 Diabetes," *American Journal of Chinese Medicine* 36, no. 4 (2008): 647–54.

24. P. W. Wilson and W. B. Kannel, "Obesity, Diabetes, and Risk of Cardiovascular Disease in the Elderly," *American Journal of Geriatric Cardiology* 11, no. 2 (2002): 119–23, 125.

25. S. S. Hui et al., "Evaluation of Energy Expenditure and Cardiovascular Health Effects from Tai Chi and Walking Exercise," *Hong Kong Medical Journal*, no. 1, 15 suppl. 2 (2009): 4; R. Song et al., "Effect of Tai Chi Self Help Program on Glucose Control, Cardiovascular Risks and Quality of Life in Type II Diabetic Patients," *Journal of Muscle and Joint Health* 12

(2007): 13–25 (in Korean); J. W. Hung et al., "Effect of 12-week Tai Chi Chuan Exercise on Peripheral Nerve Modulation in Patients with Type 2 Diabetes Mellitus," *Journal of Rehabilitation Medicine* 41 (2009): 924–29.

26. One Hong Kong study including 207 healthy adults compared 12 weeks of Tai Chi to strength and resistance training, as well as to a usual-care (control) group. The elder participants in this study had various CVD risk factors. The results show that levels of fasting glucose and other blood sugar markers in both exercise groups were not different from those in the control group: G. N. Thomas et al., "Effects of Tai Chi and Resistance Training on Cardiovascular Risk Factors in Elderly Chinese Subjects: A 12 Month Longitudinal, Randomized, Controlled Intervention Study," *Clinical Endocrinology* 63 (2005): 663–69. Also see T. Tsang et al., "Effects of Tai Chi on Glucose Homeostasis and Insulin Sensitivity in Older Adults with Type 2 Diabetes: A Randomized Double-blind Sham-controlled Exercise Trial," *Age and Ageing* 37 (2008): 64–71.

27. P. Libby et al., "Inflammation in Atherosclerosis," *Nature* 420, no. 6917 (2002): 868–74.

28. P. M. Ridker et al., "Relation of Baseline High-sensitivity C-reactive Protein Level to Cardiovascular Outcomes with Rosuvastatin in the Justification for Use of Statins in Prevention: An Intervention Trial Evaluating Rosuvastatin (JUPITER)," *American Journal of Cardiology* 106, no. 2 (2010): 204–9; B. M. Everett et al., "Rosuvastatin in the Prevention of Stroke among Men and Women with Elevated Levels of C-reactive Protein: Justification for the Use of Statins in Prevention: An Intervention Trial Evaluating Rosuvastatin (JUPITER)," *Circulation* 121, no. 1 (2010): 143–50.

29. S. C. Chen et al., "Effect of T'ai Chi Exercise on Biochemical Profiles and Oxidative Stress Indicators in Obese Patients with Type 2 Diabetes," *Journal of Alternative and Complementary Medicine* 16, no. 11 (2010): 1153–59.

30. T. W. Tsang et al., "A Randomized Controlled Trial of Kung Fu Training for Metabolic Health in Overweight/Obese Adolescents: The 'Martial Fitness' Study," *Journal of Pediatric Endocrinology and Metabolism* 22, no. 7 (2009): 595–607. Also see: C. Lan et al., "Effect of T'ai Chi Chuan Training on Cardiovascular Risk Factors in Dyslipidemic Patients," *Journal of Alternative and Complementary Medicine* 14, no. 7 (2008): 813–19.

31. S. S. Hui et al., "Evaluation of Energy Expenditure and Cardiovascular Health Effects from Tai Chi and Walking Exercise," *Hong Kong Medical Journal* 15, no. 1, suppl. 2 (2009): 4–7.

32. C. Lan et al., "Changes of Aerobic Capacity, Fat Ratio and Flexibility in Older TCC Practitioners: A Five-year Follow-up," *American Journal of Chinese Medicine* 36, no. 6 (2008): 1041–50.

33. For example, see: J. F. Audette et al., "Tai Chi versus Brisk Walking in Elderly Women," *Age and Ageing* 35, no. 4 (2006): 388–93; R. E. Taylor-Piliae

et al., "Improvement in Balance, Strength, and Flexibility after 12 Weeks of Tai Chi Exercise in Ethnic Chinese Adults with Cardiovascular Disease Risk Factors," *Alternative Therapies in Health and Medicine* 12, no. 2 (2006): 50–58; R. E. Taylor-Piliae et al., "Tai Chi as an Adjunct Physical Activity for Adults Aged 45 Years and Older Enrolled in Phase III Cardiac Rehabilitation," *European Journal of Cardiovascular Nursing* 11, no. 1 (2012): 34–43; R. E. Taylor-Piliae et al., "Hemodynamic Responses to a Community-based Tai Chi Exercise Intervention in Ethnic Chinese Adults with Cardiovascular Disease Risk Factors," *European Journal of Cardiovascular Nursing* 5, no. 2 (2006): 165–74.

34. G. Y. Yeh et al., "Effect of Tai Chi Mind-Body Movement Therapy on Functional Status and Exercise Capacity in Patients with Chronic Heart Failure: A Randomized Controlled Trial," *American Journal of Medicine* 117, no. 8 (2004): 541–48; G. Y. Yeh et al., "Enhancement of Sleep Stability with Tai Chi Exercise in Patients with Chronic Heart Failure: Preliminary Findings Using an ECG-based Spectrogram Method," *Sleep Medicine* 9, no. 5 (2008): 527–36.

35. G. Y. Yeh et al., "Tai Chi Exercise in Patients with Chronic Heart Failure: A Randomized Clinical Trial," *Archives of Internal Medicine* 117, no. 8 (2011): 750–57.

36. G. Y. Yeh et al., "Tai Chi in Patients with Heart Failure with Preserved Ejection Fraction: A Pilot Study," *Congestive Heart Failure* (e-pub October 12, 2012.

37. G. Caminiti et al., "Tai Chi Enhances the Effects of Endurance Training in the Rehabilitation of Elderly Patients with Chronic Heart Failure," *Rehabilitation Research and Practice* (2011): article ID 761958.

38. D. E. Barrow et al., "An Evaluation of the Effects of Tai Chi Chuan and Chi Kung Training in Patients with Symptomatic Heart Failure: A Randomised Controlled Pilot Study," *Postgraduate Medical Journal* 83, no. 985 (2007): 717–21; J. A. Fontana et al., "T'ai Chi Chih as an Intervention for Heart Failure," *Nursing Clinics of North America* 35, no. 4 (2000): 1031–46.

39. See reviews by G. Y. Yeh, C. C. Wang, P. M. Wayne, and R. Phillips, "Tai Chi Exercise for Patients with Cardiovascular Conditions and Risk Factors: A Systematic Review," *Journal of Cardiopulmonary Rehabilitation and Prevention* 29, no. 3 (2009): 152–60; and A. Dalusung-Angosta, "The Impact of Tai Chi Exercise on Coronary Heart Disease: A Systematic Review," *Journal of the American Academy of Nurse Practitioners* 23, no. 7 (2011): 376–81.

40. K. S. Channer et al., "Changes in Haemodynamic Parameters following Tai Chi Chuan and Aerobic Exercise in Patients Recovering from Acute Myocardial Infarction," *Postgraduate Medical Journal* 72, no. 848 (1996): 349–51.

41. R. Y. Chang et al., "The Effect of T'ai Chi Exercise on Autonomic Nervous Function of Patients with Coronary Artery Disease," *Journal of Alternative*

and Complementary Medicine 14, no. 9 (2008): 1107–13; S. Sato et al., "Effect of Tai Chi Training on Baroreflex Sensitivity and Heart Rate Variability in Patients with Coronary Heart Disease," *International Heart Journal* 51, no. 4 (2009): 238–41.

42. C. Lan et al., "The Effect of Tai Chi on Cardiorespiratory Function in Patients with Coronary Artery Bypass Surgery," *Medicine and Science in Sports and Exercise* 31, no. 5 (1999): 634–38.

43. "Post-Stroke Rehabilitation Fact Sheet," *NINDS,* October 2008, NIH Publication No. 08-4846.

44. S. S. Au-Yeung et al., "Short-form Tai Chi Improves Standing Balance of People with Chronic Stroke," *Neurorehabilitation and Neural Repair* 23, no. 5 (2009): 515–22.

45. J. Hart et al., "Tai Chi Chuan Practice in Community-dwelling Persons after Stroke," *International Journal of Rehabilitation Research* 27, no. 4 (2004): 303–4.

Chapter 7

1. H. J. Schunemann et al., "Pulmonary Function Is a Long-term Predictor of Mortality in the General Population: 29-year Follow-up of the Buffalo Health Study," *CHEST* 118, no. 3 (2000): 656–64.

2. W. B. Kannel et al., "Vital Capacity as a Predictor of Cardiovascular Disease: the Framingham Study," *American Heart Journal* 105, no. 2 (1983): 311–15.

3. H. J. Schunemann et al., "Pulmonary Function Is a Long-term Predictor of Mortality in the General Population: 29-year Follow-up of the Buffalo Health Study," *CHEST* 118, no. 3 (2000): 656–64.

4. Margaret Pisani ed., *Aging and Lung Disease: A Clinical Guide* (New York: Humana Press, 2012).

5. N. Berend, "Normal Ageing of the Lung: Implications for Diagnosis and Monitoring of Asthma in Older People," *Medical Journal of Australia* 183, suppl. 1 (2005): S28–29.

6. Ibid.

7. Ibid.

8. Given the pluralism of Tai Chi and its multiple applications (e.g., martial, health, meditative), it should not be surprising that instructions regarding how to (or not to) breath and coordinate the breath with movements varies greatly between styles, and even among individual teachers within a style. For example, in some systems, students are taught to breathe in during expanding movements, while in others, to exhale during expanding movements (e.g., during a punch). Still other instructors suggest no attempt to coordinate breathing patterns with movement, but simply to let both occur naturally. Examples of good discussions of this topic can be found in Robert

Chuckrow, *Tai Chi Dynamics* (Boston: YMAA Publications, 2008); M. Mellish, *A Tai Chi Imagery Workbook: Spirit, Intent, and Motion* (London: Singing Dragon, 2011); Mantak Chi and Juan Li, *The Inner Structure of Tai Chi: Tai Chi Chi Kung I* (New York: Healing Tai Books, 1996); J. Loupos, *Tai Chi Connections: Advancing Your Tai Chi Experience* (Boston: YMAA Publication Center, 2005).

9. T. J. Kaptchuk, J. M. Kelley, A. Deykin, P. M. Wayne, L. C. Lasagna, I. O. Epstein, I. Kirsch, M. E. Wechsler, "Do 'Placebo Responders' Exist?" *Contemporary Clinical Trials* 29, no. 4 (2008): 587–95.

10. C. Lan et al., "Changes in Aerobic Capacity, Fat Ratio, and Flexibility in Older TCC Practitioners: A Five Year Follow-up," *American Journal of Chinese Medicine* 36 (2008): 1041–50; C. Lan et al., "The Aerobic Capacity and Ventilatory Efficiency during Exercise in Qigong and Tai Chi Chuan Practitioners," *American Journal of Chinese Medicine* 32, no. 1 (2004): 141–50; C. Lan et al., "Cardiorespiratory Function, Flexibility, and Body Composition among Geriatric Tai Chi Chuan Practitioners," *Archives of Physical Medicine and Rehabilitation* 77, no. 6 (1996): 612–16; J. S. Lai et al., "Two-year Trends in Cardiorespiratory Function among Older Tai Chi Chuan Practitioners and Sedentary Subjects.," *Journal of the American Geriatrics Society* 43, no. 11 (1995): 1222–27; J. S. Lai et al., "Cardiorespiratory Responses of Tai Chi Chuan Practitioners and Sedentary Subjects during Cycle Ergometry," *Journal of the Formosan Medical Association* 92, no. 10 (October 1993): 894–99.

11. R. Taylor-Piliae et al., "Improvement in Balance, Strength, and Flexibility after 12 Weeks of Tai Chi Exercise in Ethnic Chinese Adults with Cardiovascular Disease Risk Factors," *Alternative Therapies in Health and Medicine* 12 (2006): 50–58.

12. L. Pomidori et al., "Efficacy and Tolerability of Yoga Breathing in Patients with Chronic Obstructive Pulmonary Disease: A Pilot Study," *Journal of Cardiopulmonary Rehabilitation and Prevention* 29, no. 2 (2009): 133–37; L. Bernardi et al., "Effect of Breathing Rate on Oxygen Saturation and Exercise Performance in Chronic Heart Failure," *Lancet* 351, no. 9112 (1998): 1308–11.

13. T. Raupach et al., "Slow Breathing Reduces Sympathoexcitation in COPD," *European Respiratory Journal* 32, no. 2 (2008): 387–92; L. Bernardi et al., "Effect of Rosary Prayer and Yoga Mantras on Autonomic Cardiovascular Rhythms, Comparative Study," *BMJ* 323, no. 7327 (2001): 1446–49; K. Narkiewicz et al., "Sympathetic Neural Outflow and Chemoreflex Sensitivity Are Related to Spontaneous Breathing Rate in Normal Men," *Hypertension* 47, no. 1 (2006): 51–55.

14. Kubzansky et al., "Angry Breathing: A Prospective Study of Hostility and Lung Function in the Normative Aging Study," *Thorax* 61 (2006): 863–68; Weuve et al., "Forced Expiratory Volume in 1 Second and Cognitive Aging in Men," *Journal of the American Geriatrics Society* 59 (2011): 1283–92.

15. E. Agostoni and H. Rand, "Abdominal and Thoracic Pressures at Different Lung Volumes," *Journal of Applied Physiology* 15 (1960): 1087–92; G. E. Tzelepis et al., "Transmission of Pressure within the Abdomen," *Journal of Applied Physiology* 81, no. 3 (1996): 1111–14; Mead et al., "Abdominal Breathing Transmission in Humans during Slow Breathing Maneuvers," *Journal of Applied Physiology* 68, no. 5 (1990): 1850–53.

16. T. Osada et al., "Determination of Comprehensive Arterial Inflow in Abdominal-Pelvic Organs: Impact of Respiration and Posture on Organ Perfusion," *Medical Science Monitor* 17 (2011): CR57–66.

17. Ken Rose and Yu Huan Zhang, *A Brief History of Qi* (Brookline, Mass.: Paradigm Publications, 2001).

18. Martin Mellish, *A Tai Chi Imagery Workbook: Spirit, Intent, and Motion* (London: Singing Dragon, 2011).

19. J. Menzin et al., "The Economic Burden of Chronic Obstructive Pulmonary Disease (COPD) in a U.S. Medicare Population," *Respiratory Medicine* 102, no. 9 (2008): 1248–56.

20. E. Sutherland and R. Cherniack, "Management of Chronic Obstructive Pulmonary Disease," *New England Journal of Medicine* 350 (2004): 2689–97.

21. G. Y. Yeh, D. H. Roberts, P. M. Wayne, R. B. Davis, M. T. Quilty, R. S. Phillips, "Tai Chi Exercise for Patients with Chronic Obstructive Pulmonary Disease: A Pilot Study," *Respiratory Care* 55, no. 11 (2010): 1475–82.

22. A. W. Chan et al., "Tai Chi Qigong Improves Lung Functions and Activity Tolerance in COPD Clients: A Single Blind, Randomized Controlled Trial," *Complementary Therapies in Medicine* 19, no. 1 (2011): 3–11. A. W. Chan et al., "Effectiveness of a Tai Chi Qigong Program in Promoting Health-related Quality of Life and Perceived Social Support in Chronic Obstructive Pulmonary Disease Clients," *Quality of Life Research* 19, no. 5 (2010): 653–64. Also see R. W. Leung et al., "A Study Design to Investigate the Effect of Short-form Sun-style Tai Chi in Improving Functional Exercise Capacity, Physical Performance, Balance and Health Related Quality of Life in People with Chronic Obstructive Pulmonary Disease (COPD)," *Contemporary Clinical Trials* 32, no. 2 (2011): 267–72.

23. For Qigong, see B. H. Ng et al., "Functional and Psychosocial Effects of Health Qigong in Patients with COPD: A Randomized Controlled Trial," *Journal of Alternative and Complementary Medicine* 17, no. 3 (2011): 243–51. For yoga, see A. Fulambarker et al., "Effect of Yoga in Chronic Obstructive Pulmonary Disease," *American Journal of Therapeutics* (October 22, 2012); L. Pomidori et al., "Efficacy and Tolerability of Yoga Breathing in Patients with Chronic Obstructive Pulmonary Disease: A Pilot Study," *Journal of Cardiopulmonary Rehabilitation and Prevention* 29, no. 2 (2009): 133–37; D. Donesky-Cuenco et al., "Yoga Therapy Decreases Dyspnea-related Distress

and Improves Functional Performance in People with Chronic Obstructive Pulmonary Disease: A Pilot Study," *Journal of Alternative and Complementary Medicine* 15, no. 3 (2009): 225–34.

24. Summary Health Statistics for U.S. Adults: National Health Interview Survey, 2008 and Summary Health Statistics for U.S. Children: National Health Interview Survey, 2008; World Health Organization, "Global Surveillance, Prevention and Control of Chronic Respiratory Diseases: A Comprehensive Approach," 2007; Centers for Disease Control. Surveillance for Asthma—United States, 1960–1995, *Morbidity and Mortality Weekly Report*, 47 (1998): SS-1.

25. W. Maziak, "The Asthma Epidemic and Our Artificial Habitats," *BMC Pulmonary Medicine* 5, no. 1 (2005).

26. Y. F. Chang et al., "Tai Chi Chuan Training Improves the Pulmonary Function of Asthmatic Children," *Journal of Microbiology, Immunology, and Infections* 41 (2008): 88–95.

27. S. Kiatboonsri et al., "Effects of Tai Chi Qigong Training on Exercise Performance and Airway Inflammation in Moderate to Severe Persistent Asthma," *CHEST* 134, no. 4 (2008): s54003.

Chapter 8

1. B. Horrigan, "Meditation and Neuroplasticity: Training Your Brain (Interview with Richard Davidson, PhD)," *Explore* 1 (2005): 381–88.

2. For a good discussion of the Shen-Jing continuum and the Chinese concept of mind, see E. Korngold and H. Beinfield, "Chinese Medicine and the Mind," *Explore* 2, no. 4 (2006): 321–33.

More generally, thoughts and emotions in Chinese medicine are not thought to originate in or be regulated solely by the brain, but rather, by all the visceral organs and their energetic interactions. For example, excessive anger is associated with an imbalance in liver energy, and short-term memory loss may be related to weak kidney Qi. This more holistic concept of the mind, and the idea that that memories, emotion, and other aspects of mind may not be stored or processed exclusively in the brain, but in other parts and tissues of the body as well, is also discussed in multiple Western traditions, including recent medical literature. For example, databases of case studies with transplant patients suggest that organ transplant recipients sometimes inherit the memories and behaviors of the donors—in these cases, clearly not via brain tissue; see P. Pearsall, G. E. Schwartz, L. G. Russek, *Nexus Magazine* 12, no. 3 (April–May 2005). Similarly, practitioners and patients of many forms of manual and movement therapies report that physical changes can trigger release of memories and emotions apparently "stored" in the body.

To read more about the concept of "embodiment," see F. Varela and E. Thompson, *The Embodied Mind* (Cambridge, Mass.: MIT Press, 1991); W.

E. Mehling et al., "Body Awareness: A Phenomenological Inquiry into the Common Ground of Mind-Body Therapies," *Philosophy, Ethics, and Humanities in Medicine* 7, no. 6 (2011): 6; E. Thompson, *Mind in Life; Biology, Phenomenology, and the Sciences of Mind* (Cambridge, Mass.: Belknap Press of Harvard University Press, 2007); and D. H. Johnson, *Groundworks: Narratives of Embodiment* (Berkeley: North Atlantic Books, 1997).

3. Shi Ming, *Mind Over Matter: Higher Martial Arts* (Berkeley: Blue Snake Books, 1994).

4. For an excellent review of plasticity research specifically related to meditation, see H. A. Slagter et al., "Mental Training as a Tool in the Neuroscientific Study of Brain and Cognitive Plasticity," *Frontiers in Neuroscience Research* 5 (2011): 17.

5. A. Nelson and S. Gilbert, *The Harvard Medical School Guide to Achieving Optimal Memory* (New York: McGraw Hill, 2005).

6. A. Pascual-Leone et al., "Modulation of Muscle Responses Evoked by Transcranial Magnetic Stimulation during the Acquisition of New Fine Motor Skills," *Journal of Neurophysiology* 74, no. 5 (1995): 1037–45; also see C. Papadelis et al., "Effects of Imagery Training on Cognitive Performance and Use of Physiological Measures as an Assessment Tool of Mental Effort," *Brain and Cognition* 64, no. 1 (2007): 74–85.

7. R. C. Peterson et al., "Prevalence of Mild Cognitive Impairment Is Higher in Men: The Mayo Clinic Study of Aging," *Neurology* 75, no. 10 (2010): 889–97; Alzheimer's Association, "2011 Alzheimer's Disease Facts and Figures," *Alzheimer's & Dementia* 7, no. 2 (2011): 208–44.

8. L. C. W. Lam et al. "Interim Follow-up of a Randomized Controlled Trial Comparing Chinese Style Mind-Body (Tai Chi) and Stretching Exercises on Cognitive Function in Subjects at Risk of Progressive Cognitive Decline," *International Journal of Geriatrics Psychology* 26 (2011): 733–40; L. C. W. Lam et al., "A 1-year Randomized Controlled Trial Comparing Mind-Body Exercise (Tai Chi) with Stretching and Toning Exercise on Cognitive Function in Older Chinese Adults at Risk of Cognitive Decline," *Journal of the American Medical Directors Association* (2012): e1–e6.

9. S. C. Burgener et al., "The Effects of a Multimodal Intervention on Outcomes of Persons with Early-stage Dementia," *American Journal of Alzheimer's Disease and Other Dementias* 23, no. 4 (2008): 382–94.

10. S. C. Burgener et al., "A Combined, Multimodal Intervention for Individuals with Dementia," *Research in Gerontological Nursing* 4, no. 1 (2011): 64–75.

11. R. E. Taylor-Piliae et al., "Effects of Tai Chi and Western Exercise on Physical and Cognitive Functioning in Healthy Community-dwelling Older Adults," *Journal of Aging and Physical Activity* 18, no. 3 (2010): 261–79.

12. J. Mortimer et al., "2012: Changes in Brain Volume and Cognition in a Randomized Trial of Exercise and Social Interaction in a Community-based

Sample of Non-demented Chinese Elders," *Journal of Alzheimer's Disease* 30, no. 4 (2012): 757–66.

13. M. M. Matthews and H. G. Williams, "Can Tai Chi Enhance Cognitive Vitality? A Preliminary Study of Cognitive Executive Control in Older Adults after a Tai Chi Intervention," *Journal of the South Carolina Medical Association* 104, no. 8 (2008): 255–57; C. D. Hall et al., "Effects of Tai Chi Intervention on Dual-task Ability in Older Adults: A Pilot Study," *Archives of Physical Medicine and Rehabilitation* 90 no. 3 (2009): 525–29; M. H. Nguyen and A. Kruse, "A Randomized Controlled Trial of Tai Chi for Balance, Sleep Quality and Cognitive Performance in Elderly Vietnamese," *Journal of Clinical Interventions in Aging* 7 (2012): 185–90.

14. W. K. Man et al., "Do Older Tai Chi Practitioners Have Better Attention and Memory Function?" *Journal of Alternative and Complementary Medicine* 16 (2009): 1259–64.

15. A. S. Chan et al., "Association between Mind-Body and Cardiovascular Exercises and Memory in Older Adults, *Journal of the American Geriatrics Society* 53 (2005): 1754–63. Also see L. C. Lam et al., "Modality of Physical Exercise and Cognitive Function in Hong Kong Older Chinese Community," *International Journal of Geriatric Psychiatry* 24, no. 1 (2009): 48–53.

16. C. Voelcker-Rehage et al., "Physical and Motor Fitness Are Both Related to Cognition in Old Age," *Cognitive Neuroscience* 31, no. 1 (2010): 167–76; C. Voelcker-Rehage et al., "Cardiovascular and Coordination Training Differentially Improve Cognitive Performance and Neural Processing in Older Adults," *Frontiers Human Neuroscience* 1, no. 5 (2011): 26.

17. S. Colcombe and A. F. Kramer, "Fitness Effects on the Cognitive Function of Older Adults: A Meta-Analytic Study," *Psychological Science* 14, no. 2 (2003): 125–30.

18. C. N. Tseng et al., "The Effectiveness of Exercise on Improving Cognitive Function in Older People: A Systematic Review," *Journal of Nursing Research* 19, no. 2 (2011): 119–31. Also see M. Angavaren et al., "Physical Activity and Enhanced Fitness to Improve Cognitive Function in Older People without Known Cognitive Impairment," *Cochrane Database of Systematic Reviews* 6, no. 3 (2008): CD005381.

19. K. I. Erickson et al., "Exercise Training Increases Size of Hippocampus and Improves Memory," *Proceedings of the National Academy of Sciences of the United States of America* 108, no. 7 (2010): 3017–22.

20. Among reported changes in human studies are higher levels of cerebral blood flow and blood volume [R. L. Rogers et al., "After Reaching Retirement Age Physical Activity Sustains Cerebral Perfusion and Cognition," *Journal of the American Geriatrics Society* 38, no. 2 (1990): 123–28; A. C. Periera et al., "An in Vivo Correlate of Exercise-induced Neurogenesis in the

Adult Dentate Gyrus," *Proceedings of the National Academy of Sciences of the United States of America* 104, no. 113 (2007): 5638–43]; increased activity in frontal and parietal regions of the brain, which are thought to be involved in efficient attentional control [S. J. Colcombe et al., "Cardiovascular Fitness, Cortical Plasticity, and Aging," *Proceedings of the National Academy of Sciences of the United States of America* 101, no. 9 (2004): 3316–21]; increased gray and white matter volume in the prefrontal cortex [S. J. Colcombe et al., "Aerobic Exercise Training Increases Brain Volume in Aging Humans," *Journals of Gerontology Series A: Biological Sciences and Medical Sciences* 61, no. 11 (2006): 1166–70]; and increased functioning of key nodes in the brain's executive control [Waton et al. "Executive Function, Memory, and Gait Speed Decline in Well-functioning Older Adults," *Journals of Gerontology Series A: Biological Sciences and Medical Sciences* 65, no. 10 (2010): 1093–100]; and default mode networks [M. W. Voss et al., "Plasticity of Brain Networks in a Randomized Intervention Trial of Exercise Training in Older Adults," *Frontiers in Aging Neuroscience*, 26, no. 2 (2010)].

21. E. B. Larson, "Exercise Is Associated with Reduced Risk for Incident Dementia among Persons 65 Years of Age and Older," *Annals of Internal Medicine* 144 (2006): 73–81.

22. K. Yaffe et al., "A Prospective Study of Physical Activity and Cognitive Decline in Elderly Women: Women Who Walk," *Archives of Internal Medicine* 161, no. 14 (2001): 1703–8.

23. C. Voelcker-Rehage et al., "Physical and Motor Fitness Are Both Related to Cognition in Old Age," *European Journal of Neuroscience* 31, no. 1 (2010): 167–76; C. Voelcker-Rehage et al., "Cardiovascular and Coordination Training Differentially Improve Cognitive Performance and Neural Processing in Older Adults," *Frontiers in Human Neuroscience* 5 (2011): 26.

24. M. C. Tierney et al., "Intensity of Recreational Physical Activity throughout Life and Later Life Cognitive Functioning in Women," *Journal of Alzheimer's Disease* 22, no. 4 (2010): 1331–38.

25. P. W. Landfield et al., "Hippocampal Aging and Adrenocorticoids: Quantitative Correlations," *Science* 202, no. 4372 (1978): 1098–102; R. M. Sapolsky and N. Y. Ann, "The Physiological Relevance of Glucocorticoid Endangerment of the Hippocampus," *Academy of Sciences* 746 (1994): 294–304, and discussion, 304–7.

26. S. J. Lupien et al., "Cortisol Levels during Human Aging Predict Hippocampal Atrophy and Memory Deficits," *Nature Neuroscience* 1, no. 1 (1998): 69–73; A. S. Karlamangla et al., "Urinary Cortisol Excretion as a Predictor of Incident Cognitive Impairment," *Neurobiology of Aging* 26, suppl. 1 (2005): 80–84.

27. R. S. Wilson et al., "Proneness to Psychological Distress Is Associated with Risk of Alzheimer's Disease," *Neurology* 961 (2003): 1479–85.

28. C. Wang et al., "Tai Chi on Psychological Well-being: Systematic Review and Meta-analysis," *BMC Complementary and Alternative Medicine* 21, no. 10 (2010): 23; L. Zhang et al., "A Review of the Psychological Effectiveness of Tai Chi on Different Populations," *Evidence-Based Complementary and Alternative Medicine* (2012): ID678107.

29. T. Esch et al., "Mind/Body Techniques for Physiological and Psychological Stress Reduction: Stress Management via Tai Chi Training—a Pilot Study," *Medical Science Monitor* 13, no. 11 (2007): CR488–497; P. Jin, "Changes in Heart Rate, Noradrenaline, Cortisol, and Mood during Tai Chi," *Journal of Psychosomatic Research* 33 (1989): 197–206; G. Y. Yeh et al., "Effect of Tai Chi Mind-Body Movement Therapy on Functional Status and Exercise Capacity in Patients with Chronic Heart Failure: A Randomized Controlled Trial," *American Journal of Medicine* 117, no. 8 (2004): 541–548; E. N. Lee, "The Effects of Tai Chi Exercise Program on Blood Pressure, Total Cholesterol and Cortisol Level in Patients with Essential Hypertension," *Taehan Kanho Hakhoe Chi* 34 (2004): 829–37 (in Korean).

30. M. L. Galantino et al., "The Effect of Group Aerobic Exercise and T'ai Chi on Functional Outcomes and Quality of Life for Persons Living with Acquired Immunodeficiency Syndrome," *Journal of Alternative and Complementary Medicine* 11, no. 6 (2005): 1085–92. An excellent qualitative study describing subjective experiences following Tai Chi is Y. Yang et al., "Subjective Experiences of Older Adults Practicing Taiji and Qigong," *Journal of Aging Research* (2011): ID650210.

31. H. A. Slagter et al., "Mental Training as a Tool in the Neuroscientific Study of Brain and Cognitive Plasticity," *Frontiers in Neuroscience Research* 5 (2011): 17.

32. A. Chiesa et al., "Does Mindfulness Training Improve Cognitive Abilities? A Systematic Review of Neuropsychological Findings," *Clinical Psychology Review* 31, no. 3 (2010): 449–64; A. Moore and P. Malinowski, "Meditation, Mindfulness and Cognitive Flexibility," *Consciousness and Cognition* 18 (2009): 176–86; P. A. van den Hurk, "Greater Efficiency in Attentional Processing Related to Mindfulness Meditation," *Quarterly Journal of Experimental Psychology* 63 (2010): 1168–80.

33. A. P. Jha et al., "Examining the Protective Effects of Mindfulness Training on Working Memory Capacity and Affective Experience," *Emotion* 10, no. 1 (2010): 54–64.

34. A. Mohan et al., "Effect of Meditation on Stress-induced Changes in Cognitive Functions," *Journal of Alternative and Complementary Medicine* 17 (2011): 207–12; B. K. Holzel et al., "Stress Reduction Correlates with Structural Changes in the Amygdala," *Social Cognitive and Affective Neuroscience* 5, no. 1 (2010): 11–17; P. van der Hurk et al., "Mindfulness Meditation Associated with Alterations in Bottom-up Processing: Psychophysiological Evidence for Reduced Reactivity," *International Journal of Psychophysiology*

78 (2010): 151–57; A. Lutz et al., "Attentional Regulation and Monitoring in Meditation," *Trends in Cognitive Science* 12 (2008): 163–69.

35. S. W. Lazar et al., "Functional Brain Mapping of the Relaxation Response and Meditation," *Neuroreport* 11, no. 7 (2000): 1581–85.

36. B. K. Holzel et al., "Mindfulness Practice Leads to Increases in Regional Brain Gray Matter Density," *Psychiatry Research* 191, no. 1 (2011): 36–43.

37. E. Luders et al., "The Underlying Anatomical Correlates of Long-term Meditation: Larger Hippocampal and Frontal Volumes of Gray Matter," *Neuroimage* 45, no. 3 (2009): 672–78; B. K. Holzel et al., "Investigation of Mindfulness Meditation Practitioners with Voxel-based Morphometry," *Social Cognitive and Affective Neuroscience*, 3, no. 1 (2008): 55–61.

38. N. A. Farb et al., "Attending to the Present: Mindfulness Meditation Reveals Distinct Neural Modes of Self-Reference," *Social Cognitive and Affective Neuroscience* 2, no. 4 (2007): 313–22; A. Lutz et al., "Regulation of the Neural Circuitry of Emotion by Compassion Meditation: Effects of Meditative Expertise," *PloS One* 3, no. 3 (2008): e1897.

39. L. A. Kilpatrick et al., "Impact of Mindfulness-Based Stress Reduction Training on Intrinsic Brain Connectivity," *Neuroimage* 56, no. 1: 290–98; E. Luders et al., "Enhanced Brain Connectivity in Long-term Meditation Practitioners," *Neuroimage* 57, no. 4 (2011): 1308–16.

40. J. Driemeyer et al., "Changes in Gray Matter Induced by Learning—Revisited," *PLoS One* 23 (2008): e2669; J. Boyke et al., "Training-induced Brain Structure Changes in the Elderly," *Journal of Neuroscience* 28, no. 28 (2008): 7031–35.

41. C. Voelcker-Rehage and K. Willimczik, "Motor Plasticity in a Juggling Task in Older Adults—A Developmental Study," *Age and Ageing* 35, no. 4 (2006): 422–27.

42. M. Groussard et al., "When Music and Long-term Memory Interact: Effects of Musical Expertise on Functional and Structural Plasticity in the Hippocampus," *PLoS One* 5, no. 10 (2010): pii: e13225; M. Herdener et al., "Musical Training Induces Functional Plasticity in Human Hippocampus," *Journal of Neuroscience* 30, no. 4 (2010): 1377–84.

43. J. C. Kattenstroth et al., "Superior Sensory, Motor, and Cognitive Performance in Elderly Individuals with Multi-year Dancing Activities," *Frontiers in Aging Neuroscience* 2 (2010): 31.

44. E. A. Mcguire et al., "Navigation-related Structural Change in the Hippocampi of Taxi Drivers," *Proceedings of the National Academy of Sciences of the United States of America* 97, no. 8 (2000)): 4398–403.

45. J. Verghese et al., "Leisure Activities and the Risk of Dementia in the Elderly," *New England Journal of Medicine* 348, no. 25 (2003): 2508–16. Also see: C. B. Hall et al., "Cognitive Activities Delay Onset of Memory Decline in Persons Who Develop Dementia," *Neurology* 73, no. 5 (2009): 356–61.

46. S. S. Bassuk et al., "Social Disengagement and Incident Cognitive Decline in Community-Dwelling Elderly Persons," *Annals of Internal Medicine* 131 (1999): 165–173; R. C. Sims et al., "The Influence of Functional Social Support on Executive Functioning in Middle-aged African Americans," *Neuropsychology, Development, and Cognition, Section B, Aging, Neuropsychology, and Cognition* 18, no. 4 (2011): 414–31.

47. Cheng Man Ch'ing, *Cheng-Tzu's Thirteen Treatises on Tai Chi Chuan* (Berkeley: North Atlantic Books, 1985).

48. Good discussions of being "in the zone" as related to Tai Chi and martial arts can be found in Shi Ming, *Mind Over Matter: Higher Martial Arts* (Berkeley: Blue Snake Books, 1994). Also see Rick Barrett, *Taijiquan: Through the Western Gate* (Berkeley: Blue Snake Books, 2006).

49. R. Chuckrow, "Practicing Correct Strength (Jin) in T'ai-Chi Movement," http://chuckrowtaichi.com/PracticingPengJin.html.

50. For reviews, see C. Schuster et al., "Best Practices for Motor Imagery: A Systematic Review of Motor Imagery Training Elements in Five Different Disciplines," *BMC Medicine* 9 (2011): 75.

51. V. K. Ranganathan et al., "From Mental Power to Muscle Power—Gaining Strength by Using the Mind," *Neuropsychologia* 42, no. 7 (2004): 944–56.

52. F. Bakker et al., "Changes in Muscular Activity while Imagining Weight Lifting Using Stimulus or Response Propositions," *Journal of Sport and Exercise Psychology* 18 (1996): 313–24. Also see Driskell et al., "Does Mental Practice Enhance Performance?" *Journal of Sports Psychology* 79 (1994): 481–92.

53. T. Mulder et al., "Observation, Imagination and Execution of an Effortful Movement: More Evidence for a Central Explanation of Motor Imagery," *Experimental Brain Research* 163, no. 3 (2005): 344–51. Also see M. Jeannerod, "Neural Simulation of Action: A Unifying Mechanism for Motor Cognition," *NeuroImage* 14, no. 1, pt. 2 (2001): S103–9; M. Jeannerod, "Mental Imagery in the Motor Context," *Neuropsychologia* 33, no. 11 (1995): 1419–32.

54. For motor imagery in stroke, see J. Zimmermann-Schlater et al., "Efficacy of Motor Imagery in Post-stroke Rehabilitaion: A Systematic Review," *Journal of Neuroengineering and Rehabilitation* 5 (2008): 8; S. J. Page et al., "Mental Practice in Chronic Stroke: Results of a Randomized, Placebo-controlled Trial," *Stroke* 38, no. 4 (2009): 1293–97; M. Ietswaart et al., "Mental Practice with Motor Imagery in Stroke Recovery: Randomized Controlled Trial of Efficacy," *Brain* 134, pt.5 (2011): 1373–86. For motor imagery in Parkinson's disease, see Braun et al., "Rehabilitation with Mental Practice Has Similar Effects on Mobility as Rehabilitation with Relaxation in People with Parkinson's Disease," *Journal of Physiotherapy* 57 (2001): 27–34; E. Heremans et al., "Motor Imagery Ability in Patients with Early- and Mid-stage

Parkinson Disease," *Neurorehabilitation and Neural Repair* 25, no. 2 (2011): 168–77; R. Tamir et al., "Integration of Motor Imagery and Physical Practice in Group Treatment Applied to Subjects with Parkinson's Disease," *Neurorehabilitation and Neural Repair* 21, no. 1 (2007): 68–75. Clinical evidence for the effectiveness of Tai Chi for neurological conditions includes F. Li et al. "Tai Chi and Postural Stability in Patients with Parkinson's Disease," *New England Journal of Medicine* 366, no. 6 (February 9, 2012): 511–19; S. S. Au-Yeung, "Short-form Tai Chi Improves Standing Balance of People with Chronic Stroke," *Neurorehabilitation and Neural Repair* 23, no. 5 (2009): 515–22.

Chapter 9

1. World Health Organization, "Promoting Mental Health: Concepts, Emerging Evidence, Practice: A Report of the World Health Organization," Department of Mental Health and Substance Abuse in Collaboration with the Victorian Health Promotion Foundation and the University of Melbourne (Geneva: World Health Organization, 2005).

2. "The Changing Organization of Work and the Safety and Health of Working People," Department of Health and Human Services (National Institute for Occupational Safety and Health) Publication No. 2002-116.

3. G. P. Chrousos and P. W. Gold, "The Concept of Stress and Stress System Disorders," *Journal of the American Medical Association* 267 (1992): 1244–52; R. P. Juster et al., "Allostatic Load Biomarkers of Chronic Stress and Impact on Health and Cognition," *Neuroscience and Biobehavioral Reviews* 35 (2010): 2–16; E. M. Backe et al., "The Role of Psychosocial Stress at Work for the Development of Cardiovascular Disease: A Systematic Review," *International Archives of Occupational and Environmental Health* 85 (2011): 67–79.

4. http://www.stress.org/

5. See Richard Lazarus and Susan Folkman, *Stress, Appraisal, and Coping* (New York: Springer Publishing Company, 1984) for a comprehensive review of stress appraisal.

6. S. S. Luthar et al., "The Construct of Resilience: A Critical Evaluation and Guidelines for Future Work," *Child Development* 71, no. 3 (2000): 543–62; D. Cicchetti, "Resilience under Conditions of Extreme Stress: A Multilevel Perspective," *World Psychiatry* 9, no. 3 (2010): 145–54.

7. "The Numbers Count: Mental Disorders in America," http://www.nimh.nih .gov/health/publications/the-numbers-count-mental-disorders-in-america/ index.shtml.

8. Surgeon General's Report on Mental Health, 1999. United States, Public Health Service, Office of the Surgeon General Center for Mental Health Services National Institute of Mental Health.

9. J. W. Smoller et al., "Genetics of Anxiety Disorders: The Complex Road

from DSM to DNA," *Depression and Anxiety* 26, no. 11 (2009): 965–75; A. Weiss et al., "Happiness Is a Personal(ity) Thing: The Genetics of Personality and Well-being in a Representative Sample," *Psychological Science* 19, no. 3 (2008): 205–10.

10. Anne Harrington and Arthur Zajonc, *The Dalai Lama at MIT* (Cambridge, Mass.: Harvard University Press, 2006).

11. R. Veenhoven, "Healthy Happiness: Effects of Happiness on Physical Health and the Consequences for Preventive Health Care," *Journal of Happiness Studies* 9 (2008): 449–69. Also see: C. D. Ryff et al., "Positive Health: Connecting Well-being with Biology," *Philosophical Transactions of the Royal Society of London* 359, no. 1449 (2004): 1383–94; Barbara Fredrickson, *Positivity: Groundbreaking Research Reveals How to Embrace the Hidden Strength of Positive Emotions, Overcome Negativity, and Thrive,* (New York: Crown, 2009).

12. A. Lutz et al., "Long-term Meditators Self-induce High-amplitude Gamma Synchrony during Mental Practice," *Procedures of the National Academy of Sciences of the United States of America* 101, no. 46 (2004): 16369–73.

13. A. Lutz et al., "Regulation of the Neural Circuitry of Emotion by Compassion Meditation: Effects of Meditative Expertise," *PloS One* 3, no. 3 (2008): e1897.

14. For example, in one study, Emory University researchers randomly assigned 61 healthy adults who had never meditated before to either six weeks of compassion meditation training or a health discussion group. The results of this small trial were provocative: the more those in the meditation group practiced, the less distress they experienced. More remarkably, meditation seemed to affect their immune system. The meditation group showed reductions in a marker of inflammation induced by stress called interleukin-6 or IL-6. Chronically high levels of this marker have been associated with major depression and the development of several diseases, including vascular disease and diabetes: T. W. Pace et al., "Effect of Compassion Meditation on Neuroendocrine, Innate Immune and Behavioral Responses to Psychosocial Stress," *Psychoneuroendocrinology* 34, no. 1 (2009): 87–98. Also see A. Ikeda, "Optimism in Relation to Inflammation and Endotheial Dysfunction in Older Men: The VA Normative Aging Study," *Psychosomatic Medicine* 73 (2011): 664–71; M. Matsunaga et al., "Association between Perceived Happiness Levels and Peripheral Circulating Pro-inflammatory Cytokine Levels in Middle-aged Adults in Japan," *Neuro Endocrinol Letter* 32, no. 4 (2011): 458–63.

15. See Elisa Rossi, *Shen: Psycho-Emotional Aspects of Chinese Medicine* (Philadelphia: Churchill Livingstone, 2007).

16. G. Maciocia, *The Psyche in Chinese Medicine: Treatment of Emotional and Mental Disharmonies with Acupuncture and Chinese Herbs* (Philadelphia: Churchill Livingstone, 2009).

17. Ibid.

18. C. Wang et al., "Tai Chi on Psychological Well-being: Systematic Review and Meta-analysis," *BMC Complementary and Alternative Medicine* 10 (2010): 23. For other reviews of Tai Chi for psychological well-being, see: L. Zhang et al., "A Review Focused on the Psychological Effectiveness of Tai Chi on Different Populations," *Evidence Based Complementary and Alternative Medicine* (2012): ID 678107; W. C. Wang et al., "The Effect of Tai Chi on Psychosocial Well-being: A Systematic Review of Randomized Controlled Trials," *Journal of Acupuncture and Meridian Studies* 2, no. 3 (2009): 171–81; A. Deschamps et al., "Effects of Tai Chi Exercises on Self-Efficacy and Psychological Health," *European Review of Aging and Physical Activity* 4 (2007): 25–32.

19. C. Wang et al., "Tai Chi and Rheumatic Diseases," *Rheumatic Diseases Clinic of North America*, 37, no. 1 (2011): 19–32.

20. G. Y. Yeh et al., "Tai Chi Exercise in Patients with Chronic Heart Failure: A Randomized Clinical Trial," *Archives of Internal Medicine* 171, no. 8 (2011): 750–57.

21. In one study, 112 adults with major depression, aged 60 years and older, were initially treated with escitalopram, a selective serotonin reuptake inhibitor, for approximately four weeks. The 73 patients who partially responded to the drug continued to take it daily and also randomly were assigned to 10 weeks of either Tai Chi or health education for two hours per week. After 10 weeks, those in the escitalopram and Tai Chi group were more likely to show a greater reduction of depressive symptoms or to be totally free of depression as compared with those receiving escitalopram and health education: H. Lavretsky et al., "Complementary Use of Tai Chi Chih Augments Escitalopram Treatment of Geriatric Depression: A Randomized Controlled Trial," *American Journal of Geriatric Psychiatry* 19, no. 10 (2011): 839–50. Also see K. L. Chou et al., "Effect of Tai Chi on Depressive Symptoms amongst Chinese Older Patients with Depressive Disorders: A Randomized Clinical Trial," *International Journal of Geriatric Psychiatry* 19 (2004): 1105–7.

22. A. Yeung, G. Yeh, L. Slipp, M. Fava, J. Denninger, H. Benson, G. Fricchione V. Lepoutre, and P. Wayne, "Tai Chi Treatment for Depression in Chinese Americans: A Pilot Study," *American Journal of Physical Medicine and Rehabilitation* 91, no. 10 (2012): 863–70.

23. J. C. Tsai et al., "The Beneficial Effects of Tai Chi Chuan on Blood Pressure and Lipid Profile and Anxiety Status in a Randomized Controlled Trial," *Journal of Alternative and Complementary Medicine* 9, no. 5 (2003): 747–54.

24. C. Wang et al., "Tai Chi on Psychological Well-being: Systematic Review and Meta-analysis," *BMC Complementary and Alternative Medicine* 10 (2010): 23.

25. I. Janssen and A. G. Leblanc, "Systematic Review of the Health Benefits of Physical Activity and Fitness in School-aged Children and Youth," *International Journal of Behavioral Nutrition and Physical Activity* 7 (2010): 40; L. M. Haarasilta et al., "Correlates of Depression in a Representative Nationwide Sample of Adolescents (15–19 years) and Young Adults (20–24 years)," *European Journal of Public Health* 14, no. 3 (2004): 280–85; P. Lampinen et al., "Changes in Intensity of Physical Exercise as Predictors of Depressive Symptoms among Older Adults: An Eight-year Follow-up," *Preventive Medicine* 30, no. 5 (2000): 371–80; M. E. Farmer et al., "Physical Activity and Depressive Symptoms: The NHANES I Epidemiologic Follow-up Study," *Journal of Epidemiology* 128, no. 6 (1988): 1340–51; I. Helmich et al., "Neurobiological Alterations Induced by Exercise and Their Impact on Depressive Disorders," *Clinical Practice and Epidemiololgy in Mental Health* 30, no. 6 (2010): 115–25.

26. Prospective clinical trials confirm these associations. A recent Cochrane Database Systematic Review published in 2009 summarized the results of studies evaluating exercise for depression. A meta-analysis of 23 trials found that exercise led to large positive effects in mood elevation when compared to either no treatment or to controls. E. Mead et al., "Exercise for Depression," *Cochrane Database of Systematic Reviews* 3 (July 8, 2009): CD004366. Also see Blake et al., "How Effective Are Physical Activity Interventions for Alleviating Depressive Symptoms in Older People? A Systematic Review," *Clinical Rehabilitation* 23, no. 23 (2009): 873–87; A. Strohle, "Physical Activity, Exercise, Depression and Anxiety Disorders," *Journal of Neural Transmission* 116, no. 6 (2009): 777–84.

27. A noteworthy series of studies conducted by Duke University Medical Center researchers compared the benefits of exercise versus antidepressant medications for older patients with major depressive disorders. In one randomized trial, 156 men and women over age 50 were assigned to one of three groups: exercise, medication, or a combination of exercise and medication. The exercise group rode a stationary bike, walked, or jogged for 30 minutes three times a week. After 16 weeks, all three groups showed statistically significant—and identical—improvements in standard measurements of depression: J. A. Blumenthal et al., "Effects of Exercise Training on Older Patients with Major Depression," *Archives of Internal Medicine* 159, no. 19 (1999): 2349–56.

28. J. A. Blumenthal et al., "Exercise and Pharmacotherapy in the Treatment of Major Depressive Disorder," *Psychosomatic Medicine* 69, no. 7 (2007): 587–96.

29. A. Strohle, "Physical Activity, Exercise, Depression and Anxiety Disorders," *Journal of Neural Transmission* 116, no. 6 (2009): 777–84.

30. M. P. Herring et al., "The Effect of Exercise Training on Anxiety Symptoms

among Patients: A Systematic Review," *Archives of Internal Medicine* 170, no. 4 (2010): 321–31.

31. One study in England specifically evaluated the impact of exercise on adults with anxiety symptoms. The participants were randomly assigned to either moderate aerobic training or strength and flexibility training for 10 weeks. The aerobic exercise program led to significant improvements in fitness and was also associated with significantly greater reductions in tension/anxiety, depression, and other moods, together with increases in perceived ability to cope with stress, in comparison to the strength/flexibility group. These positive effects were maintained for three months: A. Steptoe et al., "The Effects of Exercise Training on Mood and Perceived Coping Ability in Anxious Adults from the General Population," *Journal of Psychosomatic Research* 33 (1989): 537–547.

32. A. B. Diaz and R. Motta, "The Effects of an Aerobic Exercise Program on Posttraumatic Stress Disorder Symptom Severity in Adolescents," *International Journal of Emergency Mental Health* 10, no. 1 (2008): 49–59.

33. D. Meron et al., "Promoting Walking as an Adjunct Intervention to Group Cognitive Behavioral Therapy for Anxiety Disorders—A Pilot Group Randomized Trial," *Journal of Anxiety Disorders* 22, no. 6 (2008): 959–68.

34. Examples of this include the approaches developed by Alexander Lowen (e.g., *The Language of the Body*, Bioenergetics Press, 2006); Moshe Feldenkrais (e.g., *Body and Mature Behavior: A Study of Anxiety, Sex, Gravitation, and Learning*, Frog Books, 2005); Ida Rolf (e.g., *Rolfing: Reestablishing the Natural Alignment and Structural Integration of the Human Body for Vitality and Well-Being*, Healing Arts Press, 1989); and Frederick Alexander (*Body Learning: An Introduction to the Alexander Technique* by Michael Gelb, Holt Paperbacks, 1996).

35. Charles Darwin, *The Expression of the Emotions in Man and Animals* (London: John Murray, 1872). For more recent research, see F. Strack et al., "Inhibiting and Facilitating Conditions of the Human Smile: A Nonobtrusive Test of the Facial Feedback Hypothesis," *Journal of Personality and Social Psychology* 54, no. 5 (1988): 768–77; J. H. Riskind and C. C. Gotay, "Physical Posture: Could It Have Regulatory or Feedback Effects on Motivation and Emotion?" *Motivation and Emotion* 6, no. 3 (1982): 273–98.

36. D. R. Carney et al., "Power Posing: Brief Nonverbal Displays Affect Neuroendocrine Levels and Risk Tolerance," *Psychological Science* 21, no. 10 (2010): 1363–68.

37. C. Hammen, "Stress and Depression," *Annual Review of Clinical Psychology* 1 (2005): 293–319.

38. Charles Genoud, *Gesture of Awarenesss: A Radical Approach to Time, Space, and Movement* (Boston: Wisdom Publications, 2006).

39. M. A. Killingsworth and D. T. Gilbert, "A Wandering Mind Is an Unhappy Mind," *Science* 330, no. 6006 (2010): 932.

40. J. M. Greeson, "Mindfulness Research Update: 2008," *Complementary Health Practice Review* 14, no. 1 (2009): 10–18. Also see Grossman et al., "Mindfulness-Based Stress Reduction and Health Benefits: A Meta-analysis," *Journal of Psychosomatic Research* 57, no. 1 (2004): 35–43; M. Merkes, "Mindfulness-based Stress Reduction for People with Chronic Diseases," *Australian Journal of Primary Health* 16, no. 3 (2010): 200–210.

41. S. Jain et al., "A Randomized Controlled Trial of Mindfulness Meditation versus Relaxation Training: Effects on Distress, Positive States of Mind, Rumination, and Distraction," *Annals of Behavioral Medicine* 33, no. 1 (2007): 11–21.

42. J. Piet and E. Hougaard, "The Effect of Mindfulness-based Cognitive Therapy for Prevention of Relapse in Recurrent Major Depressive Disorder: A Systematic Review and Meta-analysis," *Clinical Psychology Review* 31, no. 6 (2011): 1032–40.

43. M. H. Bonnet et al., "Hyperarousal and Insomnia: State of the Science," *Sleep Medicine Reviews* 14, no. 9 (2010): 9–15; M. M. Ohayon, "Epidemiology of Insomnia: What We Know and What We Still Need to Learn," *Sleep Medicine Reviews* 6, no. 2 (2002): 97–111.

44. F. E. Cappuccio et al., "Sleep Duration Predicts Cardiovascular Outcomes: A Systematic Review and Meta-analysis of Prospective Studies," *European Heart Journal* 32, no. 12 (2011): 1484–92.; D. Foley et al., "Sleep Disturbances and Chronic Disease in Older Adults: Results of the 2003 National Sleep Foundation Sleep in America Survey," *Journal of Psychosomatic Research* 56, no. 5 (2004): 497–502; K. L. Knutson et al., "Role of Sleep Duration and Quality in the Risk and Severity of Type 2 Diabetes Mellitus," *Archives of Internal Medicine* 166 (2006): 1768–64; E. Kasasbeh et al., "Inflammatory Aspects of Sleep Apnea and Their Cardiovascular Consequences," *Southern Medical Journal* 99, no. 1 (2006): 58–67; S. Taheri, "The Link between Short Sleep Duration and Obesity: We Should Recommend More Sleep to Prevent Obesity," *Archives of Disease in Childhood* 91, no. 11 (2006): 881–84.

45. D. J. Kupfer and C. F. Reynolds III, "Management of Insomnia," *New England Journal of Medicine* 336, no. 5 (1997): 341–46; J. Glass et al., "Sedative Hypnotics in Older People with Insomnia: Meta-analysis of Risks and Benefits," *BMJ* 331, no. 7526 (2005): 1169.

46. B. Sivertsen et al., "Cognitive Behavioral Therapy vs Zopiclone for Treatment of Chronic Primary Insomnia in Older Adults: A Randomized Controlled Trial," *Journal of the American Medical Association* 295, no. 24 (2006): 2851–58; G. D. Jacobs et al., "Cognitive Behavior Therapy and Pharmacotherapy for Insomnia: A Randomized Controlled Trial and Direct Comparison," *Archives of Internal Medicine* 164, no. 17 (2004): 1888–96.

47. G. D. Jacobs, "Clinical Applications of the Relaxation Response and Mind-Body Interventions," *Journal of Alternative and Complementary Medicine* 7, suppl. 1 (2001): S93–101; W. F. Waters, "Behavioral and Hypnotic Treatments for Insomnia Subtypes," *Behavioral Sleep Medicine* 1, no. 2 (2003): 81–101; M. K. Means et al., "Relaxation Therapy for Insomnia: Nighttime and Daytime Effects," *Behaviour Research and Therapy* 38 (2000): 665–78.

48. A. N. Vgontzas et al., "Middle-aged Men Show Higher Sensitivity of Sleep to the Arousing Effects of Corticotropin-releasing Hormone than Young Men: Clinical Implications," *Journal of Clinical Endocrinology and Metabolism* 86, no. 4 (2001): 1489–95.

49. A. N. Vgontzas et al., "Chronic Insomnia Is Associated with Nyctohemeral Activation of the Hypothalamic-Pituitary-Adrenal Axis: Clinical Implications," *Journal of Clinical Endocrinology and Metabolism* 86, no. 8 (2001): 3787–94.

50. J. D. Lattimore et al., "Obstructive Sleep Apnea and Cardiovascular Disease," *Journal of American College of Cardiology* 41, no. 9 (2003): 1429–37.

51. A. Dechamps et al, "Pilot Study of a 10-Week Multidisciplinary Tai Chi Intervention in Sedentary Obese Women," *Clinical Journal of Sports Medicine* 19 (2009): 49–53.

52. M. R. Irwin et al., "Improving Sleep Quality in Older Adults with Moderate Sleep Complaints: A Randomized Controlled Trial of Tai Chi Chih," *Sleep* 31, no. 7 (2008): 1001–8.

53. F. Li et al., "Tai Chi and Self-rated Quality of Sleep and Daytime Sleepiness in Older Adults: A Randomized Controlled Trial," *Journal of the American Geriatrics Society* 52, no. 6 (2004): 892–900; also see: M. H. Nguyen and A. Kruse, "A Randomized Controlled Trial of Tai Chi for Balance, Sleep Quality and Cognitive Performance in Elderly Vietnamese," *Journal of Clinical Interventions in Aging* 7 (2012): 185–90.

54. G. Y. Yeh et al., "Enhancement of Sleep Stability with Tai Chi Exercise in Chronic Heart Failure: Preliminary Findings Using an ECG-based Spectrogram Method," *Sleep Medicine* 9, no. 5 (2008): 527–36.

55. C. Wang, "A Randomized Trial of Tai Chi for Fibromyalgia," *New England Journal of Medicine* 363, no. 8 (2010): 743–54; C. Wang, "Tai Chi and Rheumatic Diseases," *Rheumatic Diseases Clinic of North America* 37, no. 1 (2011): 19–32; C. Wang et al., "Tai Chi Exercise versus Rehabilitation for the Elderly with Cerebral Vascular Disorder: A Single-blinded Randomized Controlled Trial," *Psychogeriatrics* 10, no. 3 (2010): 160–66.

Chapter 10

1. Some books that include significant discussion on interactive Tai Chi include: Cheng Man Ch'ing et al., *Cheng Tzu's Thirteen Treatises on T'ai Chi Ch'uan* (Berkeley: Blue Snake Books, 1993); Stuart Olson, *Tai Chi Sensing*

Hands (Prescott Valley, Calif.: Unique Publications, 1999); Wolfe Lowenthal, *There Are No Secrets: Professor Cheng Man Ch'ing and His T'ai Chi Chuan* (Berkeley: North Atlantic Books, 1993); T. T. Liang, *T'ai Chi Ch'uan for Health and Self-Defense: Philosophy and Practice* (New York: Vintage, 1977); Rick Barrett, *Taijiquan: Through the Western Gate* (Berkeley: Blue Snake Books, 2006); Bruce Kumar Frantzis, *The Power of Internal Martial Arts and Chi: Combat and Energy Secrets of Ba Gua, Tai Chi and Hsing-I* (Berkeley: Blue Snake Books, 2007); Yang Jwing-Ming, *Tai Chi Chuan Martial Applications: Advanced Yang Style Tai Chi Chuan* (Boston: YMAA Publication Center, 1996).

2. For example, see R. Dunbar, "The Social Role of Touch in Humans and Primates: Behavioural Function and Neurobiological Mechanisms," *Neuroscience and Biobehavioral Reviews* 34 (2010): 260–268; A. Gallace and C. Spencer, "The Science of Interpersonal Touch: An Overview," *Neuroscience and Biobehavioral Reviews* 34 (2010): 246–259; K. M. Grewen et al., "Effects of Partner Support on Resting Oxytocin, Cortisol, Norepinephrine, and Blood Pressure before and after Warm Partner Contact," *Psychosomatic Medicine* 67 (2005): 531–538; K. C. Light et al., "More Frequent Partner Hugs and Higher Oxytocin Levels Are Linked to Lower Blood Pressure and Heart Rate in Premenopausal Women," *Biological Psychology* 69 (2005): 5–21.

3. Cabrera and L. Colosi, "The World at Our Fingertips: The Connection between Touch and Learning," *Scientific American* (September 2010).

4. K. Huang , "PianoTouch: A Wearable Haptic Piano Instruction System for Passive Learning of Piano Skills," *12th IEEE International Symposium on Wearable Computers* (2008): 41–44; J. Bluteau et al., "Haptic Guidance Improves the Visuo-Manual Tracking of Trajectories," *PLoS One* 3, no. 3 (2008): e1775.

5. W. W. Tsang et al., "Trunk Position Sense in Older Tai Chi Sword Practitioners," *Hong Kong Physiotherapy Journal* 27, no. 1 (2009): 55–60; B. H. Jacobson, "The Effect of T'ai Chi Chuan Training on Balance, Kinesthetic Sense, and Strength," *Perception and Motor Skills* 84, no. 1 (1997): 27–33.

6. C. E. Kerr et al., "Tactile Acuity in Experienced Tai Chi Practitioners: Evidence for Use Dependent Plasticity as an Effect of Sensory-Attentional Training," *Experiential Brain Research* 188, no. 2 (2008): 317–22.

7. Y. Zhou, "The Effect of Traditional Sports on the Bone Density of Menopause Women," *Journal of Beijing Sport University* 27 (2004): 354–60.

8. H. C. Chen et al., "The Defense Technique in Tai Chi Push Hands: A Case Study," *Journal of Sports Science* 28, no. 14 (2010): 1595–1604; L. H. Wang et al., "Ground Reaction Force and Postural Adaptation of the Push Movement in Tai Chi," *Journal of Biomechanics* 40 (2007): S430.

9. Angus Clark, *The Complete Illustrated Guide to Tai Chi. A Practical Approach*

to the Ancient Chinese Movement for Health and Well-being (Boston: Element Books, 2000).

10. S. M. Jourard, *Healthy Personality: An Approach from the Viewpoint of Humanistic Psychology* (New York: Macmillan, 1974).

Chapter 11

1. W. W. Tsang et al., "The Effects of Aging and Tai Chi on Fingerpoint toward Stationary and Moving Visual Targets," *Archives of Physical Medicine and Rehabilitiation* 91, no. 1 (2010): 149–55.

2. M. Timothy Gallwey, *The Inner Game of Tennis: The Classic Guide to the Mental Side of Peak Performance* (New York: Random House, 1977).

Chapter 12

1. http://www.stress.org/

2. M. M. Clark et al., "Stress Level, Health Behaviors, and Quality of Life in Employees Joining a Wellness Center," *American Journal of Health Promotion* 26, no. 1 (2011): 21–25.

3. Note, for smaller companies with 50 to 99 employees, closer to only 5 percent offer comprehensive programs. See: L. Linnan et al., "Results of the 2004 National Worksite Health Promotion Survey," *American Journal of Public Health* 98, no. 8 (2008): 1503–09.

4. L. L. Berry et al., "What's the Hard Return on Employee Wellness Programs?" *Harvard Business Review* (December 2010): http://hbr.org/2010/12/whats-the-hard-return-on-employee-wellness-programs/ar/1.

5. D. R. Anderson et al., "Conceptual Framework, Critical Questions, and Practical Challenges in Conducting Research on the Financial Impact of Worksite Health Promotion," *American Journal of Health Promotion* 15 (2001): 281–88.

6. M. Carnethon et al., "Worksite Wellness Programs for Cardiovascular Disease Prevention: A Policy Statement from the American Heart Association," *Circulation* 120 (2009): 1725–41.

7. D. R. Anderson, et al., "The Relationship between Modifiable Health Risks and Group-level Health Care Expenditures: Health Enhancement Research Organization (HERO) Research Committee," *American Journal of Health Promotion* 15, no. 1 (2000): 45–52.

8. K. S. Calderon et al., "Kennedy Space Center Cardiovascular Disease Risk Reduction Program Evaluation," *Vascular Health and Risk Management* 4, no. 2 (2008): 421–26; R. Merrill et al., "Effectiveness of a Workplace Wellness Program for Maintaining Health and Promoting Healthy Behaviors," *Journal of Occupational and Environmental Medicine* 53, no. 7 (2011): 782–87.

9. W. F. Stewart et al., "Lost Productive Work Time Costs from Health Conditions in the United States: Results from the American Productivity Audit,"

Journal of Occupational and Environmental Medicine 45, no. 12 (2003): 1234–46; W. F. Stewart et al., "Cost of Lost Productive Work Time among US Workers with Depression," *Journal of the American Medical Association* 289, no. 23 (2003): 3135–44.

10. W. N. Burton et al., "The Association between Health Risk Change and Presenteeism Change," *Journal of Occupational and Environmental Medicine* 48, no. 3 (2006): 252–63.

11. S. G. Aldana, "Financial Impact of Health Promotion Programs: A Comprehensive Review of the Literature," *American Journal of Health Promotion* 15, no. 5 (2001): 296–320.

12. N. Kawakami et al., "Effects of Perceived Job Stress on Depressive Symptoms in Blue-Collar Workers of an Electrical Factory in Japan," *Scandinavian Journal of Work, Environment, and Health*, 18 (1992): 195–200.

13. Karl H. E. Kroemer, *Office Ergonomics* (Boca Raton, Fla.: CRC Press, 2001).

14. H. Tamin et al. "Tai Chi Workplace Program for Improving Musculoskeletal Fitness among Female Computer Users," *Work* 34, no. 3 (2009): 331–38.

15. M. V. Palumbo et al., "Tai Chi for Older Nurses: A Workplace Wellness Pilot Study," *Applied Nursing Research* 25, no. 1 (2010): 54–59.

Chapter 13

1. Cheng Man Ch'ing and Mark Hennessy, *Master of Five Excellences* (Berkeley: Frog Books, 1995).

2. Tam Gibbs, "Cheng Tzu: Master of the Five Excellences: A Life Biography of Cheng Man Ching," 1978, http://www.sinobarr.com/cheng/cheng_life_bio.htm.

3. I. Foxman and B. J. Burgel, "Musician Health and Safety: Preventing Playing-related Musculoskeletal Disorders," *AAOHN* Journal 54, no. 7 (2006): 309–16.

Afterword

1. D. U. Himmelstein et al., "Medical Bankruptcy in the United States, 2007, Results of a National Study," *American Journal of Medicine* 122, no. 8 (August 2009): 699.

2. S. Blumenthal et al., "Putting Prevention into Practice in Health Care Reform," *Huffington Post,* July 18, 2009, http://www.huffingtonpost.com/susan-blumenthal/putting-prevention-into-p_b_239260.html.

3. A. Singh, et al., "Physical Activity and Performance at School: A Systematic Review of the Literature including a Methodological Quality Assessment," *Archives of Pediatric and Adolescent Medicine* 166, no. 1 (January 2012): 49–55; C. N. Rasberry et al., "The Association between School-based Physical Activity, including Physical Education, and Academic Performance: A Systematic Review of the Literature," *Preventive Medicine* 52, suppl. 1

(2011): S10–20. Also see J. Ratey, *Spark: The Revolutionary New Science of Exercise and the Brain* (New York: Little, Brown and Company, 2008).

4. See, for example, "Tai Chi for Kids" (www.taichiforkids.com); and G. Gurman "Tai Chi Animal Frolics: Introducing Tai Chi and Qigong in Public School Settings," http://imos-journal.net/?p=3511.

5. L. Baron and C. Faubert, "The Role of Tai Chi Chuan in Reducing State Anxiety and Enhancing Mood of Children with Special Needs," *Journal of Bodywork and Movement Therapies* 9, no. 2, (2005): 120–123.

6. C. Witt et al., "Qigong for Schoolchildren: A Pilot Study," *Journal of Alternative and Complementary Medicine* 11, no. 1 (February 2005): 41–47; L. S. White, "Reducing Stress in School-age Girls through Mindful Yoga,"*Journal of Pediatric Health Care* 26, no. 1 (2012): 45–56; G. S. Birdee, G. Y. Yeh, P. M. Wayne, R. S. Phillips, R. B. Davis, and P. Gardiner, "Clinical Applications of Yoga for the Pediatric Population: A Systematic Review," *Academic Pediatrics* 9 (2009): 212–20; and many others.

7. R. Wall, "Tai Chi and Mindfulness-based Stress Reduction in a Boston Public Middle School," *Journal of Pediatric Health Care* 19 (2005): 230–37.

8. J. J. Noggle, et al., "Benefits of Yoga for Psychosocial Well-being in a US High School Curriculum: A Preliminary Randomized Controlled Trial" *Journal of Developmental and Behavioral Pediatrics* 33, no. 3 (April 2012): 193–201; also see S. B. Khalsa et al., "Evaluation of the Mental Health Benefits of Yoga in a Secondary School: A Preliminary Randomized Controlled Trial," *Journal of Behavioral Health Services and Research* 39, no. 1 (2012): 80–90.

9. K. Caldwell et al., "Changes in Mindfulness, Well-being, and Sleep Quality in College Students through Taijiquan Courses: A Cohort Control Study," *Journal of Alternative and Complementary Medicine* 17, no. 10 (2011): 931–38; K. Caldwell et al., "Developing Mindfulness in College Students through Movement-based Courses: Effects on Self-regulatory Self-efficacy, Mood, Stress, and Sleep Quality," *Journal of American College Health* 58, no. 5 (2010): 433–42; K. Caldwell et al., "Effect of Pilates and Taiji Quan Training on Self-efficacy, Sleep Quality, Mood, and Physical Performance of College Students," *Journal of Bodywork Movement Therapy* 13, no. 2 (2009): 155–63; Y. T. Wang et al., "Effects of Tai Chi Exercise on Physical and Mental Health of College Students," *American Journal of Chinese Medicine* 32, no. 3 (2004): 453–59.

10. P. A. Saunders et al., "Promoting Self-awareness and Reflection through an Experiential Mind-Body Skills Course for First Year Medical Students," *Medical Teacher* 29, no. 8 (October 2007): 778–84; B. W. MacLaughlin et al., "Stress Biomarkers in Medical Students Participating in a Mind-Body Medicine Skills Program," *Evidence-Based Complementary and Alternative Medicine* (2011): ID 950461. For programs in other medical schools, see C.

Finkelstein et al., "Anxiety and Stress Reduction in Medical Education: An Intervention," *Medical Education* 41, no. 3 (2007): 258–64; S. L. Shapiro et al., "Effects of Mindfulness-based Stress Reduction on Medical and Pre-medical Students," *Journal of Behavioral Medicine* 21 (1998): 581–99.

11. S. L. Shapiro et al., "Mindfulness-Based Stress Reduction for Health Care Professionals: Results from a Randomized Trial," *International Journal of Stress Management* 12 (2005): 164–76.

12. E. Frank et al., "Physician Disclosure of Healthy Personal Behaviors Improves Credibility and Ability to Motivate," *Archives of Family Medicine* 9, no. 3 (2000): 287–90; M. Howe et al., "Patient-related Diet and Exercise Counseling: Do Providers' Own Lifestyle Habits Matter?" *Preventive Cardiology* 13, no. 4 (Fall 2010): 180–85.

Index

alignment and, 138–40
breathing and, 143
chronic, 133–34
mental factors, 133–35, 140–43
pain relief, 129–50
Qi and, 129–30
sleep and, 215–16
See also back pain
Parkinson's disease, 121–22
peripheral neuropathy, 113, 118
placebo effect, 31, 33, 42–43, 142
proprioception, 112, 118–119
Push Hands, 19, 224, 256

Qi (energy flow in the body), 2,
    14–15
    alignment and, 45–46, 138
    awareness and, 38
    belief and, 7, 60
    breathing and, 58–59, 174–75
    Chinese medicine and, 20–21
    creativity and, 253–54
    emotions and, 204–5
    heart and, 152
    intention and, 41
    pain and, 129–30
    science and, 7, 44
Qigong, 15

relaxation, 30, 50–52

70-percent rule, 73, 140–41, 228, 233,
    245, 257, 261
skiing, 238–39
sleep, 213–16
social support, 30–31, 59–61
    cognitive function and, 192
    heart health and, 156
    pain and, 143
    partner Tai Chi and, 227–28
    70-percent rule and, 228
socialism, 22
spirituality, 31, 63–65

sports, 109–10, 159–60, 195–96,
    229–39. *See also* golf; skiing;
    tennis
strengthening, 30, 53–55, 223–24
stress
    back pain and, 241
    breathing exercises and, 55, 169
    cognitive function and, 188–89
    health and, 153–55, 242–45
    mental health and, 199–201
    sleep and, 214–15
    visualization and, 210
    work and, 241–45
    See also anxiety
stroke, 163–64
Sung (relaxed, open state), 50 51, 120.
    See also relaxation

Tai Chi
    animal influences, 17, 20–21, 192
    children and, 272–74
    etymology, 14
    finding teachers, 263–67
    five excellences of, 24, 252–53
    goals, 3, 14
    history, 15–28
    integration of Tai Chi into daily
        life, 240–49, 259–69,
        272–75
    martial arts competitions, 19
    science and, 2–3, 7, 26–28, 44
    styles, 13–15, 19–20, 266
    in the West, 8, 16, 24–27
    See also Tai Chi exercises
Tai Chi exercises, 66–105
    for balance and bones, 125–28
    cool-down exercises, 104–5
    for pain, 149–50
    partner Tai Chi, 219–28
    Push Hands, 19, 224, 256
    Tai Chi Pouring, 37, 41, 45–46, 52,
        68–70
    Tai Chi Tennis, 235–36